HIV/AIDS AND THE SOUTH AFRICAN STATE

Global Health

Series Editor: Nana K. Poku,
Health Economics and AIDS Research Division (HEARD), South Africa

The benefits of globalization are potentially enormous, as a result of the increased sharing of ideas, cultures, life-saving technologies and efficient production processes. Yet globalization is under trial, partly because these benefits are not yet reaching hundreds of millions of the world's poor and partly because globalization has introduced new kinds of international problems and conflicts. Turmoil in one part of the world now spreads rapidly to others, through terrorism, armed conflict, environmental degradation or disease.

This timely series provides a robust and multi-disciplinary assessment of the asymmetrical nature of globalization. Books in the series encompass a variety of areas, including global health and the politics of governance, poverty and insecurity, gender and health and the implications of global pandemics.

Also in the series

Living with HIV and Dying with AIDS
Diversity, Inequality and Human Rights in the Global Pandemic
Lesley Doyal with Len Doyal
ISBN 978 1 4094 3110 7

Informal Norms in Global Governance
Human Rights, Intellectual Property Rules and Access to Medicines
Wolfgang Hein and Suerie Moon
ISBN 978 1 4094 2633 2

Ethics and Security Aspects of Infectious Disease Control
Interdisciplinary Perspectives
Edited by Christian Enemark and Michael J. Selgelid
ISBN 978 1 4094 2253 2

Migrants and Health
Political and Institutional Responses to
Cultural Diversity in Health Systems
Christiane Falge, Carlo Ruzza and Oliver Schmidtke
ISBN 978 0 7546 7915 8

HIV/AIDS and the South African State
Sovereignty and the Responsibility to Respond

ANNAMARIE BINDENAGEL ŠEHOVIĆ
*The Willy-Brandt School of Public Policy at
the University of Erfurt, Germany*

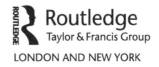

Routledge
Taylor & Francis Group

LONDON AND NEW YORK

First published 2014 by Ashgate Publishing

Published 2016 by Routledge
2 Park Square, Milton Park, Abingdon, Oxfordshire OX14 4RN
711 Third Avenue, New York, NY 10017, USA

First issued in paperback 2016

Routledge is an imprint of the Taylor & Francis Group, an informa business

British Library Cataloguing in Publication Data
A catalogue record for this book is available from the British Library

The Library of Congress has cataloged the printed edition as follows:
Bindenagel
Šehović, Annamarie.
  HIV/AIDS and the South African state : sovereignty and the responsibility to respond / by Annamarie Bindenagel Šehović.
     pages cm. -- (Global health)
  Includes bibliographical references and index.
  ISBN 978-1-4724-2337-5 (hardback)
  1. AIDS (Disease)--Government policy--South Africa. 2. HIV
Infections--Government policy--South Africa. 3. Medical policy--South Africa. I. Title.
  RA643.86.S6B56 2014
  362.19697'9200968--dc23

                                                                    2013041455

ISBN 13: 978-1-138-27931-5 (pbk)
ISBN 13: 978-1-4724-2337-5 (hbk)

Contents

List of Figures

Acknowledgments

This book is the result of a process; of exuberance and of diligence; of patience. In the fact of its being I owe a debt of gratitude towards all of those who contributed their time and effort and who offered their support. I want especially to thank: Ambassadors (ret.) Richard Barkley, who provided valuable insights into American foreign policy in South Africa during the dying day of the apartheid regime just as the HIV/AIDS epidemic was emerging and Thomas Wheeler, whose knowledge of South Africa's foreign and domestic policy and policy priorities deepened my analysis; Professor Solomon Benetar who's work on the ethics of health care provision and whose use of HIV/AIDS as a "window and a mirror" informed the analytical framework used here early on; Professor Vittorio Hösle, whose definition of sovereignty greatly influenced mine, planting the seeds for the GAP analysis; Johan Calitz, who generously shared survey data; and Fanyana Shiburi, who was there from the beginning before there were beginnings.

I also want to thank Professors Thomas Risse and Tanja Börzel, and Franklyn Lisk for bringing the beginning to an end; and Franklyn for his steadfast encouragement and mentoring.

Finally, I want to thank my parents, Ambassador (ret.) J.D. and Jean Bindenagel, and my brother, Carl, for "letting" me go to Africa, and for not minding (too much) when I did not return; Dennis Rose for the same; and all of them for being there and believing. And my daughters, Marjam and Lejla, born during this process: your being promises beginnings paved in light.

This book is for my husband, Kenan, for bringing into being a new local and global belonging.

List of Abbreviations

ANC	African National Congress
ARV	Antiretroviral
ASSA	Actuarial Society of South Africa
BEE/BBBEE	Black Economic Empowerment/Broad-Based Black Economic Empowerment
BRICS	Brazil, Russia, India, China, South Africa
CCM	Country Coordinating Mechanism
DBSA	Development Bank of Southern Africa
DIB	Demographic Information Bureau
EU	European Union
FDI	Foreign Direct Investment
GAP	Governance Accountability Problem
GBC	Global Business Coalition against AIDS, TB and Malaria
GDP	Gross Domestic Product
GEAR	Growth, Employment and Redistribution strategy
GHI	Global Health Initiative
GSK	GlaxoSmithKline
HAART	Highly Active Antiretroviral Treatment
HIV/AIDS	human immunodeficiency virus/ acquired immunodeficiency syndrome
ICISS	International Commission on Intervention and State Sovereignty
IFP	Inkatha Freedom Party
IGO	International Governmental Organization
ILO	International Labor Organization
IMF	International Monetary Fund
KZN	KwaZulu-Natal
MAP	World Bank's Multi-Country AIDS Program
MCC	Medical Control Council
MDG	Millennium Development Goals
MDR/XDR-TB	Multi-Drug/Extremely-drug Resistant Tuberculosis
MOU	Memorandum of Understanding
MSF	Médecins Sans Frontières
NACOSA	National AIDS Convention of South Africa
NEPAD	New Partnership for Africa's Development
NGO	Non-Governmental Organization
PEPFAR	US President's Emergency Plan for AIDS Relief

PMTCT	Prevention of Mother-to-Child-Transmission
R2P	Responsibility to Protect
RDP	Redistribution and Development Program
SABCOHA	South African Business Coalition against HIV/AIDS
SADC	Southern African Development Community
SANAC	South African National AIDS Council
SM(M)Es	Small, Medium (and Micro) Enterprises
TAC	Treatment Action Campaign
TB	Tuberculosis
TNC	Transnational Corporation
TRIPS	Trade-Related Aspects of Intellectual Property Rights
UN	United Nations
UNAIDS	The Joint United Nations Programme on HIV/AIDS
UNSC	United Nations Security Council
WHO	World Health Organization
WTO	World Trade Organization

Chapter 1

Introduction: The South African State and the Responsibility to Respond

The assumption of state sovereignty is convenient, persistent, but incomplete. This fact has become particularly salient in the wake of the end of the Cold War in 1989/1990, amidst the re-emergent emphasis on freedom and human rights propelled the responsibility of state protections to the fore of both sovereign debate and sovereign practice. Since then especially, both the need for state sovereignty and its apparent wane have become the topic of intense debate. The associated delimitations of sovereignty can be differentiated from three directions:

> from 'above'—that is, in terms of the claims of international organizations; from 'alongside'—that is, in terms of states, often operating in loose coalitions with others, who claim the right and/or duty to cross international borders in pursuit of specified interests; and from 'below'—that is, in terms of citizens' militias or people's armies who present themselves as defenders of justice to which established state and/or international authorities are indifferent or even actively hostile. In every case, the notion of states as political entities whose borders are sacrosanct appears to be outdated.[1]

Indeed, it can be argued that no state is, or ever was, completely sovereign. Instead, the opposite might be true—and increasingly so.

Weak states, frail states, fragile states, failing states: an increasing number of states around the world receive any one of these diagnoses. These constitute areas of limited statehood. They are unable or unwilling to enact their sovereign responsibilities to protect and provide for their populaces. Yet each bears, in principle if not in practice, the responsibility and accountability for the (human) security of its citizens: the assumption of state sovereignty in theory and practice. This represents the apparent incongruence on which I build my hypothesis for a renewed responsibility to respond.

In making this assertion, I base my theoretical argument for a re-conceptualization of sovereignty on three assumptive pillars: First, that state-based sovereignty stipulates the state as the agent responsible for awarding and enacting the rights of its constituents, most importantly, the provision of security, the promotion of welfare, and the accountability of the state to the international community of

---

1 Carlson, J.D. and Owens, E.C. eds. 2003. *The Sacred and the Sovereign*. Georgetown University Press: Washington, DC: 113.

sovereign states; Second, that this initial stipulation implies that the state is also the ultimate guarantor of those rights; and Third, that where the state cannot or does not act as the enacting agent, it becomes concomitant upon the "international community of sovereign states" to intervene/assume some responsibility. All the while, however, the erstwhile sovereign state, or state presumed to reassert sovereignty at some later stage, remains the ultimate guarantor thereof. The arrangement, however, conspicuously lacks an inverse relationship: whereas the state is accountable to the "international community," the same is not true in reverse. Despite whatever action or intervention this "international community" might take on behalf of, with or without the consent of the sovereign state, for whatever period of time, this is not subject to the same ultimate guarantee. Thus if that "international community" deigns to continue its intervention, there is little if any recourse for the state to take to reinstate a guarantee; if such intervention has undermined state provision all the worse for the state; precisely as this ultimate guarantee of sovereign rights remains with the state.

The consequences of this non-alignment in a global, state-based governance system also populated by a burgeoning number of non-state actors and agents, are manifold. The most important of these is the disconnect between agents—state, external state, or non-state—appropriating and engaging in (for good and bad) the delivery of rights without assuming the corresponding sovereign responsibility or accountability. In other words, these actors do not assume long-term or ultimate responsibility, and cannot be held to account by the recipient state or citizens for the services they deliver, or the ensuing consequences to the authority or capacity, particularly in terms of undermining of limiting these, of state sovereignty. Ultimate responsibility and accountability for human security remain with the state. This conundrum exemplifies the vital necessity of re-thinking the provision and implementation of sovereignty, and of re-tooling it towards the guarantee of the rights and responsibilities.

Precedents show that such a governance order where responsibility and accountability are divvied up and delegated has indeed existed.

> The authority of political rule also is a matter of contention between medieval and modern versions of sovereignty. The medieval archetype highlights the growing acceptance that nations must give up sovereign space and share authority with a host of other actors, including religious bodies and institutions. This account also admits that a universal ethic or regime of human rights (perhaps codified by international law) could delimit the sovereignty of states and *hold them accountable to a higher moral standard than a minimalist anarchic system would allow.*[2]

---

2   Carlson, J.D. and Owens, E.C. eds. 2003. *The Sacred and the Sovereign.* Georgetown University Press: Washington, DC: 17.

Such a rearrangement must be global, since effective sovereign responsibility already functions not only within the realm of states, but over and under these (through transnational alliances),[3] as well as across them (bilaterally and multilaterally).[4]

> We must be mindful, though, that a challenge to the sovereign authority of oppressive states is contingent on the sovereignty of states that are willing to intervene (politically or militarily) on behalf of oppressed people. This assessment suggests that as we sketch out permutations and transfigurations of sovereignty, we cannot stop thinking about the continued importance of statehood.[5]

Therefore, the foundational stone of the current international system, namely state sovereignty (in all of its imperfections), remains as such. State sovereignty is (still) the recipient of advocacy effects to get it to act according to the obligations set forth by the parameters of sovereignty; it is also the first court of appeal for (sovereign) rights' protection and provision, as well as the (final) buffer against untoward global intervention [1]. In other words, state sovereignty is likely here to stay—subject to evolution and revolution.[6]

Given these precedents, the assumption of statehood remains intact and is differentiable according to the weight placed upon sovereignty and that placed upon statehood. For it is possible to have statehood without sovereignty, as implied by areas of limited statehood. In this instance, the state exists and is recognized by the international community of likewise sovereign states, but is unable to exercise its sovereignty. Examples include Somalia during its war-torn decades, as well as Bosnia during its suzerainty under the EU following the Balkan wars of the 1990s. It is similarly possible to have (limited) sovereignty without statehood, as the case of the Palestinian Territories exemplify. Welded together into the notion of *sovereign statehood*, it is possible to assume that the state's role as the *ultimate bearer of responsibility and accountability for the security and welfare of its populace* as prescribed by the tenets of sovereignty holds. These tenets of sovereignty include, as detailed below, most importantly, the provision of security, the promotion of welfare, and the accountability of the state.

---

3   See Keck, M.E. and Sikkink, K. 1998. *Activists beyond Borders: Advocacy Networks in International Politics*. Ithaca and London: Cornell University Press, on "boomerang effect" of actors working to influence states to act to meet their sovereign responsibilities—to protect, notably human rights' norms.

4   See Rosenau, J.N. 1992. "Governance, order, and change in world politics." In Rosenau, J. and Czempiel, E.-O. eds. *Governance without Government: Order and Change in World Politics*. Cambridge: Cambridge University Press. Re: "regimes."

5   Carlson, J.D. and Owens, E.C. eds. 2003. *The Sacred and the Sovereign*. Georgetown University Press: Washington, DC: 10.

6   Philpott, D. 2001. *Revolutions in Sovereignty: How Ideas Shaped Modern International Relations*. Princeton: Princeton University Press.

The projected path to recovery depends upon the successful implementation of *the responsibility to respond.* The treatment prescribed usually involves some variant of the nominally sovereign state asking, allowing, or at least acknowledging that external state and non-state actors and entities assume some of the functions that are the remit of sovereign statehood. In theory, this might strengthen sovereign statehood, where it is able to both assert sovereignty and maintain authority and control over the responsibility to respond. In practice, however, the prognosis is often another; namely the devolution of *sovereign* responsibility whereby external state and non-state actors effectively take on some of the tasks required to enact some of the tenets of sovereign protection and welfare at least on a temporary basis; they but do not assume ultimate or final sovereign responsibility or accountability. This results in a schism between state and external state and non-state responsibility and accountability. I call it the Governance Accountability Problem, the GAP. Far from supporting sovereign statehood this can further weaken it, jeopardizing the state's *ultimate* responsibility and accountability. Even a state not normally considered fragile, such as South Africa, can be affected.

In introducing this new concept, I aim to draw attention to the confluence of the legitimacy of the sovereign state, its theoretical as well as functional role as the guarantor of the rights of its citizens, and the allocation and assumption of the execution of the responsibility of those rights by both the state and external actors. In doing so, I argue that merely allowing the latter—external actors—to assume in an ad hoc manner the execution of states whose ultimate responsibility and guarantee lies with the state is neither a legitimate nor sustainable governance solution. As such, the suggestion of the GAP has two purposes: first, to further contribute to the understanding of the idea of limited sovereignty, and second, to deepen policy analysis both theoretically and practically where it can be applied particularly to the problem of national and global allocation of human rights to (public) goods.

The newest member of the BRICS (Brazil, Russia, India, China, and South Africa) group of emerging global powers, South Africa is the largest economy on the African continent. It has been hailed as a leader in democracy and reconciliation. Yet South Africa is arguably also a weak state, struggling to exercise its ultimate responsibility and accountability to respond.

Acknowledging the fact that in practice no state is completely sovereign, the focus here is on South Africa's "domestic" sovereignty, its control over its internal affairs (even as affected by external actors), as differentiated by Stephan Krasner. His classification of sovereignty also includes international (legal), Westphalian, and interdependence sovereignty; wherein:[7] international (legal) sovereignty is the state's legal recognition by other states, Westphalian sovereignty connotes the indivisibility and inviolability of its borders under a strict hierarchy of bilateral rule, and interdependence sovereignty refers to state control over border flows.

---

7   Krasner, S. 1999. *Sovereignty: Organized Hypocrisy.* Princeton: Princeton University Press.

It is important to note that for this analysis, the responsibility to respond, though interfered with *inside* the state by non-state actors, is not subject to a breach of Westphalian sovereignty and the imposition of hierarchical norms and rules imposed from the *outside*. Likewise, the constraints this constellation imparts are not challenges to international or interdependence sovereignty, but fundamentally infractions on domestic sovereignty. This is especially evident in South Africa's decades-long response to its HIV/AIDS epidemic.

The case of HIV/AIDS in South Africa is an apt departure of analysis of the responsibility to respond in terms of sovereign statehood for three reasons: first (as noted above), because South Africa is rarely thought of as a weak state dependent upon external assistance to meet its responsibility to respond; second, because HIV/AIDS is a complex problem—long-term, with social, economic, and political dimensions all bringing with them repercussions for sovereign statehood—that not only requires an individual medical response, but also demands local, national and global governance mobilization and intervention; and third, because the lessons to be learned from South Africa's experience responding to the demands of health rights, notably as related to HIV/AIDS response, are applicable beyond that incisive case study.

The World Health Organization (WHO) defines the right to health as "*the enjoyment of the highest attainable standard of health is one of the fundamental rights of every human being ...*" which is increasingly read to mean not only access to preventive and primary care, but to tertiary care and complicated medical regimens for communicable disease, as well as treatments against non-communicable and chronic illnesses, as well as mental health care. Providing not only access to such comprehensive care but also ensuring its sustainable provision is a behemoth task. A number of instruments attempt to regulate and reinforce this sentiment, including the Trade-Related Aspects of Intellectual Property Rights (TRIPS) Agreement, signed under the auspices of the World Trade Organization in 1995, which provides protection for states invoking a national emergency to access vital patented medications—

> While the WTO Doha Declaration on TRIPS affirmed its members' right to protect public health, access to affordable pharmaceuticals was blocked by the requirement that the drug in question only have its patent removed if the state proved that the disease in question was of epidemic and emergency proportions[8]—

and the International Covenant on Economic, Social and Cultural Rights' (ICESCR), whose Article 12 stipulates that the right to health requires states to recognize the right of everyone to the enjoyment of the highest attainable standard of physical and mental health, meaning that states have the obligation to respect, protect, and fulfill the right to health.[9]

---

8   Davies, S.E. 2010. *Global Politics of Health*. Cambridge: Polity Press.
9   See General Comment 14.

> Governments have a responsibility for the health of their people which can be fulfilled only by the provision of adequate health and social measures. A main social target of governments, international organizations and the whole world community in the coming decades should be the attainment by all peoples of the world by the year 2000 of a level of health that will permit them to lead a socially and economically productive life.[10]

Of course, fulfilling this right, in other words meeting this obligation, requires a state to possess the "necessary means for individuals to access health care." But whether that means that the state has to provide healthcare beyond access, and to what extent it is obligated to provide it, remains unclear. Indeed, how to deliver upon how much of this mandate has been a debate for the past 30 years, most notably surrounding contested space of the HIV/AIDS response, particularly in South Africa.

As a medical crisis, HIV/AIDS threatens the lives of individual human beings as well as the livelihoods of families, the transfer of knowledge across generations, and the integrity and stability of communities forced to cope with the burden of the sick and dying, as well as with those left behind by a disease that incapacitates and kills people in their prime. Likewise, the disease and its ramifications negatively impact business performance, with small-, and medium-sized enterprises crippled by the loss of labor, and even larger businesses budgeting to train two or three workers for each position under the working assumption that only one will live long enough to assume it; money that might have been used in innovation and production instead. The compounded effects of such socio-economic dissolution cripple political institutions dependent upon amassed knowledge and accumulated tax revenue, and legitimized by voter participation. Where these components are lacking, domestic sovereignty lacks both the capacity and (eventually) the authority to implement its associated responsibility to respond. This arguably became the case in South Africa.

As a consequence, in order to enact its responsibility to respond, the state depends upon non-state actors; at times willingly and by invitation and at times not. There are referred to here as "local-global alliances." They operate by "creating constraining institutions and bringing states into more routinized contacts" of "transnational activist networks," "enabling them to use both these institutions and the state resources behind them to contact and assist domestic groups in conflict with their own states," reaching "across and within societies and authority for the implementation of policies;" and their impact occurs not on a cloud of global governance, but at the very concrete level of local and state governance.[11]

Such entities have included internal actors, such as advocacy (for example, South Africa's Treatment Action Campaign, TAC) and non-governmental

---

10   From the Declaration of Alma-Ata, paragraph V.

11   Tarrow, S. 1999. "International Institutions and Contentious Policies: Does Internationalization Make Agents Freer—or Weaker?" ASA Presentation: 4.

organizations (NGOs) which form local-global alliances with external advocacy (such as the US's ACT-UP) with and non-governmental organizations (for instance Médecins Sans Frontières (MSF)/Doctors without Borders) to put pressure on the state to take up its responsibility to respond. Multilateral assistance programs such as those implemented by international governmental organizations (IGOs), principally the World Bank's Multi-Country AIDS Program (MAP) and the UN and UNAIDS, provide educational and prevention campaigns as well as technical support to countries to address the epidemic. They also count among them and their advocates and enablers, bilateral programs, most prominently the US President's Emergency Plan for AIDS Relief (PEPFAR), and transnational corporations (TNCs), notably Anglo Group, DeBeers, Daimler (Chrysler), Eli Lilly, and VW, as well as global philanthropies, including the Bill and Melinda Gates Foundation, enter the fray with their own intervention programs, creating response systems parallel to that of the state.

The evolution of the response to HIV/AIDS in South Africa designated by both the state and a host of external state and non-state actors and entities resulted in a plethora of actions to fight the epidemic. These, while addressing the demands of the HIV/AIDS epidemic, served to decouple the tactical from the ultimate responsibility to respond of the South African state. This decoupling progressed because the state does not formally *shed* responsibility; whereas doing so would have vouchsafed its accountability. Failing that, the state did not span, but rather expanded, the schism implied in the GAP. Instead, it increasingly relied upon external actors to enact its response, without accounting for the (transfer of) its ultimate responsibility, which remains under the purview of the state.

In identifying the GAP, this book builds on the inheritance of the constructivist ideas presented in *The Power of Principles: International Human Rights Norms and Domestic Change*,[12] which argues that the adoption of new norms depends upon the constellation of the domestic political scene and access of policy advocates to it, as well as that of *The Power of Human Rights: International Norms and Domestic Change*, which explores the conditions "under which networks of domestic and international actors are able to change these domestic structures themselves."[13] It moves a step beyond that of Keck and Sikkink's "boomerang effect" hypothesis,[14] in which transnational advocacy networks exert their influence upon states who execute the desired response, to assert that transnational alliances are not only changing domestic structures, but are supplanting them. In this instance, such transnational alliances of non-state actors are not merely *advocating* state action and sourcing the power of their activism from both within

12   Risse-Kappen, T. 1994. *The Power of Principles: International Human Rights Norms and Domestic Change*. Cambridge: Cambridge University Press.

13   Risse, T., Ropp, S.C. and Sikkink, K. eds. 1999. *The Power of Human Rights: International Norms and Domestic Change*. Cambridge: Cambridge University Press: 8–9.

14   Keck, M.E. and Sikkink, K. 1999. *Transnational Advocacy Networks in International and Regional Politics*. Blackwell Publishers, UNESCO, ISSJ 159: 90–103.

and outside of the state to *boomerang* back to the state to compel it to act,[15] but are, in fact, themselves actively engaging in the targeted action. The crucial caveat is that these usurpers—intentionally or unintentionally—are doing so without assuming ultimate responsibility or accountability. In making this distinction, this book draws on Krasner (cited above), and Vittorio Hösle's seminal work, *Morals and Politics*, as well as Daniel Philpott's *Revolutions in Sovereignty*,[16] to grapple with and construct a new understanding of the relationship between rights, responsibility and accountability from the vantage point of evolutions in sovereignty. This *ultimate* responsibility and accountability remains within the remit of the (contested) domestic sovereignty of the state.

Bearing this in mind, and in order to pursue the analysis, this book makes three formal assumptions. First, that HIV/AIDS does indeed pose a problem for the South African state and its responsibility to respond. Second, that this problem is actually transnational, and that local-global alliances of non-state actors, multi- and bilateral programs, IGOs, and TNCs are assuming not only advocacy and agenda-setting and financing roles in the face of it, but are also increasingly taking on tactical roles in response. In the case of HIV/AIDS, this includes not only challenging the state's responsibility to respond in court, but also importing and prescribing medicines, and building and staffing clinics. In doing so, they are supplementing or supplanting the role of the state in terms of response, but without assuming ultimate responsibility and accountability.

Increasingly, non-state actors are (also) taking on some of the functions formerly reserved for the realm of sovereignty. They are persuading states to act, or even bullying them, assuming some of erstwhile state functions and poaching some of state capacity to do so, in effect creating a parallel system of sorts—one that proffers at least as much possibility as it portends danger.

Daimler (Chrysler)'s initial policy outlining the company's response to HIV/AIDS treatment stipulated that after two years of the company providing treatment to its employees and a limited number of dependents, it would transfer their care to the state. AngloGroup arguably forswore some of its responsibility by firing its salaried miners and (re)hiring contract workers for whom the company bears no liability.[17] Neither is a prescription for the responsibility to respond. These are examples of the operational assumption: that the state will assume the burden of that responsibility.

---

15   "Many activities of advocacy networks follow the 'boomerang pattern': State A blocks redress to organizations within it; they activate networks, whose members pressure their own state and (if relevant) a third-party organization, which in turn pressure State A." Keck, M.E. and Sikkink, K. 1998. *Activists beyond Borders: Advocacy Networks in International Politics*. Ithaca and London: Cornell University Press: 13.

16   Philpott, D. 2001. *Revolutions in Sovereignty: How Ideas Shaped Modern International Relations*. Princeton: Princeton University Press.

17   Personal communication with Fanyana Shiburi, in his capacity as healthcare consultant with CompleteMed, Midrand, South Africa, 2006.

A society in which the piling up of special interests replaces a single strong voice for the common good is unlikely to fare well. Single-issue voters, as Americans know all too well, polarize and freeze public debate. In the longer run, a stronger civil society could also be more fragmented, producing a weakened sense of common identity and purpose and less willingness to invest in public goods, whether health and education or roads and ports. More and more groups promoting worthy but narrow causes could ultimately threaten democratic government.[18]

And so some of them came, and they said [sic] we'll form our own NGOs to drive it. And so the system was in serious tension. And new sources of funding like the philanthropies who were coming up, the Gates Foundations, et cetera, all came with a—with a project. And all of them were worthy. You [the state] couldn't argue against someone wanting to come and fight malaria or HIV.[19]

There are roles that only the state—at least among today's polities (as actors responsible for the guarantee of sovereign protections)—can perform. Mathews' analysis even foreshadows such a reality:

It maybe that only the nation-state can meet crucial social needs that markets do not value. Providing a modicum of job security, avoiding higher unemployment, preserving a livable environmental and a stable climate, and protecting consumer health and safety are but a few of the tasks that could be left dangling in a world of expanding markets and retreating states.[20]

Who then, and how then, can the ultimate responsibility to respond be guaranteed? That is the question.

In order to arrive at the answer in the case of HIV/AIDS in South Africa, this one overarching question can be broken down into three parts. How did South Africa meet its responsibility to respond to its HIV/AIDS epidemic between 1981 and 2011? The answer must be divided into two: the direct state response to the epidemic, including the early identification of the problem coupled with an initial policy response against the backdrop of the country's democratic transition, followed lately by the provision of antiretroviral medicines; and the parallel transnational and non-state efforts to steer South Africa's response.

Where to, then, the ultimate responsibility to respond? Arguably, it is a victim of the GAP. On the one hand, the state and the parallel alliances each stepped in to respond to HIV/AIDS and assumed various operational responsibilities. Nonetheless, state sovereignty dictates that it harbor the ultimate responsibility and

---

18   Ibid.
19   Rasool, E. 2012. Remarks to CFR, 9 January. Available at: www.cfr.org/.
20   Mathews, J.T. 1997. "Power Shift." *Foreign Affairs*, January/February.

accountability. Therefore, on the other hand, there is a void—widening—between a weak(ening) state without recourse to share its responsibility and accountability: the GAP.

Two solutions stand out. First, that a state of necessity relying on external, non-state actors to assume capacity and to deliver a response should be able to *shed* not only functions and responsibility but also the associated accountability. Second, that since a state having to so delegate is unlikely to have the ability to enforce the breach of such delegation, a system of coordinated *shared* governance, consisting of legal delineation of responsibility and accountability among all participating actors at the local, national and global governance levels, is required to sustain sovereign statehood and the responsibility to respond.

By analyzing the responsibility to respond to the HIV/AIDS crisis in South Africa though the lens of sovereign statehood, this dissertation makes two contributions to political science. First, it analyzes the contemporary constellation of responsibility and accountability vis-à-vis the responsibility to respond on the part of the sovereign state and its interlopers, and identifies a GAP in both theory and practice. Second, it proposes both theoretical and practical solutions to bridge this GAP.

1.1 State Sovereignty

Sovereign statehood as defined above implicates three central tenets subsumed under the rubric of the responsibility to respond. These are generally understood as the obligations to (a) ensure the territorial and physical security of citizens; (b) protect lives and livelihoods by providing basic economic stability, health, and welfare; and (c) bear accountability to itself and to the international community.[21] All three encoded responsibilities are intrinsically tied to a state's domestic sovereignty. The final tenet foreshadows the GAP as it holds the state to account to the international community of states, and arguably the non-state entities they support, but lacks an inverse stipulation.

This is especially evident in the trajectory of South Africa's response to its HIV/AIDS epidemic, which unfolded in three phases and mirror the three tenets of sovereignty outlined above. The first (ca. 1981–1998) acknowledged the problem, but was accompanied by a limited interpretation of the responsibility to respond, particularly as the state balanced competing priorities, including the basic security of its citizens in the state of emergency that marked the end of apartheid and in the first uncertain years after the transition to democratic rule. The second (ca. 1998–2003) was characterized by a fierce debate, even battle, over

---

21 Hösle, V. 2004. *Morals and Politics.* Notre Dame: University of Notre Dame Press; and Risse, T. 2007. "Paradoxien der Souveränität. Die konstituive Norm, auf der die heutige Staatenwelt gründet—dass nämlich Staaten souverän sind—gilt uneingeschränkt nicht mehr. Was heisst das?" *Internationale Politik,* July/August: 40–47.

the components of a broader responsibility to respond, pitting the state against alliances of external state and non-state actors both locally and globally, to provide medical treatment and economic welfare. The third (ca. 2003–2011) is the struggle for ultimate responsibility, as the state and external actors who intervened with tactical solutions in the second phase now must sort out where the necessarily associated sovereign responsibility and accountability lie. The challenges they face affirm not only the GAP but also highlight the broader phenomenon of limited statehood.

1.2 (Limited) State Sovereignty in South Africa

As posited above, though it is not usually considered a weak state or more specifically one limited in its sovereign statehood, South Africa does show some of the designating characteristics. This is especially evident with regard to the state's responsibility to respond and to account in terms of its own domestic sovereignty as well as in relation to the international community of sovereign states in the case of its HIV/AIDS epidemic. There, South Africa did not respond to HIV/AIDS in a manner designated by its local advocates and activists in alliance with global state and non-state actors. Its weakness in failing to respond as such opened the gates for those alliances and the 'international community of sovereign states' to which South Africa is in essence accountable as well as non-state actors, to intervene. These interventions did not constitute a breach of Westphalian sovereignty, as they did not impose an external, rule-based hierarchy upon South Africa, but their assumption of tactical response without ultimate accountability nonetheless further weakened the South African state—limiting its state sovereignty.

Is this weakness a one-way street?

According to the third tenet of sovereignty, the state is accountable to itself and to that international community of sovereign states, but the latter is not likewise accountable to the former. In very extreme cases of state failure to enact its responsibility to respond, notably in cases of genocide, crimes against humanity and ethnic cleansing, states external to that committing unable to stop or itself perpetrating such atrocities would be called upon to invoke the "responsibility to protect" (R2P) and to intervene to deliver the erstwhile sovereign responsibility for security. This happened, retroactively, in Kosovo in 1999, and arguably in Libya in 2011; the verdict is out on whether the doctrine will be invoked with repercussions in Syria in 2012. R2P asserts an international responsibility and accountability for security in weak states only begrudgingly accepted. Whether R2P interventions strengthen or weaken the states they "protect" (given that Kosovo is now an independent country, having seceded from Serbia) is debatable. However, what becomes obvious is that while this "international community of sovereign states" can pursue an intervention to respond to the lack of responsibility and accountability of the erstwhile sovereign state, no mechanism holds that same "international community of sovereign states," let alone non-state actors, to account for such an intervention. Whether then their intervention strengthens or weakens the target state, or even successfully or unsuccessfully responds to the problem at hand, remains outside of the realm of accounting.

Thus, the evolution of South Africa's responsibility to respond to its HIV/ AIDS epidemic is invariably tied to that of its limited statehood.[22] What came first, South Africa's limited statehood and therefore its necessary reliance on external state and non-state actors to enact its responsibility to respond? Or the intervention of external state and non-state actors to assume the state's responsibility to respond, thereby weakening its statehood? The source of South Africa's limited statehood is not (only) the weakness of the state itself, but (also) the consequence of dissociating sovereign functions while leaving the state to guarantee ultimate responsibility and accountability.[23]

This divergence between tactical responsibility and ultimate responsibility and accountability in sovereign statehood is not only a problem for South Africa. No state is completely sovereign. Every one relies to differing degrees on local and external and global partners to define priorities and set agendas. They "breed new ideas; advocate, protest, and mobilize public support; do legal, scientific, technical, and policy analysis; provide services; shape, implement, monitor, and enforce national and international commitments; and change institutions and norms."[24] "They" include individuals empowered by globalizing technologies; international governance bodies such at the UN, and the G8 and G20, and the BRICS association; as well as civil society organizations (CSOs), NGOs, (international governmental organizations) IGOs, transnational corporations (TNCs), and global philanthropies such as the Bill and Melinda Gates Foundation, and others.

> Where governments are unresponsive to groups whose claims may none the less resonate elsewhere, international contacts can 'amplify' the demands of domestic groups, pry open space for new issues, then echo these demands back into the domestic arena. Needless to say, in such cases the use of a boomerang strategy is politically sensitive, and is subject to charges of foreign interference into domestic affairs.[25]

---

22   See for example, Risse, T. 2007. "Paradoxien der Souveränität. Die konstitutive Norm, auf der die heutige Staatenwelt gründet—dass nämlich Staaten souverän sind—gilt uneingeschränkt nicht mehr. Was heisst das?" *Internationale Politik*, July/August: 40–47.

23   "It is no accident that 'rights' claims may be the prototypical language of advocacy networks. Governments are the primary 'guarantors' of rights, but also among their primary violators. When a government violates or refuses to recognize rights, individuals and domestic groups often have no recourse within domestic political or judicial arenas. They may seek international connections to express their concerns or even to protect their lives." Keck, M.E. and Sikkink, K. 1999. *Transnational Advocacy Networks in International and Regional Politics*. Blackwell Publishers, UNESCO, ISSJ 159: 90–103.

24   Mathews, J.T. 1997. "Power Shift." *Foreign Affairs*, January/February.

25   Keck, M.E. and Sikkink, K. 1999. *Transnational Advocacy Networks in International and Regional Politics*. Blackwell Publishers, UNESCO, ISSJ 159: 94.

In some instances, they even deliver the response.

In doing so, these non-state actors simultaneously support and supplement state action, but also circumvent and curtail it.[26] On the one hand, they are persuading states to act, or even bullying them.

> Many transnational advocacy networks link activists in developed countries with others in or from less developed countries. These kinds of linkages are most commonly intended to affect the behavior of states. When the links between state and domestic actors are severed (or at least strained) domestic NGOs may directly seek international allies to try to bring pressure on their states from outside (external). This is the 'boomerang' pattern of influence characteristic of transnational networks where the target of their activity is to change a state's behavior.[27]

On the other hand they are assuming, as in enacting, some of erstwhile state functions and poaching some of state capacity to do so, in effect creating a parallel system of sorts—one that proffers at least as much possibility as it portends danger. Possibility where the responsibility to respond might be enhanced and states of limited statehood shored up; danger where the responsibility to respond is devolved among a series of unaccountable actors further limiting statehood.

Counter-intuitive to the post-modern notion that states are interdependent and integrated to the point of irrelevance, is the verdict premised on this contextual analysis that states are and remain the inherent building blocks of the current (global) governance system. Their viability therefore, most especially including their ability to assume ultimate responsibility and accountability is fundamentally necessary.

> The Westphalian system and an evolving one will exist side by side. States will set the rules by which all the others operate, but outside forces will increasingly make decisions for them. In using business, NGOs, and international organizations to address problems they cannot or do not want to take on, states will, more often than not, inadvertently weaken themselves further … At least for a time, the transition [to global governance] is likely to weaken rather than bolster the

---

26   See also Tarrow, S. 1999. "International Institutions and Contentious Policies: Does Internationalization Make Agents Freer—or Weaker?" 6. "Analysts like Peter Katzenstein focus on the loss of control involved in internationalization; Although internationalization can take many different forms, virtually all analysts agree that the openness of national economies to a variety of cross-border flows … is its defining characteristic. Internationalization can lead to a loss of control and accountability as markets and social processes circumvent state borders and government policies."

27   Keck, M.E. and Sikkink, K. 1999. *Transnational Advocacy Networks in International and Regional Politics*. Blackwell Publishers, UNESCO, ISSJ 159: 94.

world's capacity to solve its problems. If states, with the overwhelming share of power, wealth, and capacity, can do less, less will get done.[28]

It is the international community of sovereign states and non-state actors which must be folded into an emerging order of shared governance delineating responsibility and accountability to counter the chaos which currently pervades the system.

1.3 The GAP

The premise offered above is derived directly from the concept of the Governance Accountability Problem. For without recourse and means of accounting, which still ends with the state—although trends in global accountability are emerging—both the validity and the practical reality of rights remain theoretical. So the GAP offers a lens through which to evaluate the delineation of such accounting for rights' responsibility at the national and global levels. It is not enough merely for problems to be solved in an ad hoc manner as long as that "works"; it is vitally necessary to prepare for the contingency and to provide the means of protecting rights precisely in the cases where they are most threatened and when problem-solving fails. In the current (inter)national system, the final port of call for such arbitration is and remains the state.

Indeed, state-centric global governance is just that: state-centric. States, under the auspices of their sovereign statehood, assume the responsibility and accountability for the security and welfare of their realm. That accountability is checked by the international community of sovereign states, which like the legion of non-state actors which populate local and global political space, paradoxically, bear no comparable responsibility or accountability to states in which they intervene. In other words, in the current system where the implementation of sovereign responsibilities is scattered between state/s and non-state actors, it is unclear who has the authority to determine and decide upon the policies of governance, and who bears the final accountability. Who is the sovereign, who is the guarantor? This question goes to the heart of the GAP between state and external state and non-state responsibility and accountability for which no clear bridge exists.

As South African Ambassador to the US, Ebrahim Rasool, said in 2012 in a statement applicable to the case study of South Africa's response to the HIV/AIDS epidemic analyzed here,

> And so some of them [external state, and non-state actors] came, and they said [sic] we'll form our own NGOs to drive it. And so the system was in serious tension. And new sources of funding like the philanthropies who were coming

---

28   Ibid.

up, the Gates Foundations, et cetera, all came with a—with a project. And all of them were worthy. You [the state] couldn't argue against someone wanting to come and fight malaria or HIV.[29]

But perhaps the state, given that "someone wanting to come and fight malaria or HIV," might not assume the corresponding responsibility and accountability for their response, could in fact argue against such intervention? Or find ways and means of legally transferring such responsibility and accountability in such a way that supports instead of limits sovereign statehood? This is the dilemma that South Africa faced, and on which the viewpoint of the GAP sheds new light.

1.4 State Sovereignty, HIV/AIDS and the Responsibility to Respond in South Africa

So what is the relationship between the South African state, its HIV/AIDS epidemic and its responsibility to respond? How has South Africa' responded? It addressed its HIV/AIDS epidemic in three phrases reflective of the three tenets of sovereignty outlined above. In doing so, the sovereign state both assumed its responsibility to respond, and challenged the GAP to find amenable ways and means of allocating responsibility and accountability amongst the litany of state and non-state players in the HIV/AIDS sphere. But it has not yet implemented a fourth (final) phase.

As epitomized in South Africa's experience, from its political transition from apartheid to democracy to its HIV/AIDS crisis, "more and more frequently today, governments have only the appearance of free choice."[30] "Markets are setting de facto rules enforced by their own power,"[31] the "often intractable rules of the global economy" and "populist and redistributive rules"[32] often backed by state governments,[33] as evidenced in the US Government backing of pharmaceutical companies involved in HIV/AIDS response, and in the epic state-financed bailouts of private financial entities in the 2007 crisis and beyond. "States can flout [such market regulations], but the penalties are severe—loss of vital foreign capital,

---

29 Rasool, E. 2012. Remarks to CFR, 9 January. Available at: www.cfr.org/.

30 Keck, M.E. and Sikkink, K. 1999. *Transnational Advocacy Networks in International and Regional Politics*. Blackwell Publishers, UNESCO, ISSJ 159: 94.

31 Ibid.

32 Thomas Friedman quoted in Booysen, S. 2001. "Transitions and trends in policy making in democratic South Africa." *Journal of Public Administration*, 36(2): 125–144.

33 See also Tarrow, S. 1999. "International Institutions and Contentious Policies: Does Internationalization Make Agents Freer—or Weaker?" 4. "These relations often involve nonstate actors directly in the internal business of target states; but they frequently turn on the power of other states and international institutions."

foreign technology, and domestic jobs,"[34] to say nothing of access to desperately needed medicines, as in the case of HIV/AIDS in South Africa.

So what did the South African state do, and why did it do it, to respond to its HIV/AIDS epidemic between 1981 and 2011?

The three phases of South Africa's response to HIV/AIDS mirror the incomplete transformation from limited sovereignty—focusing only on territorial security—to limited sovereign statehood that can account, to itself and the international community of sovereign states, for its responsibility to respond.

In this process, the state's initially cautious and limited response to its burgeoning HIV/AIDS epidemic is to be seen in light of its pursuit of the integrity of the country's territorial security after years of emergency rule and violent struggle. Amidst the spread of HIV/AIDS in the meantime, this 'misplaced' prioritization served as an impetus for a loose coalition of local and global non-state actors initially try to elicit, as per the boomerang hypothesis, a prompt response to the epidemic. Despite political awareness of the impending epidemic, this did not succeed.

The second phase, coinciding roughly with the entry then of anti-AIDS medications, antiretrovirals (ARVs), onto the global market in 1996, parallels the sovereign tenet to provide for the well-being and welfare of a sovereign state's populace. The South African state sought access to medicines without sacrificing its independence in exchange. In the meantime, in seemingly apparent reaction to this stance, local-global alliances, with significant state-backing external to South Africa, changed their approach. They shifted from advocacy to action. This shift is also evidenced in the UN General Assembly adopted Resolution 60/262, entitled "Political Declaration on HIV/AIDS" adopted on 15 June 2006. It reiterated many of the stipulations of UN Security Council Resolution S-26/2 of 2001, with one significant exception: whereas S-26/2 focused its attention on strategies on local, *national*, regional and global governmental responses to HIV/AIDS, resolution 60/262 all but ignored the role of state governments in shaping and enacting the response to the pandemic, instead highlighting the role of non-governmental organizations, many of which bypass the structural authority of national governments.

These developments had two consequences. First, as a *du jour* arrangement, it appropriated functions of the responsibility to respond formally subsumed under state sovereignty. It did not assume associated responsibility or accountability that remained under the rubric of South Africa's sovereign statehood. Second, lacking this authority, the arrangement did not foster the South African states ability to deliver upon its sovereign responsibility to respond, but instead actually undermined it. This contributed to the GAP.

---

34   Keck, M.E. and Sikkink, K. 1999. *Transnational Advocacy Networks in International and Regional Politics*. Blackwell Publishers, UNESCO, ISSJ 159: 91.

Why, after pitched legal battles and protracted stalling in providing access to antiretroviral medicines, did South Africa relent to this tactical-ultimate accountability schism? What changed?

In this third phase, South Africa rose to the occasion to meet its accountability to the international community of sovereign states as spelled out under the third tenet of sovereignty. By 2003, the South African Government recalibrated its response to the epidemic in collaboration with local-global pressure. That year, it promulgated the first national strategic plan to fight HIV/AIDS complete with provision for antiretroviral drugs. In adopting that initial strategic plan, the country's leadership attempted to corral the sovereign responsibility and ability to respond to the burgeoning HIV/AIDS epidemic. Its efforts were matched, even outmatched, by the launch of various international HIV/AIDS programs (notably the US President's Emergency Fund against AIDS (PEPFAR)), on whose financial prowess South Africa's HIV/AIDS response also drew. The alliance has two key consequences. First, it illustrates the possibility of providing complex treatment in a resource-poor setting. It also showcases one effect of local-global cooperation, for instance through non-state networks or alliances or through more formal bilateral or multilateral institutions, which appears to assume some of the traditional tasks of national government. As a result, the control sphere of the government becomes yet more circumscribed. Consequently, when the global financial crisis commenced in 2007, the country lost some of the external funding necessary to enact its commitments related to the HIV/AIDS response. This again scuttled its ability to guarantee its enactment of sovereign commitments while leaving it carrying the ultimate burden of its responsibility to respond.

What lessons can be learned from the South African experience to facilitate the bridging of the GAP between national and global responsibility and accountability to respond?

The trajectory of this evolution of a renegotiated allocation of responsibility and accountability flows to its ultimate repository in the sovereign state. As such, only the state can reallocate, or delegate, that responsibility and accountability: if it does so, it maintains its authority and power, but allows the instruments thereof to be wielded by partners. This enables the bridging of the GAP between the state's theoretical and practical sovereignty.

1.5 Analyzing South Africa's Response to HIV/AIDS

This analysis has two aims. The first is to dissect the South African policy response to its HIV/AIDS epidemic with a view toward how and why the state sought to act upon its sovereign responsibility to respond. The second is to discern theoretical insights from this case study that can be applied to the GAP between tactical and ultimate responsibility and accountability of sovereign statehood.

Towards this end, three things are vital to bear in mind: these are, the three tenets of sovereignty, notably the provision of security, of welfare, and of accountability; the limits of sovereign statehood and the state as the ultimate repository of responsibility and accountability; and the differentiation between the un-delineated allocation and assumption of the responsibility to respond that leads to the GAP in weak states and states compromised by limited statehood, and the complete capacity void suggested by the notion of "hollow states."[35]

According to Poku and Whiteside, "hollow states" are "unable to fulfil their core responsibilities and functions," and "could not provide sustained leadership across society or adequately interact with citizens through democratic institutions—and would thus be at risk for greater political instability."[36] An assertion of such sweeping inability is not the assumption of this analysis, which rather posits that the state possesses and retains legitimacy, and that the source of its limitation is instead a function both of circumscribed capacity per se, as well as of intervention visited upon it by local-global alliances of extra-state actors (both state and non-state) relieving it of some tactical responsibility—but in neither instance assuming accompanying responsibility and accountability to respond. This becomes a circular equation in which one element reinforces the other. As such, the state's sovereign statehood is in the essence of its theory untouched, while its practical exercise is increasingly circumscribed. Yet, as noted above, "there are roles that only the state" can perform, responsibilities that lie exclusively within its remit. Therefore, any solution to this systemic GAP requires states. Therefore this analysis focuses primarily on the South African national governmental response to the HIV/AIDS epidemic as it navigates its domestic sovereign statehood responsibility to respond amidst competing local-global priorities and pressures.

This book proceeds from a public policy analysis and develops the emergent evidence into a new theory of the GAP in sovereign statehood's responsibility to respond and its ability to do so. This analytical approach stands in contrast to the policy analysis of management presented by scholar Pieter Fourie,[37] which focuses on the 'what' of South Africa's leaders, notably former President Mandela's reluctance while in office to address the crisis and former President Mbeki's ostensible "denialist" stance, as well as that of Nicoli Nattrass,[38] which focuses on the anti-AIDS drug debased in isolation of competing national and international priorities and policy impositions which influence positively or limit South Africa's response and its responsibility to respond to HIV/AIDS.

---

35   Poku, N. and Whiteside, A. 2006. "25 years: Challenges and prospects." *International Affairs HIV/AIDS Special Issue*, 82(2). Oxford: Chatham House (March).

36   Ibid.

37   Fourie, P. 2006. *The Political Management of HIV and AIDS in South Africa: One Burden Too Many?* London: Palgrave Macmillan; see also Fourie, P. 2007. "The Relationship between the AIDS Pandemic and State Fragility." *Global Change, Peace & Security* (Australia), 19(3).

38   Nattrass, N. 2007. *Mortal Combat: AIDS Denialism and the Struggle for Antiretrovirals in South Africa.* Scottsville: University of KwaZulu-Natal Press.

It is divided into five main sections. The first defines the dimensions of the problem of the HIV/AIDS epidemic in South Africa. This section consists of chapters two and three, which present a background analysis of the HIV/AIDS situation in South Africa. They explore the scope of the problem relying on both published and unpublished, primary-source, empirical epidemiological and demographic data, and employing statistics and qualitative analysis of the initial trajectory of the spread of the HI-virus into South Africa. They also locate the point in time when the burgeoning epidemic registered on the radar screens of policy-makers responsible for a response, and indicate the initial how and why of that reaction.

The second section analyses the phases of agenda-setting and option consideration, as influenced by the international and domestic circumstances prevalent in the HIV/AIDS policy arena in South Africa between 1990 and 2007. These profile South Africa's initial prioritization with the integrity of its security, the first tenet of implementing sovereign statehood. Going into detail, Chapters four and five focus on the international and national policy environments respectively, paying particular attention to the political and economic factors that compete for the South African Government's attention alongside and concomitant to the intensifying assertion of the presence of the HIV/AIDS epidemic.

The third section of this book is the step-by-step analysis of South Africa's litany of responses directly to its HIV/AIDS epidemic primed by the conditions presented in the above chapters. This constitutes the state's actions towards providing for the welfare and well-being of its citizens. As such, it begins with policy initiation, prompted (late) by the inauspicious encroaching of the epidemic, and advances to the initial identification of the problem. Agenda-setting and initial implementation of a policy follow, spurred not by state planning, but by non-state advocacy and activism, illustrating the complexity of policy-making in an area of limited statehood and portending toward the GAP.[39]

Section four offers an evaluation of the consequences of the fact that emerges from this case study of South Africa's responsibility to respond to its HIV/AIDS epidemic, and relates this to the state's accountability, as per tenet three of sovereign statehood, to the international community of sovereign states. It emerges that neither the national state nor non-bindingly responsible global governance, are conclusively endowed with or able to assume and act upon the protective tenets of sovereignty with complete and comprehensive responsibility and accountability. Based on its insights, chapter seven confirms both the existence of and the necessity

---

39   This refers notably to a system of global governance that relies on and cultivates local footprints which in turn serve to aid and abet that global system in bypassing the state apparatus: undermining sovereign statehood, and for a time perhaps, filling its shoes, but as this analysis will show, not assuming the long-term, sustainable responsibility and accountability for either its actions or for the protection of citizens, which remains the onus of the (crippled) state.

of closing the GAP due to limited statehood and a lack of delineation or delegation of sovereign responsibility that might bridge it.

Finally, section five proposes policy recommendations relating specifically to the responsibility to respond to HIV/AIDS at the national and global governance levels as a practical means of bridging the GAP on this particular issue, and more broadly to the responsibility to respond in light of the required reform of the systems and structures of global governance to accrue and achieve greater responsibility and accountability.

1.6 Conclusion

A new era of sovereign statehood is dawning: one where states and non-state actors are increasingly intertwined in implementing the sovereign responsibility to respond. Yet the allocation and assumption of associated accountability remains unclear, causing a GAP to form between tactical responsibility and ultimate accountability. This diagnosis, which left untreated, threatens increased state weakness and instability in a global governance system that relies upon states to shoulder the burdens of security and the responsibility to respond, requires a remedy.

That in turn entails a system alignment in which states assert their sovereign authority not only to enact the tenets of sovereignty but to delegate those they cannot meet alone while retaining their ultimate responsibility and accountability. Of course, this assumes that the state has the power to hold these actors and entities with which it entrusts the delivery of elemental sovereign functions to account in the event that they should fail. If these two criteria can be met, the GAP will be closed.

Ambassador Rasool calls this "shared governance" and declares that

> This change from an international system which was multinational, needing coordination for certain things, to a global health system in which national had to *cede some autonomy and take on transnational responsibility* was driven by the impact of globalization on health at that point; that *suddenly the tension between the national state and the globalizing world needed to be dealt with.*[40]

This is not a sudden development; all the more reason that the GAP needs to be addressed.

HIV/AIDS and the crises in global health—stemming not only from communicable diseases but increases from non-communicable diseases—as well as in governance areas such as global migration and associated rights and responsibilities with regard to healthcare and taxation, for example, and likewise

---

40   Rasool, E. 2012. Remarks to CFR, 9 January. Available at: www.cfr.org/ (emphasis added).

the regulation of water, are such that an ever increasing litany of states must regard themselves as weak and requiring ever more state and inter-state and non-state support to meet their responsibility to respond.

Therefore, given the particular and general applicability of this analysis, this dissertation aims to contribute two new insights to both the theoretical and practical political science debate on sovereign statehood and the public policy response to attendant crises. First, it offers an evidenced-based analysis of the GAP as illuminated by the case of HIV/AIDS in South Africa. Second, it provides a possible response of overlapping governance structures to bridge that gap in South Africa and HIV/AIDS, and beyond.

Chapter 2

Situational Analysis of HIV/AIDS in South Africa

This and the following chapter trace the historic and geographic trajectory of the HIV/AIDS crisis into and in South Africa. Relying on published and unpublished, primary-source, empirical epidemiological and demographic data, these inaugural chapters of this book analyze the scope and significance of the epidemic for South Africa. They also sketch South Africa's initial attempts at formulating a response.

The HIV/AIDS situation in South Africa is serious. Statistical analysis, whether at the local, national, or global levels, indicates that South Africa's epidemic remains the epicenter of the global pandemic. Forecasts are equally bleak. The historical trajectory of HIV/AIDS, as it traversed into South Africa, contains clues to the present crisis—and possibly to its future evolution. It also tracks the individual, social, economic and political repercussions. Arguably from the outset, political awareness existed, even if action, notably political and governmental action against HIV/AIDS lagged or lacked.

What are the characteristics of the HIV/AIDS epidemic crisis in South Africa? What are its social, economic and political attributes and impacts? What kind of challenge, or threat, does HIV/AIDS pose to the state?[1] Have these inspired a political response?

2.1 State of HIV/AIDS: Statistics

According to the December 2006 UNAIDS Epidemic report, South and sub-Saharan Africa together continue to bear the brunt of the epidemic impact, which shows no sign of abating. Two thirds (63 percent) of all adults and children with HIV globally live in sub-Saharan Africa, and 72 percent of all AIDS deaths globally

---

1 Some have argued that HIV/AIDS pose an "existential" threat to South Africa; I argue that the threat is one of myriad dimensions, from not quite a "hollowing out" of the state, to a "gap" between national and international governance, particularly of responsibility—in action—to respond; but not necessarily an existential threat per se. Nonetheless, indicating the continued relevance of the "exceptionalism" of HIV/AIDS, on 20 April 2009, Dr Alan Whiteside from South Africa's University of Natal Health Economics and HIV/AIDS Research Division (HEARD) presented on that topic at the Center for Global Development in Washington, DC.

occurred at the epidemic's epicenter in southern Africa.[2] These percentages translate into roughly 24.7 million people living with HIV/AIDS, including 2.8 million newly infected in 2006, with 2.1 million deaths in the sub-Saharan region in 2006 alone.

An era of HIV/AIDS has dawned and is here to stay.

Statistics offer a first glimpse into the divergent and yet interdependent local and global insights and responses to HIV/AIDS, which are the focus of later parts of this analysis. However, it is important to take these numbers with a grain of salt. Statistics, by their very nature, notably their methodology, cause significant controversy. They are continuously updated and revised. Nonetheless, they remain estimates, as statisticians are unable to test and assess the infection of each individual—though that is an aim of newer HIV/AIDS programs. Even if they could, by the time they did, more people would be infected, raising the incidence rate; others would have died, decreasing some prevalence; and still others would have accessed ARVs and increased their life expectancy. All these chances together would raise prevalence and perhaps contribute to increased incidence as the virus continues to spread. Plus, statistics are generally retrospective: released a number of years after the situation they assess. Furthermore, statistical data gathering is often constrained by access to clinics, testing-sites, and sources, and compounded by stigma, which tends to reduce the numbers of those being tested. Finally, the farther removed the statistical surveys from the afflicted, i.e. the individual test results in this case, the more unreliable their estimates.

Bearing this in mind, it comes as no surprise that there is contradictory statistical evidence as to HIV/AIDS in South Africa. Those discussed here are taken from four main sources: the Joint United Nations Programme on HIV/AIDS (UNAIDS) at the global level; the Department of Health at the national level; the Actuarial Society of South Africa's (ASSA) theoretical simulation and prediction also at the national level; and the Demographic Information Bureau (DIB) of the Development Bank of Southern Africa (DBSA) at the local level. True to the above statistical caveats, those from UNAIDS at the global level tend to posit higher levels of infection than does the national Department of Health. Interestingly, while ASSA's theoretical approach projects higher incidence and prevalence rates than those of the Department of Health, those attributed to the DIB, which uses a household survey and thus the most local approach to its statistical collection, are even higher—though not surpassing those of UNAIDS. It should be noted, too, that due to its methodology, DIB also has the most up-to-date data.[3]

Notwithstanding their shortcomings, these statistics all confirm the stark portrait of HIV/AIDS in South Africa. In its December 2006 report, UNAIDS estimated a prevalence rate of 18.8 percent, which corresponded to roughly nine

---

2   UNAIDS. 2006. AIDS Epidemic Update 2005. Geneva: UNAIDS: 10–23; main findings reiterated in 2009 and 2011 as well.

3   DIB Comparison Population Projections (3). Obtained from Johan Calitz at DIB/DBSA via private communication, 27 May 2008.

million HIV-infected South Africans. Bearing out the correlation between global distance and higher statistics, when compared with the national Department of Health's report, the difference is over seven percent and nearly four million people. According to the Demographic Impact Report of HIV/AIDS in South Africa—National and Provincial Indicators for 2006, the Department of Health calculated that out of a population of 48 million, 11 percent, or 5.4 million South Africans were HIV-positive. Of those, the Department estimated that 600,000 were living with AIDS, of whom 225,000 were receiving antiretroviral treatment. Of the other 3.5 million HIV-infected individuals, some 1.3 were estimated to be under 25 years of age. Furthermore, using an erstwhile popular indicator—HIV status as measured at antenatal clinics (despite these being self-selecting, and therefore poor sources from which to generalize, as at the time such testing was both officially encouraged and an act of courage in the face of potential familial and social rejection, with imperfect guarantees of treatment and assistance)[4]—for extrapolating upon population infection rates, UNAIDS estimates HIV prevalence of women attending public antenatal clinics to be roughly 35 percent in 2005.[5] The Department of Health's Demographic Impact Report records women's peak infection rate at 32.5 percent between the ages of 25 and 29, and that of men at 26.5 percent between the ages of 30 and 34. DIB statistics for 2007 showed that women's HIV prevalence as measured at antenatal clinics increased to 31.67 percent, up two percent on the previous year. DIB also estimated that 27 percent of both men and women between the ages of 20 and 64 were HIV-positive.[6] Illustrating the long-wave impact of the epidemic, the Demographic Impact Report estimates that 64,000 babies will be infected either at birth or through breastfeeding. DIB puts that number at 92,000. Furthermore, infant and under-five mortality are on the increase, to 48 and 73 per 1000 live births, respectively. Concurrently, life expectancy is falling. ASSA pins it at around 41 years, though expects a rise again by 2008 to 50 years; DIB estimates it to be only 44.[7]

By contrast, ASSA's 2000s model predicted an overall prevalence of 16.6 percent for 2006, falling to 15.96 percent by 2008, premised on falling incidence and rising deaths. ASSA's 2003 model revised those predications to estimate overall prevalence of 11.2 percent and 11.6 percent respectively, almost perfectly

---

4   As Mercy Makhalemele (personal communication, 2003–2004), founder of Tsa-Botsogo Community Development in Soweto, discovered upon testing positive and being thrown out of her home by her husband and her family; as women were given a once-off treatment of Nevirapine to limit the vertical transmission of HIV to their babies, but not afforded antiretroviral treatment upon their hospital release; and as some women were able to access disability grants due to their HIV status, a grant they often lost again if they became well enough to be deemed able to work (more on this in later chapters).

5   UNAIDS. 2006. AIDS Epidemic Update 2005.

6   Comparison Population Projections (3). Obtained from Johan Calitz at DIB/DBSA via private communication, 27 May 2008.

7   Ibid.

reflecting the Department of Health's findings. However, the newer ASSA figures revised again in 2008 predict higher prevalence, of 14.7 percent and 13.8 percent, respectively.[8]

Perhaps most revealing are the statistics of the DIB. While indicating the same slight dip in prevalence plausibly attributable to falling incidence and rising deaths, these trump ASSA's and the Department of Health's numbers. For 2006, DIB estimates prevalence at 16.26 percent, and for 2008 at 15.98 percent. These rates correspond to 7.2 million HIV-infected South Africans, 1,636,338 of whom DIB calculates were AIDS-sick by the middle of 2008. In addition, it estimates that over 911,000 died through the first half of 2008.[9] That translates to more than 2,500 deaths a day: about the same number as died in the 9/11 terrorist attacks in New York City. DIB attributes its higher rates of prevalence to its bottom-up approach, as it conducted household surveys, and also to the fact that it includes 17 million illegal immigrants. These can access antiretroviral medication once they have obtained South Africa identity documents, which many of them—legally or illegally—do.

Broken down beyond overall prevalence, these statistics reveal a nuanced image of HIV/AIDS in South Africa. Further attesting to this is the uneven spread of the epidemic prevalence across South Africa's provinces, which carries its own complex social, economic, and political implications. The province with the highest prevalence rates, ranked by the Department of Health's Demographic Impact Report, is KwaZulu-Natal, where 40 percent of women attending antenatal clinics are infected. The other provinces follow, with Gauteng, which includes Pretoria and Johannesburg, the Eastern Cape, Mpumalanga, the Free State, and North-West recording prevalence rates between 30 and 35 percent; the Northern Cape and Limpopo rates in the high teens and low 20s, and the Western Cape the lowest prevalence, 17 percent.[10]

The exceptionally high prevalence of HIV in KwaZulu-Natal (KZN) demands attention, as it sheds light on the power of political images and perceptions and the associated consequences that characterize and complicate the HIV/AIDS epidemic in South Africa. The shocking reality of KZN's prevalence rates is inextricably wedded to the trajectory of the epidemic's spread, both in terms of its transmission and its political pedigree, and to the province's economic and political impoverishment.

KZN's prevalence may be attributed, at least in part, to the vast numbers of miners who migrated north from that province during and at the end of apartheid, increasing their exposure to the virus in countries where the epidemic was further developed.[11] It might also be correlated to the cessation of Zulu circumcision

---

    8   Ibid.

    9   Personal correspondence with Johan Calitz, senior demographer at DIB/DBSA, 27 May 2008, and DIB Comparison Population Projections.

    10   Statistics taken from the Department of Health's Demographic Report 2006.

    11   More detail on this below.

rites.[12] These are—as of 2010/2011—being resumed under the chief's own stewardship. Yet KZN's predicament is seemingly inextricable from the particular fate of the Zulus, the state's majority population, who are more politically and economically impoverished, less well-educated and more likely to have remained in South Africa under apartheid (inciles)[13] than their better-educated, more likely to have been in exile, wealthier and well-connected Xhosa cousins. The first two presidents of the democratic era, Nelson Mandela and Thabo Mbeki, are Xhosa. Jacob Zuma, the third such president, is a Zulu. Furthermore, during the struggle for freedom, Zulus aligned with the Inkatha Freedom Party (IFP) constituted the most significant and notably internal competition to the African National Congress (ANC). These divisions have deep historical roots linking them to the educational preferences of colonial powers: the English codified and educated Xhosas along the Eastern Cape coast, preparing their elite for service governance in institutions such as Fort Hare, which both Mandela and Mbeki attended. The French, per contrast, codified and educated the Sotho, though did not groom this particular group for government. In addition, Zulus, apart from both of these, and although powerful and numerically, remained somewhat ostracized from these hierarchies.

The result, reflected in the perception and response to the HIV/AIDS epidemic, is of a group failing to dispel the disease, a group powerless and disaffected; itself a perception that feeds an insecurity which fuels the fire of the epidemic, and yet invoking adamancy to fight against this foregone conclusion. This paradoxical situation is not unique to KwaZulu-Natal, but is evident across South Africa, particularly in its political response, rhetorical and practical, to the HIV/AIDS epidemic.[14]

---

12   Recent studies have shown that circumcision reduces the transmission rate of HIV. See also Iliffe, J. 2006. *A History: The African AIDS Epidemic*. Athens, Ohio: Ohio University Press: 45.

13   Calland, R. 2006. *Anatomy of South Africa: Who Holds the Power?* Cape Town: Zebra Press.

14   The May 2007 xenophobic attacks that crisscrossed South Africa included hints at internecine strife. Predominantly foreigners were attacked, and a National Intelligence Agency member alleged the role of a "third force" in provoking the violence. Though later refuted, the comment invoked images of apartheid-era violence, in which the "third force," constituted by apartheid security forces, exploited interethnic black tensions. Suspected "informers" were famously "necklaced": a burning tire was thrown around their necks and they burned to death. Similar images captured worldwide media attention in the May 2007 xenophobic attacks. Both anti-foreigner and interethnic tensions characterize a South Africa at times still tense from the past and in the present. This mistrust bodes ill for South Africa's cohesion. The uneven occurrence of HIV/AIDS and the equally uneven response to it offer insight into these currents. A more thorough discussion and analysis will follow in Chapter 3.

2.2 Assessment of HIV/AIDS: A Crisis

The path to this perilous juncture was not paved—or eroded—overnight.

The crisis presented by HIV/AIDS is critical at three levels: existential, as a threat to the life of infected individuals; social, as concerned with or involving human co-existence in terms of social order over the course of its long-wave arc; and as a crisis of governability, of governance, of the capacity and ability of the national sovereign state to provide both protection for individual life and for its own sustainable functioning throughout and beyond the long-wave event. The first two levels concern HIV/AIDS as a specific crisis portending death for millions and decimating numerous generations by virtue of its intergenerational impact. These levels are, however, of less interest in the case of this analysis, which is primarily concerned as to the role of HIV/AIDS as it and interventions against it impact the sovereign responsibility of the government, of the national state, to protect the lives and livelihoods of its citizens. It assesses whether the state is to some extent hollowed out by HIV/AIDS at the level of its individual citizenry and social fabric. It asks whether local-global alliances of activists and actors are complementing the state's sovereign responsibility to the citizens of its polity, or whether the effect of these two developments is resulting in the South African state reneging on or being relieved of its responsibility; and whereto the attendant accountability?

2.3 HIV/AIDS as a Long-wave Event

As noted above, HIV/AIDS can be described as a long-wave event.[15] By affecting both current and future generations, it constricts economic productivity, human capital development, and political participation. It does so in a selective way:[16] killing adults in their reproductive and working prime, robbing children of parents, and depriving the state of revenue and economic growth. HIV/AIDS weakens or even "wreck[s] the mechanisms that generate human capital formation: ... if one or, worse, both parents die while their offspring are still children, the transmission or knowledge and potential productive capacity across the two generations will be weakened."[17]

---

15   Barnett, T. 2006. "A Long-Wave Event. HIV/AIDS, Politics, Governance and 'Security'." *International Affairs HIV/AIDS*, Special Issue, 82(2): 297–313.

16   Bell, C., Devarajan, S. and Gersbach, H. 2004. "Thinking about the Long-Run Economic Costs of AIDS" (ed.) Haacker, M. Washington, DC: International Monetary Fund.

17   Ibid. and Lisk, F. 2009. *Global Institutions and the HIV/AIDS Epidemic*. London: Routledge: 105: "Global estimates of the impact of HIV/AIDS on labor made by the ILO indicate that over two-thirds of the losses in human resource capacity worldwide have occurred in sub- Saharan Africa."

In HIV/AIDS, African countries face a challenge that is simultaneously a tragedy for individuals, families and communities and a threat to sustainable development. HIV/AIDS brings three processes together in a unique and devastating combination. First, it kills people in the prime of their working lives (typically those aged between 15 and 49). This has the effect of sharply reducing life expectancy, eroding the labor force and destroying intergenerational socio-cultural capital formation. Second, by destroying intergenerational capital formation is also weakens the ability of succeeding generations to maintain the development achievements of the past; and third, the net effect of the preceding two processes is the systemic erosion of societies' ability to replenish the stock and flow of vital human capital needed to sustain socio-economic development and political governance.[18]

Defining orphans as those who have lost their mothers, the DIB estimated there to be 765,280 AIDS orphans in 2006 and 1,440,624 in 2008. The loss of income due to disability and early death reduces the lifetime resources available to the family, which may well result in the children spending much less time (if any) at school. In its December 2006 Report, UNAIDS calculated that 21 percent of South African teachers were HIV-positive. Thus the long-wave event becomes a compound problem.

A consequence of this long-wave trend is likely to be that "as the children of AIDS victims become adults with little education and limited knowledge received from their parents, they are in turn less likely to raise their own children and to invest in their education."[19] This vicious cycle stymies not only the potential of individual lives, but also the sustainability of social and economic development. Suitably, and insightfully, the HIV epidemic is itself a consequence of social and economic change. In tracing its trajectory, plausible aides and abettors become clear, as do possible—remaining—points of intervention, and lessons for similar crises.

2.4 Historical Trajectory

The history of the HI-virus is complex, and coincides with changes in human history. From an inauspicious, silent, beginning in the Congo, specifically at the gestation of urbanization in Kinshasa,[20] HIV/AIDS spread across the African continent, streaming, along with waves of wanderers, into southern and South Africa.

---

18   Poku, N.K. 2006. "Financing: improving aid." *International Affairs HIV/AIDS,* Special Issue, 82(2): 346.

19   Bell, C., Devarajan, S. and Gersbach, H. 2004. "Thinking about the Long-Run Economic Costs of AIDS" (ed.) Haacker, M. Washington, DC: International Monetary Fund.

20   See also Timberg, C. and Halperin, D. 2012. *Tinderbox: How the West Sparked the AIDS Epidemic and How the World Can Finally Overcome it.* New York: The Penguin Press.

HIV-1 first became epidemic during the 1970s in western equatorial Africa, its place of origin. It was at first a silent epidemic, unnoticed until established too firmly to be stopped. In this region, also, during the mid 1980s, the epidemiology of heterosexual HIV/AIDS was first determined, exposing a pattern whose main features were to extend through sub-Saharan Africa but whose local peculiarities were also to limit epidemic growth within the western equatorial region itself. From this region, moreover, variants of the virus were carried to the rest of the continent.[21]

By 2004, over 20 years into the AIDS epidemic, the southern African region, "had 2 percent of the world's population and nearly 30 percent of its HIV cases, with no evidence of overall decline in any national prevalence."[22] This concentration might be attributed in part to the "region's history of white domination and the dramatic economic change and social inequality it has wrought [and yet ...] the scale of the epidemic was chiefly due to the long incubation period that enabled it to spread silently beyond hope of rapid suppression."[23] These few historical observations set the scene for understanding the unique HIV/AIDS epidemic and its existential threat in South Africa: its stealthy and widespread heterosexual transmission, bound to social and economic change, and associated movement and migration, which would wreak upheaval and impart profound personal and political implications.

The intersection of these social, economic, and political trends and their consequences exacerbates the crisis of HIV/AIDS most notably in South Africa. In particular,

> Not only did the socio-economic structures of Apartheid make the country an almost perfect environment for HIV, but the beginning of the epidemic coincided with the township revolt of the mid 1980s and its peak took place a decade later during the transition to majority rule, which compelled ordinary people to concentrate on survival and distracted both the outgoing regime and its nationalist successor from making HIV their chief priority.[24]

Given the historical circumstances, Iliffe argues that "it would be naïve to think that even the most vigorous, stable, and popular government could have protected South Africa from a major epidemic."[25] This sentiment is echoed by South African experts on the ground, too. For one thing, South Africa's epidemic "bordered a massive continental epidemic, had no identifiable core group [such as prostitutes,

---

21   Iliffe, J. 2006. *A History: The African AIDS Epidemic*. Athens, Ohio: Ohio University Press: 10.
22   Ibid., 33.
23   Ibid.
24   Ibid., 43.
25   Ibid.

intravenous drug users, or homosexuals] but a great diversity of cross-border contacts."[26] In Iliffe's picturesque words, "trying to prevent the extensive infection of South Africa would have been like sweeping back the ocean with a broom."[27] Certainly, keeping HIV/AIDS out of South Africa would have been a behemoth task bound to fail, particularly given the volume of cross-border traffic, which escalated with the end of apartheid and the return to South Africa of thousands of exiles. In hindsight, this indeed became the case. Whether it was a foregone conclusion is debatable.

HIV/AIDS did not cross the border in 1994, but much earlier. As early as the 1980s the virus was detected and identified inside the country. By the mid-1980s, preliminary indications of a possible epidemic were available. In early 1983, the first two AIDS-related deaths of two white South African Airlines crew members were reported. This announced the presence of the disease in South Africa. In Johannesburg at the same time, Professor Ruben Sher began noticing HIV among the white, homosexual population. Later it would be shown that this population became infected mostly with HIV-1, subtype B, a different version of HIV to that which would afflict the majority, black, heterosexual population. The differences are due to the evolution and spread of the virus initially in Central Africa across the globe, and play an important role with regard to treatment. At the time, however, the virus was mostly thought to be a "gay plague," infected individuals derided, including by then US President Ronald Reagan, and its impact dismissed.

This perception began to change already a few years later. In 1985, Professor Sher visited AIDS co-discoverer Dr Robert Gallo's laboratory at the National Institutes of Health in Washington, DC.[28] There he was given a culture of the virus in a number of culture bottles to bring back to South Africa.

> I strapped them to my waist wrapped in newspapers to maintain adequate temperature. Had the pilot or fellow travelers known what I had strapped to my waist, I would probably have been thrown out of the aircraft! With the help of Professor Barry Schoub arrangements were made to collect the packages from me at Jan Smuts Airport [later renamed first the Johannesburg International Airport, and now Oliver Tambo International Airport]. I handed over the samples into the care of Dr Sue Lyons, who subsequently developed an indirect fluorescent antibody test.[29]

By the end of 1985, South Africa had ELIZA kits, developed by Abbott Laboratories, to detect of HIV antibodies. With those tools, Professor Sher and his

26   Ibid.
27   Ibid.
28   Interview with Professor Ruben Sher, 8 March 2005.
29   Interview with Professor Ruben Sher, 8 March 2005, and Professor Sher's private notes.

colleagues could identify HIV-infection. The initial tests they conducted pointed to the impending epidemic.

The first cases of HIV were white homosexual men and hemophiliacs who received blood, as well as others who had had blood transfusions. The situation affecting hemophiliacs was particularly tragic: when the necessary blood factor 8 could no longer be sourced in Durban, South Africa, imported [vials] from the United States, of which a number turned out to be HIV-infected. As a result some 86 percent of the hemophiliac community in Johannesburg became HIV-positive.[30]

Then, in 1986 and 1987, along with his colleague Dr Dennis Sifris and the ELIZA test, Sher conducted the first wider testing under the auspices of the newly-established AIDS unit of the South African Institute for Medical Research. The testing focused on miners in South Africa, the largest pool of migrant labor in the country. By then, Sher and Sifris had already identified mobility as a potential factor in HIV/AIDS transmission:

> We worked with the Chamber of Mines, we worked very closely, and they were interested to know [the HIV prevalence] and of course many of the miners didn't have their wives here [in South Africa], so there [in South Africa] they all had girlfriends, so they were all promiscuous and we know that HIV was present in the countries to the north.[31]

Along with Dr Brian Brink, now at Anglo American, Sher and Sifris took blood samples from 50,000 miners from Malawi, Zambia, Zimbabwe, and Mozambique, where the epidemic was already established. The finding indicated the following prevalence rates, from highest to lowest; reflecting geographic location as well: Malawi, 3.76 percent; Botswana, 0.34 percent; Mozambique, 0.09 percent; Lesotho, 0.9 percent; Swaziland, 0.05 percent; and South Africa, 0.02 percent.

These prevalence rates indicated HIV/AIDS's presence throughout sub-Saharan Africa. It would soon spread further and drastically increase its prevalence. In fact, the epidemic, along with migrants, would travel south, and concentrate itself at the now-epicenter of the epidemic in South Africa. Given this route and its consequences, it is pertinent to take a more detailed look at the modes of that transmission.

2.4.1 Migration

Migrants moving between rural homesteads and towns and mines also moved between wives and families and sex workers or girlfriends. When one link in this human chain became infected with HIV, all were at risk. This same pattern, though initially observed in miners, repeated itself amongst a wide array of sexual

---

30   Interview with Professor Ruben Sher, 8 March 2005.
31   Ibid.

networks, notably featuring concurrent sexual partnerships. As the epidemic progressed, Professor Sher attributed the spread of HIV/AIDS to two factors: "it was obvious to us that in order for an epidemic to occur you needed two things, you needed an agent, which was the HIV and you needed promiscuity."[32] Both are amply present in South Africa, and both have accelerated the HIV/AIDS epidemic.

Professor Sher recounts how in black, African culture, distorted by the apartheid regime's Bantustan or native homeland policies coupled with coercive labor migration, it was accepted that "a man who came from [KwaZulu-Natal], of which there were thousands or millions, would come up [to Johannesburg] and work" and "could have a sexual partner here [in Johannesburg], where he works." Simultaneously, "the woman, his wife back home [likely rural KZN]—and he was away from home for a year—that was a difficult problem [raising the likelihood that she would also likely acquire another sexual partner, adding risky links to the chain]."[33] This back-and-forth migration would play a pivotal role in fostering the spread of HIV/AIDS.

Indeed, that spread is due, among other factors, significantly to networks of simultaneous sexual liaisons and migration which spurred HIV transmission initially from northern countries nearer the center of origin, southwards.

> The virus seemed to have come down South, the same as you look at the incidence of the northern provinces versus the southern [provinces]. The Western Cape has a smaller percentage of people [infected] because the virus was coming down. You know there were things like truckers, long distance truckers that were picking up the virus in those various [northern] countries. There were [also] ANC freedom fighters that came down here [into South Africa] for military purposes; and they were living in the camps there [in those northern countries] where the HIV rate was very high, we thought it was about 30 percent at one stage. And they would come to see their girlfriends and so the virus began to spread in a silent manner.

> There was a lot of migrant labor because of the mines, and industries that grew up here. And long-haul distance drivers: they would be away from home, they would seek sexual favors which they paid for by money or petrol that they had in the car or in the truck, etc. and they were obviously picking up the virus in countries to the north and bringing it back to their wives.[34]

Some of those wives and girlfriends acquired and transmitted the virus, too. This includes those wives whose husbands worked in the mines and ceased sending money home, and so took another sexual partner as a means of subsistence, as well

---

32   Ibid.
33   Ibid.
34   Interview with Professor Ruben Sher, 8 March 2005, and Professor Sher's private notes, acquired March 2005.

as women who generally relied on sexual favors or transactional sex to support themselves and their families.

Further attesting to the relationship between HIV and mobility in southern Africa, by 1991, a correlation emerged between pregnant women testing HIV-positive at Baragwaneth Hospital in Soweto, and those with partners who traveled or came from countries north of South Africa. Also, by "the late 1990s sex workers were often heavily infected—60 percent in the Hillbrow area of Johannesburg, 56 percent at truck stops in the Natal midlands—but this was not the case earlier in the decade and professional sex workers were rare in African townships."[35]

As the above statistics reveal, initial routes of transmission followed the migration patterns of miners from northern to southern Sub-Saharan countries. The same trajectory transmitted HIV into and within South Africa, spreading through the dying days of the apartheid regime in the 1980s and expanding exponentially at the transition to democracy in the early 1990s—and to today.

> Today [2005] with the taxis, he [a miner or town worker, likely with a permanent home in a rural area] gets around much easier, and he may go home six times a year. Ok, so that facilitated that spread of the virus, the taxis. Same as the airplane did between different continents. You know what taxi drivers tell you, for sexual favors give a person a free lift. All these things were done and stopovers of trucks on the road to Durban and most truck drivers who went into North Africa stopped in Johannesburg and didn't have a different route going to Durban. It's difficult to explain why some of these things spread like that but the taxi permitted people to go more frequently. Therefore the chances of contact became easier and greater.[36]

Later studies have shown that once prevalence exceeds one percent of the general population, the HIV/AIDS epidemic explodes. Further blood screening done in 1987 indicated that HIV prevalence among black Africans was already eight times higher than among whites, and was doubling every six months. The pieces were in place for South Africa's HIV/AIDS crisis.

2.4.2 Biological and Cultural Fueling Factors

Accompanying co-factors that further facilitate the virus's spread are embedded in and exacerbated by social, economic, and lastly, political, conditions. Biological and social factors include the vulnerability of women's vaginas to infection, the non-visibility of the initial infection, the prevalence of simultaneous, as opposed to sequential, liaisons among several partners, and increasing mobility as noted above, which is conducive to wider transmission. Additional factors are economic

---

35   Iliffe, J. 2006. *A History: The African AIDS Epidemic*. Athens, Ohio: Ohio University Press: 44.

36   Interview with Professor Ruben Sher, 8 March 2005.

in nature, and include the prevalence of poverty and the associated practice of transactional sex, where sex is exchanged for survivalist support such as rent and food as well as gifts; the disempowerment of men and their inability to pay the traditional bride price, *lobola*, to set up a household and pass on their paternal name to their children;[37] the desire for children, and high incidence of rape.

All of these factors fuel the transmission of HIV throughout South Africa. Though identified by Professor Sher and colleagues already in the early 1980s, HIV transmission continued more or less unabated. As South Africa began negotiating its transition from the era of apartheid to a democratic dispensation, HIV continued its insidious spread while newly-free South Africans and the inaugural state largely focused elsewhere. In the meantime, the impact of the virus, on individual lives, but also on South Africa's fragile economy, increased.

2.5 Economic Situation—Status of the South African Economy

South Africa's current economic situation is inextricably tied to HIV/AIDS; and the country's epidemic a consequence, too, of its economics. Since the epidemic's spread gathered steam before it became a registered reality, it is not possible to measure the precise impact of HIV/AIDS by comparing probable scenarios without and with its presence. However, varying degrees of its economic effects can be deduced. This section attempts to tease out the relationship between the economic conditions in which South Africa confronted the epidemic and the influence of the epidemic itself on those economic conditions.

The mid-term spread of HIV/AIDS, when it really gained traction, coincided with a slowdown in worldwide growth between 1989 and 1993: precisely the time period during which South Africa embarked on its transition from the apartheid era to a democratic dispensation. Poor economic management coupled with increasing international credit isolation of the apartheid government saw real GDP growth decline from 3.3 percent between 1970 and 1979, to 2.2 percent between 1980 and 1989, and 0.2 percent between 1990 and 1994. Inflation during the same time period rose to an average of 14.6 percent between 1980 and 1989.[38] This led to a situation in which the South African Government, in the waning days of the apartheid regime[39] and in the early hours of democracy faced

---

37   Thus establishing their manhood and taking their place in adult society, an achievement increasingly elusive. See also Iliffe, J. 2006. *A History: The African AIDS Epidemic*. Athens, Ohio: Ohio University Press: 46.

38   Hamilton, L. and Viegib, N. 2007. "The Nation's Debt and the Birth of the New South Africa." Work in Progress (September).

39   There have been assertions that the apartheid regime deliberately sought to bankrupt South Africa in order to hinder and hamper the governance of the new leadership; though this did not happen, the economic and fiscal situation that the new government inherited severely constricted its room to maneuver.

the possibility of bankruptcy, and an abrupt termination of the long fought-for freedoms the latter purportedly entailed. The realization of those freedoms rested on a solvent state, a functioning economy, (re-)integrated into the international economy, and a thriving business sector; and left no room for the threat posed by HIV/AIDS. "The end of apartheid could not reverse the economic decline, which vastly limited the Mandela and Mbeki governments' ability to secure sufficient economic expansion to fund their programs, and that of course, was also true of the HIV issue."[40] Economic priorities, particularly pertaining to rendering South Africa an independent sovereign state, both politically and fiscally, emerged as paramount. Concerns over the HIV/AIDS epidemic took a back seat. The idea was to get the groundwork right and then to deal with special-issues. However, the path there was riddled with hurdles, competing local, national, international and global priorities. If the government jumped one, it bypassed others. Even a perfect play or play-off of priority interests, pressure and power could not defy the impossibility of leaping every hurdle.

South Africa's first democratic government initially promulgated the Reconstruction and Development Act (RDP), followed by the Growth, Employment and Redistribution strategy (GEAR) designed to attract business and investment into South Africa. GEAR in particular banked on a strict program of fiscal discipline to attract foreign direct investment and to infuse growth into the fragile economy. "The ANC leadership knew of the need for rapidly expanding growth and more resources, [but they] were totally unprepared to handle that segment of the economy."[41] Though Mandela told US companies that had left South Africa during the apartheid era to return "he clearly did not understand how businesses work. The companies had sustained terrific losses and were not about to return to an uncertain future."[42] Nonetheless, in the interim, South Africa made significant progress in promoting economic growth and delivering upon such constitutionally-guaranteed rights as access to housing, water and electricity for the majority of South Africans who had lacked these basic amenities under the previous regime. While the government focused on resuscitating the economy and reconstituting South Africa as a sovereign, democratic state, HIV/AIDS silently seeped into its fabric, challenging its newly assumed responsibility to respond.

2.6 Political Situation

That responsibility, to respond to HIV/AIDS as well as any other political and governmental challenge, lies within the contested terrain of political power. In South Africa, political association has long been tied to tribes: the two white tribes which ruled for centuries, and the numerous black tribes, whose authority

---

40   Personal correspondence with Ambassador Barkley, 11 February 2008.
41   Ibid.
42   Ibid.

stretches back further but which are only now being tested throughout the entire country, plus the colored (of whom former Finance Minister and current Minister of Planning Trevor Manuel is perhaps the most famous) and Indian cohorts who have had to make their allegiances and strike deals to survive.

The lines of power and patronage are not split squarely along ethnic lines, but are delineated among those with anti-apartheid credentials, particularly in exile, combined at times with ethnic ties particularly Xhosa or Zulu, and by derivation, access to Black Economic Empowerment (BEE) and Broad-Based Black Economic Empowerment (BBBEE) opportunities. This was evidenced in the battle for succession in the ANC in 2007, an effective repeat of the contest that Mbeki won to succeed Mandela in 1998, and eerily, again surfacing in 2012 as corruption charges against Zuma make the case for a strong deputy president imperative. Pitched between Mbeki, a former exile and a Xhosa, and Zuma, an incile and a Zulu, and further contested by Zulu business tycoon Tokyo Sexwale, and Cyril Ramaphosa, a Venda, a small group sometimes referred to as the 'Jews' of South Africa, the lines were drawn.[43] The latter two, both inciles, have benefitted enormously from BEE/BBBEE, if not from exile credentials and political ties. Zuma won in 2007; but the fight for political and economic clout is far from over. In the interim, the struggle against HIV/AIDS's spread and its associated impacts has arguably been sidelined by pride and political-economic expediencies.

At the same time, and unremittingly, the stipulations of South Africa's political transition vied with the rising transmission of HIV, as well as international market prescriptions and local labor demands for policy attention. The prioritization of these interrelated issues remains largely unresolved. Consequently, and with special regard to HIV/AIDS, Professor Sher minces no words when he says that "there has been one major defect running through the previous and the current [ANC] government, and that is, the failure to prioritize HIV/AIDS. It should have been at the top of the list and not at the bottom."[44] Sher elucidates upon the situations in which both governments were making decisions. First, referring to the apartheid government, he argues that it sought excuses: "who were the people who were being involved? People in the fringes of society, gay men, sex workers, they were black."[45] In other words, they—these people[46]—were expendable. Second, with regard to the democratic regime, Sher asserts that

> Government didn't appreciate the extent of the epidemic. I don't think they understood how it was transmitted. I think government, certainly in the mid-1990s [was] more concerned about apartheid then they were about the HIV,

---

43   Fanyana Shiburi, personal communication, 2005.
44   Interview with Professor Sher, 8 March 2005.
45   Ibid.
46   This phrase, "these people" would have unfortunate reverberations when iterated by the democratic government referring to those infected with HIV.

cause even at that stage it was predominantly gay men. They were not aware of this undercurrent spread of the HIV epidemic.[47]

While it is evidenced that the incoming democratic regime was more concerned with economics and independence, in the sense of being free from notably financial dependency, than with HIV/AIDS, its leaders, especially those in exile, were well aware of the rapidly spreading epidemic and its potential impact. However, their concerns lost out in policy agenda-setting.

Indeed, as Sher laments, the prioritization of HIV/AIDS continues to rank below the top five in South Africa, despite his and colleagues' article published in the *South African Medical Journal* in 1988, outlining a strategy to respond to the impending epidemic.

Nonetheless, Chris Hani, guerilla leader of Umkhonto we Sizwe (MK), in particular, took heed of HIV/AIDS. Noting the epidemic's prevalence in the countries north of South Africa, hosts to the majority of exiled South Africans, he acknowledged early the potential of the further spread of the virus fueled by those returning.

> Those of us in exile are especially in the unfortunate situation of being in the areas where the incidence of disease is high. We cannot afford to allow the AIDS epidemic to ruin the realization of our dreams. Existing statistics indicate that we are still at the beginning of the AIDS epidemic in our country. Unattended, however, this will result in untold damage and suffering by the end of the century.[48]

At an April 1990 conference in Maputo, the returning exiles together with what would form the nucleus of the new democratic government agreed to establish a task force to prepare an HIV/AIDS program.[49] Numerous preparations, plans, programs, strategies and interventions later the HIV/AIDS epidemic continues to rage.

In 1991, Sher met with Mangosutho Buthelezi. Buthelezi, a prominent Zulu chief, was leader of the Inkatha Freedom Party and head of the Bantustan KwaZulu that would become the province of KwaZulu-Natal. Though Buthelezi recognized the decimation being wreaked by HIV/AIDS, he did little politically or practically to stem the tide; perhaps preferring to prioritize the battle for political power. As noted above, KwaZulu-Natal remains the South African province hardest-hit by the epidemic.

In 1992, prior to the first free democratic elections in 1994, the transitional government created the National AIDS Convention of South Africa (NACOSA).

---

47   Professor Ruben Sher's private notes, acquired March 2005.

48   Nattrass, N. 2007. *Mortal Combat: AIDS Denialism and the Struggle for Antiretrovirals in South Africa.* Scottsville: University of KwaZulu-Natal Press: 39.

49   Iliffe, J. 2006. *A History: The African AIDS Epidemic*. Athens, Ohio: Ohio University Press: 73.

NACOSA comprised of the ANC, government health bodies and representatives of trade unions, business, churches and NGOs. The plan the body drew up and presented to the ANC government in July 1994 was "drafted with WHO assistance and embodied all the current international priorities."[50] Still these plans and policies did not make a dent in the spread of the epidemic.

Also in 1994, as the elections were imminent, Sher met with Nelson Mandela. Mandela showed concern about the epidemic, but subordinated this to politics: "I wanted to win and I didn't talk about AIDS" and "had no time to concentrate on the issue" while President.[51] Mandela's decision to demote HIV/AIDS from any list of priorities had a profound impact on policy, and on the spread of the epidemic. Not the only political leader to desist from dealing with HIV/AIDS directly, Mandela's initial silence stands in stark contrast to his later outspokenness on the issue.

> For political leaders, moreover, HIV/AIDS was a profoundly distasteful subject to mention in public. It questioned their competence because they had no remedy, it threatened to raise demands for assistance that they could not afford to give, it distracted them from more pressing anxieties, it was potentially divisive, its victims had as yet no political voice, and it might damage their country's image and tourist industry.[52]

The initial costs of addressing HIV/AIDS appeared high, while those of ignoring it relatively low.

Subsequently the policy decisions pertaining to HIV/AIDS that Mandela and Mbeki to Zuma and their governments made reflect a political calculation between on the one hand the political gain of prioritization of issues that could be controlled—and HIV could not be controlled; and on the other, the political costs associated with rising internal and external pressure to respond, or not, to HIV/AIDS. In the balance of this equation, the internal dynamics of a country are important; but, "it is the stance of the external world [with] respect [to] these countries with serious current HIV epidemics and looming AIDS epidemics"[53] that will matter most. In fact, it's not quite so simple. South Africa arguably tried to protect and implement the tenets of its domestic sovereignty with regard to the requisites of its responsibility and accountability. It attempted simultaneously to heed and adhere to the requirements of global market economics.

At the same time, ardent local-global alliances advocated for and then took concrete action to respond to South Africa's HIV/AIDS epidemic. The resulting interventions did not take into account the South African state's ability to assume ultimate responsibility and accountability. It also made no provision for the

---

50 Ibid.

51 Ibid., 67.

52 Ibid.

53 Barnett, T. 2006. "A Long-Wave Event. HIV/AIDS, Politics, Governance and 'Security'." *International Affairs HIV/AIDS,* Special Issue, 82(2): 297–313.

transfer of that responsibility and accountability. What transpired was not, as will this analysis will show, a boomerang effect in which this alliance advocacy and action resulted in state action. Instead, alliance activism eventually circumvented the state apparatus, supplanting it. The pressure fractured the fault line between state and non-state actors on South Africa's responsibility to respond, which led to the GAP.

2.7 Conclusion

As this chapter illustrates, South Africa faced a formidable challenge in acknowledging and addressing the emerging HIV/AIDS epidemic at the dawning of its democratic era. Despite hopes to the contrary, HIV/AIDS has resulted in the infection and death of millions of South Africans, whose shortened life-spans impact negatively on the country's inter-generational transfer of knowledge, its economic potential, and its political stability. The implications for the state's decision-making ability and for its social cohesion, economic viability, and sovereign statehood are profound. The reverberations and the repercussions thereof are analyzed in more detail in the following chapter.

Chapter 3
Social, Economic, and Political Consequences of HIV/AIDS in South Africa

As illustrated in Chapter 2, the HIV/AIDS epidemic constitutes a crisis for South African society, economy, and polity. This chapter evaluates the ensuing consequences of HIV/AIDS on each of those levels in South Africa. It asks the questions: are the costs of not addressing the epidemic at its outset as high as it appeared in chapter two and do these costs, both of addressing and of failing to respond to the epidemic, affect the state's ability to enact its sovereign responsibilities?[1]

3.1 Social Level—The Price of Freedom, the Cost of HIV

On the social level, HIV/AIDS is closely associated with broader political-economic trends related to South Africa's transition from the apartheid to the democratic era. The transition heralded freedom and liberty, but also brought death and destruction. HIV/AIDS is an individual and medical disease; and a social, economic, and political dilemma at the same time. Steeped as it is in sexuality and morality, and imbued with judgments, it is also a disease with especially profound *political* implications.

By harnessing the basic human desire for sexual intimacy [and the breastfeeding of babies] as the prime means of transmission, the virus can gain a fast and extensive grip on an entire population, leaving heartbreak and socio-economic devastation in its wake.[2] "A new democracy is an era of resurging life. Sex is the most life-giving of activities. That a new nation's citizens are dying from sex seems to be an attack both on ordinary people's and a nation's generative

---

1　See Brühl, T. and Rittberger, V. 2001. "From International to Global Governance: Actors, Collective Decision-making, and the United Nations in the Twenty-First Century." In *Global Governance and the United Nations System* (ed.) Rittberger, V. Tokyo: United Nations University Press; International Commission on Intervention and State Sovereignty (ICISS). "The Responsibility to Protect": 2.15; Hösle, V. 2004. *Morals and Politics*. Notre Dame: University of Notre Dame Press; and Risse, T. 2007. "Paradoxien der Souveränität. Die konstituive Norm, auf der die heutige Staatenwelt gründet—dass nämlich Staaten souverän sind—gilt uneingeschränkt nicht mehr. Was heisst das?" 40–47.

2　Nattrass, N. 2004. *The Moral Economy of HIV/AIDS*. Cambridge: Cambridge University Press: 23.

capacities, an insult too ghastly to stomach."[3] Consequently, as will be shown repeatedly, amidst other dire and pressing concerns, South Africans, in opinion polls, and the South African Government, in its political prioritizations, as well as rhetoric and resource allocation, did not afford HIV/AIDS the rank concomitant to that expected to be accorded a deadly disease whose spread endangers the capacity of the state to enact its sovereign responsibilities to respond.

For indeed HIV/AIDS is also a disease of freedom and democracy. Coinciding with South Africa's first decades of democracy and political freedom, the spread of HIV/AIDS represents fettering chains not fledgling freedom: a seemingly impossible incongruence and cruelty in a country that has already suffered for centuries. The implications are manifold: a liberation movement unable to liberate; an African Century populated by dying citizens; an independent, sovereign, national democracy made dependent on other nations and the global community; a revolution unraveling: all transmitted by the essential life-giving force of the politically touchy and often still taboo subject of sex.

> When dying is transmitted by sex, the politics get more difficult still. And when the dead were voters in a brand-new democracy, sons and daughters of people just liberated from a while dictatorship, the spectacle appears cynical in the extreme, as if guided by an evil hand.

> AIDS has given rise to accusation. Nowhere is this more evident than in the politics of South Africa's president, Thabo Mbeki, who questioned with bitterness whether the dying was caused by a sexually transmitted disease after all, and who asked caustically whether antiretroviral drugs were for the benefit of Africans or pharmaceutical companies.[4]

This paradox of competing freedoms and fetters characterizes not only the emergence of HIV/AIDS at the dawn of South Africa's democracy, but also the pattern of reaction to it by the state. This led most notably and notoriously to South Africa, in the throes of its historical transition, to downplay and deferral of adequate responses to the epidemic, both in the public consciousness and the political arena. "Arguably, post-Apartheid South Africa is in the throes of such an historical moment, in which the politicization of sexuality is perhaps the most revealing marker of the complexities and vulnerabilities of the drive to produce a newly democratic, unified nation."[5] Preoccupied with the transition from the apartheid era to democracy, and piqued by sexual freedoms across formerly rigid color and cultural lines, public prioritization of HIV/AIDS has long remained low.

---

3   Steinberg, J. 2008. *Sizwe's Test: A Young Man's Journey through Africa's AIDS Epidemic*. New York: Simon & Schuster: 6.
4   Ibid.
5   Posel, D. 2005. "Sex, Death and the Fate of the Nation: Reflections on the Politicization of Sexuality in Post-Apartheid South Africa." *Africa*, 75, 125–153.

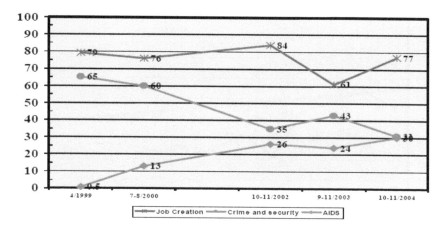

Figure 3.1   AIDS and the public agenda in South Africa, 1999–2004

Note: Afrobarometer 2005. "HIV/AIDS and the Public Agenda." No. 14. Available at: http://www.afrobarometer.org [accessed: 17 July 2012].

Though consistently ranking behind other priorities in the public domain, HIV/AIDS and the necessity of a response steadily climbed in the public estimation. It was ranked as a priority by still only 30 percent of the public surveyed in 2006, up from 26 percent in 2003, 13 percent in 2000 and 1 percent in 1994.

This almost matched the level of public concern over crime and security, at 31 percent, but still fell far short of the primary issue: employment, cited by 77 percent. This public elevation has played an important role in the parallel prioritization of that of the South African Government, with its broad remit to protect and more importantly to respond to and implement the rights of its citizens.[6]

However, the prioritization of HIV/AIDS then stagnated, hovering between concerns over crime and security, housing, and poverty. It continued to be ranked consistently lower than the prioritization of employment and job creation.

It is possible to attribute the initial lag in and lack of prioritization of HIV/AIDS to both the myriad other demands vying for public and political attention especially in the first decade of democracy, including housing, water and electricity provision, education, employment, and healthcare generally. In addition, the higher ranking of HIV/AIDS response is undoubtedly also attributable to the increased international and global attention paid to the disease and associated media coverage and local activism. The "collective, society-wide scope of the pandemic is difficult for less politically literate people to grasp … The higher a

---

6   The relationship between South African rights and state responsibilities will be analyzed in detail in Chapter 5.

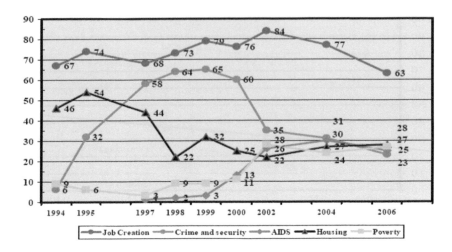

Figure 3.2   South Africa's public agenda over time, 1999–2006

Note: Afrobarometer 2006. "HIV/AIDS and the Public Agenda." No. 45. Available at: http://
www.afrobarometer.org [accessed: 17 July 2012].

person's level of formal education and the more often they read newspapers, the
more likely they are to cite 'AIDS' as an important issue."[7]

At this point in time, the relative importance ascribed to these priorities seems
to be stabilizing: as noted briefly in Chapter 2, the significance of unemployment
and its relationship to HIV/AIDS should not be ignored. Indeed, the overwhelming
issue of unemployment can be interpreted in two main ways over the course
of the social impact of HIV/AIDS and the responses to it. First, the issue of
unemployment is itself critical. Second, with regard to HIV/AIDS, unemployment
both affects and is affected by the spread of the epidemic. Both before and after
the emergence and even circumscribed availability of antiretrovirals, there appears
to be a relationship between HIV/AIDS and unemployment in South Africa.
This insight will be explored further in the depiction of the consequences of the
epidemic at the economic level.

3.2 Economic Level

The economic effects of HIV/AIDS on South Africa are often the subject of
speculation and projection, but are hard to measure precisely. Some models try
to extrapolate South Africa's rate of growth without AIDS. However, even the
base numbers taken as early as the late 1970s or early 1980s cannot foreswear the

---

7   Afrobarometer 2004. "HIV/AIDS and the Public Agenda." No. 12 (April). Available
at: http://www.afrobarometer.org [accessed: 17 July 2012].

presence of the emerging epidemic, and often do not incorporate the effects on the economy of all of the subsequent social, economic, and political changes in South Africa and the global arena that have occurred in the interim. In addition, by the late 1980s the presence of the HI-virus was known, even if no full-fledged response was forthcoming, or even, given the absence of prevention knowledge or treatment options, possible.

As the long-wave description indicates, the course of HIV/AIDS impacts and plays out across generations. From a microeconomic point of view, rising HIV/AIDS incidence leads to increases in employer costs of training, and sick, and funeral leave. In parts of southern Africa, three people are trained for each available position as companies adjust to the likelihood that two of the three will succumb to AIDS. The impacts of the virus on workers ability to work and on productivity also arguably deplete taxes and thus diminish state revenue.[8] From a macroeconomic viewpoint, the resulting insecurity and rising risk aversion due to diminishing anticipated returns on investments, threaten South Africa's desperately sought economic growth and stability. This section will delve more deeply into the detailed economic followed by political implications of the HIV/ AIDS epidemic in South Africa.

During the global downturn lasting roughly from 1989 to 1993, South Africa suffered a fall in gross domestic savings as part of Gross Domestic Product (GDP) from an average of 24.5 percent in the early 1980s to 18 percent in 1994. In an attempt to forestall the impending debt crisis, the South African Reserve Bank enacted currency controls and long-term currency transactions, which allowed the exchange of South African rand in return for US dollars on a commitment to repay the dollar liability at the forward rate once the contract matured. While this allowed the Reserve Bank to operate in foreign exchange markets in excess of its reserves, it contributed to the depreciation of the rand, increasing the value of the country's debt burden. The policy caused significant losses, which would eventually undermine South Africa's credit rating in the international marketplace. In addition, in the run-up to the first democratic elections, also in 1994, a total of 20.4 billion rand in capital fled the country. The new democratic South Africa inherited this un-dealt with debt as well as the by then surging spread of the HIV/ AIDS epidemic and its compound economic effects.

---

8   As of 2007, seemingly despite the costs of high HIV/AIDS incidence and prevalence in South Africa, the Minister of Finance announced a budget surplus. This likely indicates three things, both removed from and masking the economic impact of HIV/AIDS. First, it indicates better tax collecting methods of the South African Revenue Service (SARS). Second, embedded in the rising tax rates is an increasing disparity between the very wealthy and the very poor in South Africa and their corresponding tax contributions. Third, although the surplus is in some circles lauded as the reward for tight fiscal policies pursued since 1994, it is also the result of arguably inadequate public investments, including in electricity, healthcare, and infrastructure.

Those effects are indeed significant. Various models predict the negative impact of HIV/AIDS on South Africa's and other sub-Saharan countries' economies:

> If nothing changes in countries where prevalence is 10 percent or more, their economies could be 18 percent smaller by 2020. Even with conservative assumptions, the commission concluded that HIV/AIDS-related mortality and morbidity cost Africa about 15 percent of its GDP in 2000. This translates into a decline in income of 1.7 percent per year between 1990 and 2000, an amount greater than previous estimates based solely on the loss of output due to the epidemic.[9]

Furthermore, in high HIV-prevalence countries [such as South Africa has become], the associated socio-economic impacts are expected to be non-linear. In other words, the higher the prevalence, "the more difficult and costly the recovery will be. [...]" The decline in economic activity takes place against a background of rising social services expenditures, both private and public, which further strains government budgets as well as contributes to increases in poverty.[10] Despite South Africa's strong economic growth through 2007, the country has seen its Gini coefficient of inequality rise, and the number of South Africans living in poverty increase.

In the associated debates around the HIV/AIDS response, a number of suggestions—both in terms of intervention and in terms of negligence—have been made to address the economic impacts of the epidemic in particular. These are worth noting in brief, to situate the thinking of the South African political leaders in relation to the responses to the epidemic which ensued.

Perhaps the most controversial proposal to deal with the epidemic involved negligence: literally doing nothing and allowing the virus to cull the population. The argument assumed that the resulting devastation would leave South African society and its economy devoid of "excess," rendering it in effect more efficient, raising its growth potential and thereby its gross domestic product (GDP). Since this approach assumed that HIV/AIDS would only eliminate those individuals deemed superfluous, in society and to the economy; but as seen above in the discussion of HIV/AIDS as a long-wave event, the virus does not differentiate. Though a disproportionate number of unskilled and under-skilled people are infected with HIV/AIDS in South Africa, the virus afflicts the skilled as well. For example, HIV infection rates rose to 23 percent of skilled and 13 percent of highly skilled workers in 2006. By 2015 these infection rates are projected to reduce the skilled work force by 18 percent and the highly skilled force by 11 percent, percentages which portend dire consequences for social and economic

---

9   United Nations 2008. Report of the Commission HIV/AIDS and Governance in Africa: An Initiative of the Secretary-General of the United Nations. "Securing our Future." Geneva: United Nations Economic Commission for Africa.

10   Ibid.

development,[11] as well as for the polity. In addition, unlike the rapid decimation caused by the Black Plague for example, the trajectory of HIV infection to AIDS death can be lengthy, as measured in years, not months, weeks or days.

This prolongs the impact of the economic costs of sickness and death and reduces incentives and available resources for investment. This pertains to incentives for personal and domestic saving and investing, as well as to those on the international level. On the domestic front, "the act of saving ... requires individuals to forgo consumption. With time at a premium, the incentive to save diminishes. Investment, which involves the commitment of current resources in the expectation of some future benefit, becomes less attractive ... Evidence suggests that families and businesses are shifting spending from productive activities to medical care and related services, reducing both savings and government revenues."[12] The resulting

> Decline in savings reduces the resources available for investment. As investment falls, the rate of economic growth can decline, reducing savings. As a result, we can expect national revenues to diminish in comparative terms and the productivity and profitability of businesses to fall. As production and service delivery is disrupted, income is also likely to fall.[13]

Negative correlations emerge between the prevalence of the disease, the levels of individual and national savings, taxes and state revenues, rates of growth, and those of national and international investments. Indeed, the mere suggestion and the ensuing reality of the economic consequences of the epidemic have reduced expectations of return on investments, and lowered South Africa's rating on international capital markets, further hampering the country's ability to attract capital to promote domestic growth.

Despite this dire situation, at the end of 2007 a glimmer of light seemed emerge at the end of the tunnel. In late 2007, South Africa boasted economic growth between five and six percent, a budget surplus of 0.5 percent, low inflation, and a strong rand. Finance Minister Trevor Manual stated in his mid-term budget speech in October 2007 that all income groups were earning roughly 22 percent more than in 1999, and that overall the country was on its way to achieving an unemployment rate of below 14 percent by 2014: still high, but significantly lower than the current official rate of 26 percent, and the unofficial rate of nearly 40 percent. Manuel added that while in 1996 just over 50 percent of South Africans lacked access to clean water in their homes, and only 64 percent lived in formal housing, by 2007, over 88 percent had access to piped water, and over 70 percent lived in formal housing. However, this progress appeared short-lived as the electricity crisis that hit South Africa at the beginning of 2008 turned the lights out. This crisis coincided

---

11   Ibid.
12   Ibid.
13   Ibid.

with an increased inflation rate reaching 11 percent and a precipitous decline in the value of the rand, set to fall further as the ripples of the global financial crisis began to be felt in South Africa in late 2009 and 2010. Combined with stubbornly high HIV/AIDS incidence and prevalence rates, business coffers, political capital and confidence have suffered additional setbacks and shrunk.

3.2.1 HIV/AIDS and Business

The HIV/AIDS epidemic in South Africa has neither bypassed businesses, nor affected all uniformly. In response, businesses have both shirked and risen to the occasion to assume a role in addressing the epidemic. At the same time, business has been responding to new national rules-of-the-game in the form of first RDP and then GEAR, as well as BEE and BBBEE; rules that have been promulgated with a sweeping sense of addressing historic wrongs, a response with a zeal unseen in the response to the HIV/AIDS epidemic.

As early as 1986, some companies registered the presence and spread of HIV. That was the year that Sher and colleagues conducted their survey mentioned in chapter two of HIV prevalence at Anglo Group mines. While the infection rate then was negligible, subsequent surveys confirmed the expected rise in incidence and prevalence. In the meantime, in addition to Anglo Group, other large multinationals, such as BMW, Daimler (Chrysler),[14] DeBeers, Ford and VW, and others recognized the impending impact of the coming epidemic. Realizing that when the epidemic asserted itself their workforces and profits would be vulnerable, one after the other these companies instituted and promulgated what would become "best practice" models to address the epidemic. These models included education campaigns, prevention interventions, voluntary counseling and testing, and eventually treatment. Starting in 2001, these efforts were further promoted through organizations such as the Global Business Coalition against AIDS, Tuberculosis, and Malaria (GBC), and the South African Business Coalition against HIV/AIDS (SABCOHA). In 2002, DaimlerChrysler won the "best practice" award from the GBC for its workplace program. These initiatives served to raise the international profile both of HIV/AIDS and of global business responses.

Treatment posed a more difficult adoption, and has been instituted to greater and lesser degrees by different companies. Some company programs include treatment coverage for family members. The specified number of family members is generally a partner and two children, regardless of how many children requiring treatment and care an employee has. In theory, once the South African Government launched its first HIV/AIDS program in 2004, all South Africans not covered for AIDS-treatment under medical insurance or through company provisions were to be able to access care through the public sector. This development notably took place in the era of ascending notions of "good governance" and "corporate social responsibility." It also makes economic sense. Though initially, then

---

14   Later DaimlerChrysler, currently Daimler.

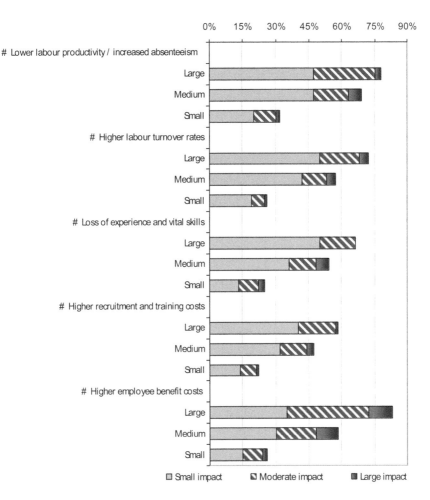

Figure 3.3   Reported impact of HIV/AIDS on productivity, per company size, 2005

Note: South African Business Coalition against HIV/AIDS (SABCOHA), "The Impact of HIV/AIDS on Selected Business Sectors in South Africa, 2005," A Survey Conducted by the Bureau for Economic Research (BER) (2005).

DaimlerChrysler expected the South African Government to take over its program after an initial two years,[15] this did not come to pass.

Small, medium and micro-enterprises (SMMEs), which employ the vast majority of South Africans working in the formal economy, however, generally lack the resources and capacity to offer such comprehensive prevention and

---

15   As cited in DaimlerChrysler HIV/AIDS policy, obtained in South Africa, 2003.

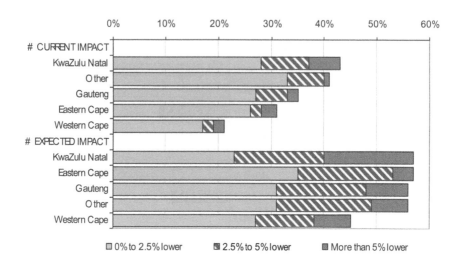

Figure 3.4   Reported impact of HIV/AIDS on profits, per province, 2005
Note: SABCOHA 2005. "The Impact of HIV/AIDS on Selected Business Sectors in South Africa, 2005."

treatment. Thus while large companies report the biggest impact of HIV/AIDS, SMMEs have not been spared. The overall impact of the epidemic on business across the country mirrors the geographic prevalence outlined in chapter two, with KwaZulu-Natal showing the highest and the Western Cape the lowest rates, as illustrated in Figure 3.4 below.

Broken down by further sector, the SABCOHA 2005 survey reports that 55 percent of mines, 46 percent of transport companies, 38 percent of manufacturers, and 35 percent of financial services companies cite an adverse effect on profitability due to HIV/AIDS.

In response, the interventions instituted by the multinational companies listed above should reverse these trends associated with the spread of HIV/AIDS, and contribute to reduced incidence, decreased AIDS-related disability, and to the protection of business productivity and profitability. In practice, however, incidence has continued to climb, and is projected to climb further until at least 2013, according to the Actuarial Society of South Africa (ASSA) 2003 model.

This predicted rise not only in AIDS deaths but also of HIV incidence (new infections) anticipates an elongated process of responding to the epidemic. It corresponds to increasing numbers of people needing to be trained for each position,[16] to rising numbers on sick leave and receiving disability pay,[17] which in turn correlates to loss of productivity and profits, negatively impacting investment. Furthermore, higher incidence rates mean that more people will require treatment for HIV/AIDS, an exorbitantly expensive endeavor, which becomes more so as more people also live longer due to access to medicine. This longer lifespan, fortified by access to medicines, increases the likelihood of further epidemic spread, including of strains resistant to currently available drugs and even those under development meant to counter it.[18] Further evidence for this is in the fight against tuberculosis (TB), multi-drug resistant tuberculosis (MDR-TB) and even extremely multi-drug resistant tuberculosis (XDR-TB). South Africa has the most cases of the latter in the world, a consequence—and facilitator—of its HIV/AIDS epidemic. The (dual) challenge is also one for business, and perhaps an impetus for private-public partnerships, confronting as they are accelerating epidemic threats to labor force and local and global markets.

3.2.2 Advent of Antiretrovirals (ARVs)

The issue of access to ARVs is fraught with friction. On the one hand they constitute a sea change in the course of the HIV/AIDS epidemic. As Sher notes, the biggest change in the fight against HIV/AIDS was the "advent of ARVs. Prior to them the diagnosis of HIV was like a judge passing a death sentence."[19] While not a cure for the virus and requiring life-long adherence, ARVs do prolong the lives of those with access to them. Individuals on ARVs are often well enough to be able to work, to contribute to the productivity of the economy, to provide for their families and thereby to ensure human capital transfer, as well as to save or invest. On the other hand ARVs present a host of complications, foremost among them being their generally high prices and their potential to foster drug resistance and inadvertently, by undermining behavioral change and contributing to resistance, the spread of the

---

16   In some cases, three people are being trained for every open position, in anticipation that two will fall sick or die of HIV/AIDS. This situation is also leading to an increase in the practice of contract labor, which includes no obligations on the part of companies to contribute to healthcare costs or other benefits, including severance pay, for hired—and fired—workers.

17   Costing both companies and the government, which must budget for disability pay in the case of the former, and disability grants in that of the latter.

18   Indeed, initial budget estimates for antiretroviral treatment (ARV) against HIV/AIDS (2003) were done with incidence estimates declining after 2004: this is emphatically not the case. Indeed, as the epidemic has spread unabated, despite—or even because of—the increased access to ARVs, prevention has, especially after 2005 with UNAIDS' Peter Piot reemphasized it, a renewed priority in the fight against HIV/AIDS; and it needs to continue to be at the center of the epicenter.

19   Interview with Professor Ruben Sher, 8 March 2005.

epidemic.[20] "In 1996 HAART [Highly Active Antiretroviral Therapy][21] became available in this country. Expensive."[22] The longer an infected individual lives, the greater the chances of spreading infection. This includes drug-resistant strains of HIV cultivated in the environment of ARVs, which can lead to "supra-infections." At present, though first-line therapy is increasingly accessible, second- and third-line treatments remain prohibitively expensive, and current patent contests before Indian courts threaten to cut off the supply of generic alternatives.[23]

These issues, of price and of the potential of ARVs to foster drug resistance and even to fuel the HIV/AIDS epidemic, are of particular importance from a state-centered, political-economic perspective. The price of treatment with ARVs is difficult to estimate as it includes not only the cost of the drugs themselves, but also that of the necessary associated clinical infrastructure,[24] and human as well as logistical capacity. Only 31.5 percent of nurses trained in South Africa between 1996 and 2004, for instance, registered with the South African Nursing Council over that period. This means that "unsustainably large numbers of trained nurses are either choosing not to pursue nursing careers in South Africa, or are leaving the country to work abroad"[25] at a substantial cost, financial and human, to South Africa and to its ability to respond to HIV/AIDS. Similarly, logistical infrastructure—from import through delivery (with refrigeration) to dispensing—is fraught with weaknesses.

---

20   For new research and commentary on HIV drug resistance, see Kambugu, A. 2012. "Pre-ART HIV resistance testing in Africa: are we there yet?" *The Lancet Infectious Diseases*, 12(4) (April): 261.

21   HAART is a combination of multiple antiretroviral drugs, rendering treatment more effective than the one-drug regimen of AZT, that was also highly toxic, that had become available a few years prior.

22   Interview with Professor Ruben Sher, 8 March 2005.

23   Pharmaceutical company Novartis is winding down six-plus years of court challenges in India whose outcome will help determine the continuing status of patents, including 'ever-greening' and therefore that of access to medicines and generics for much of the developing and emerging world.

24   A new study by Peter, T., Blair, D., Reid, M. and Justman, J. 2010. "DART and laboratory monitoring of HIV treatment." *The Lancet*, 375(9719) (20 March): 979, argues that laboratory work is much more important to monitoring and treating HIV/AIDS that has previously been accepted and employed.

25   Nattrass, N. 2004. *The Moral Economy of HIV/AIDS*. Cambridge: Cambridge University Press: "South Africa's 'Roll-Out' of Highly Active Anti-Retroviral Therapy: A Critical Assessment." In addition, some NGOs fly nurses into South Africa, a practice that is unsustainable and which undermines local capacity-building. For example, the US President's Emergency Plan to Fight AIDS (PEPFAR) first-round legislation even makes provisions for loan-relief for American medical practitioners who serve for limited times in HIV-affected counties, such as South Africa. This might serve to support American students in repaying their medical school loans, but it does little to support the education, capacity-building, and deployment of long-term professionals within South Africa.

Another factor in the cost of ARV treatment is the consequence of price fluctuations related to the varying value of the South African rand. ARVs are generally purchased in US dollars on the international market.[26] Given the difficulties associated with South Africa's access to capital markets and investment outlined above, this is not a negligible concern in the country's response to the epidemic. When the rand devalues, the prices become prohibitive. Furthermore, most cost calculations are based on an assumption that the incidence and prevalence rates of HIV/AIDS in South Africa will stagnate at a certain date, such as in the ASSA model cited above. Most models assume that the costs of ARV treatment will continue to fall based on price calculations for first-line drugs increasingly available as generics. However, as noted above, as incidence and prevalence continue to rise, so, too, does the need for second- and even third-line drugs,[27] which remain largely out of reach and which have not been put under pressure to reduce their prices. As such, the cost of treatment might not decline overall.

One study calculates that an antiretroviral program that covers 26 percent of the population in need of such treatment would pay for itself, though it would require a "willing" household sacrifice amounting to 12 percent of GDP:[28] hardly reasonable in a country where up to 40 percent of the population is unemployed, unable to save, and likely unwilling to make an additional, long-term sacrifice. Also, what about the other 74 percent of the population needing treatment?

An example illustrates some of the relevant social and economic challenges complicating ARV access and HIV/AIDS control. Take the scene at Kalafong Hospital, a public facility north of Pretoria in South Africa. There in November 2004, just as the ASSA model and the calculations cited above were published predicting decreasing incidence and cost-efficiencies, a nurse, Elizabeth, was witnessing other predictors of the course of the epidemic. Working in an HIV/AIDS unit with patients lined up all along the corridor, she saw no sign of an abating epidemic. According to the then-current treatment guidelines, she could only initiate treatment in patients whose CD4 immune cell counts had fallen below 200 per milliliter (mL).[29] At this low CD4 count (the normal range being between 500–1000), marking them as ill, patients also qualified for a government disability grant, roughly 700 rand per month. This was often their only source of income and supported, on average, 10 people. However, the initiation of ARVs

---

26   Personal correspondence with Fanyana Shiburi in his capacity as former director of government relations and policy at DaimlerChrysler SA.

27   Within the coming years, some 70 percent of those needing anti-retroviral treatment will require these more expensive treatments.

28   Johansson, L.M. 2006. "Fiscal Implications of AIDS in South Africa," Department of Economics, Stockholm University (14 June).

29   New World Health Organization (WHO) guidelines, released in November 2009 recommend initiating treatment at 350CD4/mL; South Africa has only adopted these in part however, for pregnant women and infants, and for those co-infected with tuberculosis. Thus this scenario still holds true.

carried with it the implication that the patient's CD4 count would rise above 200 per mL, disqualifying him for the disability grant, and depriving him of a source of income. This often led to a vicious cycle of patients beginning ARV treatment, but not returning for periodic CD4 count tests in order to retain their disability grants, or of ceasing ARVs to retain the grant or even sharing ARVs among other infected individuals, reducing their efficacy and increasing the risk of the development of resistance.[30] Of patients who return for CD4 count tests and lose their disability grants, in some cases continue treatment, but also engage in survivalist practices such as transactional sex in order to earn an income. "Given South Africa's high unemployment rates, many will not be able to find work, and hence will face a trade-off between health (taking HAART [highly active antiretroviral therapy]) and income (keeping the disability grant)."[31] Managing this relationship between South Africa's HIV/AIDS epidemic and its economy, including that of poverty, is critical. It is a *governance* challenge that mandates actions by the sovereign state to enact its responsibility to respond.

3.3 Political Level

The response to and the eventual eradication of HIV/AIDS must include medical, social and economic intervention, political action, responsibility and accountability. As such, it represents a particular challenge for South Africa's governance in terms of its sovereign statehood. The associated political calculations involved are, however, also at least as complex as the economic ones, involving factors of confidence, perceived and real impact of the epidemic, prioritization and ability to respond.

Mandela's reluctance to address HIV/AIDS at the outset of the democratic era stalled the process of response. Mbeki, though he did initiate interventions against the epidemic, put other priorities first. In particular, acknowledging and acquiescing to the global "rules of the game," then President Mbeki stated: "South Africa had no choice but to play by the rules of the global economy."[32] By "no choice," Mbeki internalized and embodied—and in the ensuing policy debate externalized—the verdict that South Africa must attempt to capitalize on fiscal discipline with the aim of attracting investor confidence and accessing capital to promote the country's economic and social development, including any possible response against HIV/AIDS. At the same time, incompatibly, the former

---

30   HIV-infected persons can additionally become infected with more than one mutation of the virus, resulting in "supra-infections," which are especially difficult to treat.

31   Nattrass, N. 2005. "Trading off Income and Health: AIDS and the Disability Grant in South Africa." *Journal of Social Policy*, 35(1): 3–19.

32   Gumede, W. 2005. *Thabo Mbeki and the Battle for the Soul of the ANC.* Cape Town: Zebra Publishers: 91.

president was striving to keep South Africa independent, especially of external financial dependencies.

However, the HIV/AIDS epidemic was already undermining that effort. As argued above, failing to adequately address HIV/AIDS slows growth, "reduces the tax capacity of the economy. It undermines the potential developmental role for the state."[33]

Voter rolls highlight this impact. Changes on the rolls between 1999 and 2003 indicate that almost 1.5 million of South Africa's 20,674,926 registered voters were removed from the roll because they had died. "Over this period, the number of deaths among registered voters increased by 66 percent. In some municipalities mortality increased by more than 300 percent over the four years for women between 30 and 39 years of age. In Limpopo Province it increased by 160 percent. Mortality in the age group 30–49 increased at a higher rate than in the other age groups,"[34] as clear an indicator as is available (since most deaths are not registered as HIV or AIDS deaths) of death attributable to the epidemic. This further highlights the fact that the epidemic targets those of working and reproductive age, their deaths again emphasizing the virus's impact on South Africa's immediate and long-term economic potential. These consequences crystallize the importance of the state to assume its responsibility to respond.

3.3.1 AIDS and the African Renaissance

As noted in the section on the social impact of HIV/AIDS in this chapter, sex is a key driver of the AIDS epidemic. Consequently, what should be a vehicle of life, and of freedom, of independence and sovereignty, inspiration and the source of President Thabo Mbeki's African Renaissance,[35] becomes a scourge of death for the individual and for the polity.

> If HIV is sexually transmitted, then sex itself has become the vector of death. Within this symbolic universe, to concede the scientific orthodoxy would be to recognize that once HIV infiltrates the social body, it snuffs out the fragile promise of new life; if sex produces death, then the infant nation is stillborn. Moreover, if the real issue in respect of HIV/AIDS is sexual, this would admit to other symbolic registers similarly disruptive of the effort to 'imagine' the nation's 'renewal.' The fatality of sex is anchored in the family itself—the crucible of

---

33 Nattrass, N. 2004. *The Moral Economy of HIV/AIDS*. Cambridge: Cambridge University Press: 33.

34 Barnett, T. 2006. "A Long-Wave Event. HIV/AIDS, Politics, Governance and 'Security'." *International Affairs HIV/AIDS*, Special Issue, 82(2): 297–313.

35 "The word Renaissance means rebirth, renewal, springing anew, even eternal. Therefore we speak of the rebirth and renewal of our continent." Mbeki quoted in Posel, "Sex, Death and the Fate of the Nation: Reflections on the Politicization of Sexuality in Post-Apartheid South Africa."

the nation. Metaphorically, it is the very intimacy of the home—mother, father and children—which has become contaminated. And it is men particularly—the fathers and sons of the nation—whose moral credibility is most acutely called into question.[36]

Mbeki pleads against the conflating of (African) life and AIDS death. Yet the two are intertwined; and that presents a crisis for South Africa's perception of itself and its confidence. It also influences its practice of power and independence. Finally, it impacts the state's response to the epidemic.

As this book argues in greater detail in Chapter 5, South Africa's reluctance, under Presidents Mandela and Mbeki, to accept and acknowledge and to effectively act against this unpalatable convergence, is derived from both the dungeons of the past and the dreams for the future. Thus,

To concede the sexual transmission of HIV would be to revitalize the racist stereotypes of rampant and unruly sex ('the things in the African bush'). It would be tantamount to acknowledging the unruliness of sex, on a catastrophic scale—bringing back [from apartheid-inspired imagery] the 'black hordes ... against which ferocious dogs must be kept on the leash.[37]

Interpreted from this angle, Mbeki's reluctance to address the atrocity of HIV/AIDS becomes a deliberate if mangled political calculation: "to admit to the enormity of the epidemic would be to reinstate the imagery of the 'abyss,' the 'African nightmare' ... Therefore, in order to succeed, to stay out of the abyss, South Africa cannot succumb to the disease."[38] In making this assertion, Mbeki vaulted over the immediate problem of responding to HIV/AIDS directly and launched instead into a more epic battle for (African) identity and independence, particularly in the inviolability of its domestic sovereignty. He encased this vision in the African Renaissance, an "admirably creative [initiative]—against the anxieties of the dream deferred; the willing of a self-determination that was not always possible in the real world he [Mbeki] came to govern."[39] Despite these valiant efforts to outshine—perhaps to blind it—however, the HIV/AIDS epidemic shattered the window and the mirror.

Similar in imagery to the African Renaissance and in fact related to it in practice, Mbeki also conceived of and established the New Partnership for African Development (NEPAD). It likewise brokered no room for the epidemic crouching in its midst. In negotiations over NEPAD and a "new deal for Africa with leaders

---

36   Posel, "Sex, Death and the Fate of the Nation: Reflections on the Politicization of Sexuality in Post-Apartheid South Africa."

37   Ibid.

38   Ibid.

39   Gevisser, M. 2007. *Thabo Mbeki: The Dream Deferred*. Jeppestown: Jonathan Ball Publishers (Pty) Ltd: xxiii and xxxiii.

of the G8 [Group of 8],"[40] and concerned in particular with the role and power of the pharmaceutical industry in proscribing rules-of-the-game in the global (HIV-related) marketplace, thereby dictating the 'appropriate' response to the epidemic, particularly in Africa, Mbeki wrote in 2002,

> We [Africans] will not be intimidated, terrorized, bludgeoned, manipulated, stampeded, or in any other way forced to adopt policies and programs inimical to the health of our people. That we are poor and black does not mean that we cannot think for ourselves and determine what is good for us. Neither does it mean that we are available to be bought, whatever the price.[41]

Explicitly referring to the repercussions of Mbeki's thinking about and policies to address HIV/AIDS a year after the UN Security Council elevated concern over the epidemic to an international security crisis, a spokesman for then-President Mbeki agreed. The epidemic constitutes "political problem that has reached the proportion of an international crisis. It threatens to destroy nations and continents."[42] Yet for all of the rhetoric against it, the epidemic continued to ravage the South African population and to challenge the ability of its state to assume and enact its responsibility to respond.

Mbeki found himself and post-apartheid governance in South Africa constrained by reality, and "having to make one of those terrible calculations of power; to sacrifice the lives of those who, he was convinced, would die from taking antiretrovirals."[43] He wanted foremost to "safeguard his government, his country, [and] the ANC's project of transformation."[44] Mbeki feared that even if those infected with HIV did not die, South Africa would, in the process of saving them by providing life-long access to ARVs, become beholden to the global pharmaceutical industry, undermining the independence he so fervently sought in order to protect lives in the first place.

Thus Mbeki's (pre)occupation with South Africa's independence and its domestic sovereignty forms part of a cyclical relationship. It is a relationship not only in his head, but a real link between the spread of the epidemic. According to this verdict, the epidemic is fostered by state failure to respond as well as HIV/AIDS' own impact on political calculations; and vice versa. In South Africa, the

---

40   Ibid., 741.

41   Ibid., 750.

42   See Altman, D. 2003. "AIDS and Security." *International Relations*, 17(4): 417–427.

43   Though ARVs do not cause death, patients who begin them very late in the stages of the disease progression from HIV to full-blown AIDS do tend to die soon after treatment initiation, giving the impression that ARVs are the culprit, when in fact, the advance progression of the disease is.

44   Gevisser, M. 2007. *Thabo Mbeki: The Dream Deferred.* Jeppestown: Jonathan Ball Publishers (Pty) Ltd: 758.

politics of sovereign statehood and its responsibility to respond to HIV/AIDS cannot be seen in isolation of each other.

3.3.2 Independence and State Sovereignty

Mbeki's main focus was on South Africa's domestic sovereignty and sovereign statehood, as detailed in the introduction. While no state in the contemporary international, state-centric system is completely sovereign, the independence each possesses, most especially in the realm of domestic sovereignty, is often jealously guarded. This leads to varying results.

As Ebrahim Rasool stated, as quoted in the introduction, external interventions, such as "programs by major international financial institutions" [as well as those imposed or implemented by pharmaceutical companies, or foreign government sponsored organizations such as PEPFAR leave their recipients often feeling that "they have no choice but to accept."[45] These conditions arguably led South Africa to adopt GEAR and likewise promulgate its ARV roll-out in the way that it did. Both represent voluntarily conceded policy positions,[46] in the face of enormous internal and external pressure, at times exercised in unison between external state and non-state, local-global alliances of actors intervening indirectly to encourage or coerce state action. By their actions, these actors assumed some interim responsibility for interventions that the state refused to perform which they took did instead. The fate of the South African state's main concern, namely, its ultimate responsibility and accountability, hung in the balance.

This transcription of responsibility and accountability lost some significant information in the encoding of state DNA into local-global alliance RNA. By impinging upon the state's domestic sovereignty,[47] and undercutting the government's ability to act without translating and transferring the conferring responsibility and accountability it created the GAP. Taken into account together, it becomes obvious that the South African state is caught between end- and exogenous conditions, amongst them the HIV/AIDS epidemic itself, which constrain the remit of its sovereign statehood. The result is the GAP in the responsibility to respond.

3.4 Conclusion

As evidenced above, HIV/AIDS inextricably impacts South Africa's society, economy, and polity: conversely, the spread of the epidemic is influenced by the confluence of social, economic and political factors. While the virus destroys individual lives and distributes its repercussions on present and future generations,

---

45   ICISS, "The Responsibility to Protect," 1.37.
46   See Krasner, S. 1999. *Sovereignty: Organized Hypocrisy.* Princeton: Princeton University Press.
47   Ibid.

ARVs can prolong the lives of HIV infected individuals, and possibly contribute to prevention as well. This complex reality renders the epidemic, and any response to it, a multi-dimensional and multi-generational problem.

It is a political and governance problem, made all the more difficult to solve due to the effective division between tactical and ultimate sovereign responsibility amongst a host of local-global alliances, state and non-state actors. This exposes the GAP which will necessarily have to be bridged if the HIV/AIDS crisis is to be resolved. The following two chapters will analyze the external and the internal influences factors and the decision-making context which characterize the international and domestic scenes surrounding South Africa's HIV/AIDS response.

Chapter 4

The (Inter)national Framework of South Africa's Policy-Making

As seen in the analysis of preceding chapters, HIV/AIDS poses a critical problem in and for South Africa. The epidemic's individual, social, economic and political dimensions span not only the local, but also the national, and spread even into the international spheres, provoking angst but also heralding a new era of global policy-making. The focus here on the latter showcases both the international and the national policy influences and implications of the response and the responsibility to respond to HIV/AIDS.

4.1 The International Scene

HIV/AIDS emerged as an international issue only in 2000. Previously, the remit to stem it belonged exclusively to national governments in Africa. South Africa did—intermittently—respond; but it did so almost solely within its self-determined policy process as befitting a national challenge. This changed significantly on 17 July 2000, the day the United Nations Security Council debated and passed Resolution 1308, entitled the "Responsibility of the Security Council in the Maintenance of International Peace and Security: HIV/AIDS and International Peace-keeping Operations." That resolution culminated in United Nations General Assembly resolution S-26/2, "Declaration of Commitment on HIV/AIDS," of 27 June 2001.

In his attendant speech, then US Vice-President Al Gore emphasized three key points with reference to HIV/AIDS and global security. He argued that the heart of the security agenda is to protect lives; that when a single disease, HIV/AIDS, threatens everything from economic strength to peacekeeping it clearly constitutes a crisis of the "greatest magnitude"; and consequently designated HIV/AIDS a security concern because it threatens not only individual lives but the essential institutions of a society such as the South African state. UN Secretary-General Kofi Annan added that states are understood to be instruments at the service of their populaces and not vice-versa. This means that states are responsible and accountable for providing protection not only against military security threats, but also against (cross-border flows of) disease. When a schism emerges wherein the state and external state and non-state actors are not aligned in guaranteeing such responsibility, the GAP emerges. R2P is at the furthest end of the spectrum of response in this instance, allocating that responsibility and its associated accountability to the international community in the event that a state should fail to protect, or itself threaten all or part of its population.

Thus this first UN Security Council resolution to concern itself with HIV/AIDS paved the way for further international attention and action against the pandemic. While that initial resolution declared HIV/AIDS an international security threat and paid particular attention to the impact of the epidemic on peace-keeping missions,[1] others would cast the focus more widely. The UN Security Council discussed the pandemic again in January 2001 and in July 2005. In 2004, the United Nations High-level Panel on Threats, Challenges and Change viewed the pandemic as a threat to international security,[2] a type of threat it defined as "any event or process that leads to large-scale death or lessening of life expectancy, and undermines States as the basic unit of the international system."[3] These meetings did two things: raised awareness about HIV/AIDS and the threat to security it constituted at the international level, and significantly, "legitimized the basis for intervention by the United Nations to combat this particular threat" posed by the epidemic.[4] Though not—yet—invoked as a ground for UN security intervention in South Africa, or elsewhere, the thinking behind the rationale presented here arguably finds expression in the external state and non-state local-global alliances and pressures brought to bear on South Africa. This rule-making, though not

---

1   Though various militaries, including South Africa's, test soldiers for HIV, in some instances barring them from external missions and from promotions, there is little consistent evidence that soldiers bring HIV/AIDS to the places where they perform peace-keeping. Furthermore, despite some dire warnings, HIV/AIDS has yet to be concretely linked to terrorism. After the September 11th, terrorist attacks on New York and Washington, DC, US strategic concerns centered around and broadened to include factors associated with weakened states, including global infectious diseases such as HIV/AIDS and threats of international terrorism. These are also reflected in a report by the UN National Intelligence Council in 2002, entitled, "The Next Wave of HIV/AIDS: Nigeria, Ethiopia, Russia, India, and China," which "presented evidence of rising trends in HIV infection in the five countries covered, each of which has a large population and was considered as strategic for different reasons by the USA," as well as in the concept of "human security" which expanded the concept of "security" to include the components of "safe, secure, healthy and productive lives, and included the implications for state security." See Lisk, F. 2009. *Global Institutions and the HIV/AIDS Epidemic.* New York: Routledge Global Institutions: 86.

2   See also Pharaoh, R. and Schoenteich, M. 2003. "AIDS, Security and Governance in South Africa. Exploring the Impact." Occasional Paper No. 65. Johannesburg: Institute for Security Studies.

3   Lisk, F. 2009. *Global Institutions and the HIV/AIDS Epidemic.* New York: Routledge Global Institutions: 85.

4   See Lisk, F. 2009. *Global Institutions and the HIV/AIDS Epidemic.* New York: Routledge Global Institutions: 85. In 2005, "a presidential statement was made on progress achieved in addressing the impact of HIV/AIDS on UN peacekeepers globally. In 2004, the United Nations High-level Panel on Threats, Challenges and Change, established by the secretary-general to examine present and potential threat to international security in a changing world, identified HIV/AIDS and other infectious diseases as a "bio-security threat."

hierarchical as in Westphalian sovereignty, but circular, surrounding the affected state, pertains not only to the fact of a response to the epidemic, but also to its particular manner. Failure to accede resulted in enormous psychological stress for the country's leadership and imparted real consequences for the state's political and economic clout.

Nonetheless, South Africa resisted this. Thus even as the prioritization of HIV/AIDS ascended policy agendas around the world, South Africa was largely preoccupied with other pressures and priorities that ranked higher, as evidenced, on its national agenda.[5] Primary among these were economic concerns and political rights. As Nelson Mandela said in his first speech to the newly elected South African Parliament, on 24 May 1994,

> Our single most important challenge is to help establish a social order in which the freedom of the individual will truly mean the freedom of the individual. We must construct that people-centered society of freedom in such a manner that it guarantees the political liberties and the human rights of all our citizens ... My government's commitment to create a people-centered society of liberty binds us to the pursuit of the goals of freedom from want, freedom from hunger, freedom from deprivation, freedom from ignorance, freedom from suppression and freedom from fear.[6]

Deprivation and dependence were the concerns that the South African state identified as its highest priorities. It wanted to ensure that its (majority) populace would no longer live in want, and that the state similarly would not operate on disadvantageous terms particularly on the international market. Influencing these priorities were not only South Africa's recent emergence from its apartheid past, but also the prescriptions, both codified and not, of global finance. This would, seemingly contradictorily, provide both the influence for South Africa's conformance with international "norms" and the impetus, revealed through the GAP analysis presented here, for its non-conformity.

4.1.1 External Economic Elements

As outlined in the preceding chapters, South Africa negotiated its transition from apartheid to democracy, as well as its response to HIV/AIDS, within the confines

---

5   See also Cox, R.W. 1992. "Towards a Post-Hegemonic Conceptualization of World Order: Reflections on the Relevancy of Ibn Khaldun." In *Governance without Government: Order and Change in World Politics* (ed.) Rosenau, J. and Czempiel, E.-O. Cambridge: Cambridge University Press: 143–144, on how domestic policies around the globe are increasingly made based on the global economy. The current global financial crisis also starkly brings this into focus.

6   Terreblanche, S. 2002. *A History of Inequality in South Africa 1652–2002.* Pietermaritzburg: University of Natal Press: 442.

not only of global market rules regarding macroeconomic and fiscal policies, but particular expectations for interventions how to tackle the epidemic. The two were and are intertwined, and depending upon the point of view—and priority—of the policy-maker, either complementary or (mutually) exclusive. This analysis argues that, unwilling to assume external dependencies that would further compromise its already limited sovereign statehood and negate its ability to assume and act upon its responsibility to respond—not only to HIV/AIDS, but across the policy spectrum—South Africa tended to view the two sets of prescriptions as mutually exclusive. So South Africa found itself wedged between the prerogative of those external state and non-state actors more single-mindedly focused on HIV/AIDS response on the one and the market stipulations of foreign direct investment it sought on the other.

Rosenau points out that states' domestic sovereignty is increasingly influenced by external material and political influence.[7] Foreign direct investment (FDI) is one example of material influence; further material and political influence will be examined below. As indicated above, South Africa's relationship to FDI is not a straight-forward tale.

The overall trend is one that calls for caution. Global FDI flows to Africa declined from six percent (of all global FDI) in the 1970s to between two and three percent in 2001. In the same time period, Africa's share of world trade also fell, from 3.1 percent to 1.8 percent. The continent's share of FDI as a percentage of GDP likewise declined precipitously, falling from close to 25 percent in the late 1970s to 17.2 in the late 1990s, with a further drop in the early twenty-first century.[8] These negative trends have certainly contributed to South Africa's sense of urgency around attracting and maintaining whatever FDI inflows it could.

Then in 2004, Africa and South Africa experienced an estimated FDI growth rate of six percent, a positive event which was repeated in 2005, 2006, and 2007. Indeed, in 2005, South Africa "was the largest FDI recipient in the region … experiencing a sharp jump in inflows to US$6.4 billion from only US$0.8 billion in 2004."[9] South Africa accounted for about 21 percent of the region's total FDI inflows, though due to a once-off acquisition.[10] This unprecedented purchase was however followed another, that of the Industrial and Commercial Bank of China

---

7   Rosenau, J.N. 1992. "Governance, order, and change in world politics." In *Governance without Government: Order and Change in World Politics* (ed.) Rosenau, J. and Czempiel, E.-O. Cambridge: Cambridge University Press.

8   See UNCTAD 2006. "Global FDI Inflows Rise for Second Consecutive Year." UNCTAD (16 October); UNCTAD 2006. "World Investment Report 2006—FDI from Developing and Transition Economies: Implications for Development." UNCTAD; and IMF 2007. "Board Concludes Article IV Consultation with South Africa," Public Information Notice (PIN) No. 07/94. The International Monetary Fund (6 August).

9   UNCTAD 2006. "World Investment Report 2006—FDI from Developing and Transition Economies: Implications for Development." UNCTAD.

10   Reuters 2007. "ICBC to buy $5.6 billion stake in South African Bank" (25 October).

(ICBC) buying 20 percent of South Africa's Standard Bank for US$5.6 billion in the fall of 2007. Commenting on the ICBC investment, Standard Bank Chief Executive Officer Jacko Maree said, "we think it is an enormous vote of confidence in South Africa and in Africa."[11] Since then, credit flows to the private sector have remained largely buoyant.[12] In addition to the financial sector, facilitated by South Africa's adoption of the Basel II international banking accords, other beneficiaries of FDI in South Africa included energy, machinery, and mining.

These developments are worth noting for two reasons. First, South Africa continues to align its macroeconomic policies to GEAR, despite evidence that the state's enactment of its constitutional responsibilities to its citizens is circumscribed, particularly those related to the response to HIV/AIDS. Second, the FDI rise in the early 2000s coincided with South Africa's abrogated challenge to intellectual property rights around ARVs and initial launch of the country's first public roll-out.

Contrary to expectations, instead of enhancing South Africa's negotiating powers and abilities to deliver upon its sovereign responsibilities particularly pertaining to HIV/AIDS, these developments, coupled with the continued focus on FDI and associated influence of international actors, had the adverse effect of limiting its domestic sovereignty and of increasing its external dependence.

4.1.2 External Actors and Roles in the HIV/AIDS Arena

Much of the circumspection of South Africa's domestic sovereignty can be ascribed to the convergence and in some instances the overlap of two kinds of influence. First, that of local-global alliances, which as shown here in the realm of HIV/AIDS can lead to voluntary circumvention of South Africa's domestic sovereignty. Second, that of South African policy decisions which involuntarily constrict the state's domestic sovereignty and more importantly its sovereign statehood per se, primarily by compelling it into accepting dependency.

Two critical examples illustrate this. First is the South African Government's attempt to invoke its rights and then voluntary rejection thereof under the Trade-Related Aspects of Intellectual Property legislation (TRIPS) of the World Trade Organization (WTO). When this did not function as intended, by enabling the country to access antiretroviral medications by issuing voluntary or compulsory licenses and conducting parallel imports, the state found itself settling to voluntarily circumscribing its sovereignty by agreeing to alternative terms of access. Second is the emergence of local-global alliances between external state and non-state actors in the HIV/AIDS arena whose advocacy and action involuntarily (on the part of the state) circumvented the authority, responsibility and accountability of the South African state.

---

11   "ICBC to buy $5.6 billion stake in South African Bank."
12   "Board Concludes Article IV Consultation with South Africa."

These alliances operate slightly differently from the boomerang effect posited by Sikkink and Keck because though they lobbied the South African Government for access to ARVs, they failed. In response, they mounted their own intervention, circumventing the state's authority and imposing a separate—and unequal—solution, notably because they did not assume ultimate responsibility and accountability for the response, which remained within the remit of the state. Therefore, though their lobbying was in effect an example of the boomerang effect, their later action was not: they assumed actual functions of intervention in South Africa's HIV/AIDS arena, circumventing, supplanting, and supplementing the role of the state. In so doing, their presence serves to emphasize and then arguably to widen the GAP in responsibility and accountability between non-state and state actors.

No bridge exists between the two spheres. This was on display in the wake of the 2008 global financial crisis, which resulted in the reduction of much funding and thereby contributed to the evaporation of capacity to the detriment of the implementation of both the tactical and the ultimate responsibility and accountability to respond. As a consequence, these local-global alliances contributed to the further—non-voluntary—erosion of South Africa's domestic sovereignty.

Each of these examples will be explored in more detail in chapter six. Here, the relevant actors and their associated actions in the HIV/AIDS arena impacting upon South Africa are introduced and explored.

4.2 International Political Prioritization of HIV/AIDS

HIV/AIDS first emerged on the international political scene as a security issue. The pandemic was brought to the attention of the United Nation's Security Council (UNSC) by US Ambassador Richard Holbrooke and the US Government on 10 January 2000. The initial concern was over the impact of the epidemic on peacekeeping operations and state security such in conflict zones across the African continent, such as that in northern Uganda. Following this first discussion of the disease threat, UN General Assembly resolution S-26/2, entitled "Declaration of Commitment on HIV/AIDS," passed on 27 June 2001. Its pledges were soon borne out in practical commitments to the fight against HIV/AIDS, accompanied also by additional UN resolutions.

What does this say about international priority and agenda-setting? What does it reveal about the relationship between international and national actors in the HIV/AIDS arena? What can be deduced with regard to the appropriation of sovereign responsibility and accountability between states and non-state entities?

Resolution S-26/2, initiated at the behest of the US, called for local, national, regional and global action against the HIV/AIDS epidemic. The resolution acknowledged the mitigating roles played by poverty, lack of access to and affordability of medications, crippling effects of external debt and debt-servicing, and strain on human resources and national health systems. In response it requested leadership, coordinated multi-sectoral strategies in prevention, care, support, and treatment—strategies undoubtedly based on the experience of the private sector noted above—as well as initiatives to alleviate the economic and social impacts of HIV/AIDS.[13] However, it did not stipulate who should be held responsible and accountable for which interventions. Instead it established a loophole through which South Africa's domestic sovereignty could be impinged upon, without a bridge across the ensuing GAP between tactical and ultimate responsibility and accountability. Spurred by the political clout associated with the passage of the resolution, interventions against HIV/AIDS grew exponentially in its wake, the establishment of the Global Fund and the initiation of PEPFAR among them: but these were all created without a clear delineation of sovereign authority.

A second UN General Assembly resolution cemented the presence of the HIV/AIDS epidemic on the international global governance agenda, moving beyond the security dimension, but likewise neglected to define the lines of responsibility and accountability. The "Political Declaration" 60/262 of 2006 reiterated many of the stipulations of resolution S-26/2, with one significant exception. Significantly, the latter asserted the role—and right—of non-governmental and civic organizations, such as groups of people living with HIV, medical, scientific, and educational institutions, the business sector, including generic and research-based pharmaceutical companies, trade unions, the media, parliamentarians, foundations, faith-based organizations and traditional leaders, other community organizations, and the United Nations agencies, to carry out the tasks of oversight and monitoring of the interventions against HIV/AIDS.[14] The resolution's support for the involvement of and intervention by these non-state organizations in the HIV/AIDS arena paved the way for the ensuing acceleration of local-global special interest alliances in the HIV/AIDS arena, many of which bypass state governments. Though the resolution promoted the response to the crisis of HIV/AIDS according to particular prescriptions and expectations deemed most applicable at the time, it did nothing to clarify the final harbor of responsibility and accountability, the consequence of which is the GAP.

Instead, it actually helped to create the GAP between state and external state and non-state responsibility and accountability. In so doing, it also gave a political

---

13   United Nations General Assembly 2001. Resolution S-26/2, "Declaration of Commitment on HIV/AIDS" (27 June).

14   For instance, United Nations General Assembly 2006. Resolution 60/262, "Political Declaration on HIV/AIDS (15 June), paragraph 19, declares: "Recognize the importance, and encourage the implementation, of the recommendations of the inclusive, country-driven processes and regional consultations facilitated by the Secretariat and the Co-sponsors of the Joint United Nations Program on HIV/AIDS for scaling up HIV prevention, treatment, care and support, and strongly recommend that this approach be continued." This provision essentially prescribed UN strategy as national policy, despite the fact outlined above that these UN strategies have thus far showed little success in curbing the epidemic or its effects. Also as illustrated above, the reality of such strategy being "country-driven" is up for dispute.

underpinning for circumscribing South Africa's domestic sovereignty while doing nothing to resolve the dilemma in which the sovereign state remained the ultimate bearer of responsibility and accountability.

For instance, resolution 60/262 further promoted "access to HIV/AIDS education, voluntary counselling and testing and related services"[15] at the "international, national and local levels."[16] Signatories affirmed their commitment to "finding appropriate solutions to overcome barriers in pricing, tariffs and trade agreements, and to making improvements to legislation, regulatory policy, procurement and supply chain management in order to accelerate and intensify access to affordable and quality HIV/AIDS prevention products, diagnostics, medicines and treatment commodities."[17] In addition, they pledged to accept and honor provisions contained in the TRIPS legislation to not "prevent members from taking measures now and in the future to protect public health," and to allow the "production of generic antiretroviral drugs and other essential drugs for AIDS-related infections."[18] These were codified in the TRIPS agreement's Article 31 itself, reiterated in the Doha Declaration on the TRIPS Agreement and Public Health and in the WTO's General Council Decision of 2005.[19] Being part of the original TRIPS agreement, indeed, these safeguards for public health existed, but were repudiated during South Africa's 1998–2001 court challenge over access to antiretroviral drugs. Brazil and Thailand were more successful in invoking Article 31. This notwithstanding, resolution acknowledged no right for action in the HIV/AIDS arena on the part of national governments, but carved out such a role for non-state actors. As such, it revealed the evolving circumvention of domestic sovereignty, and the GAP.

The third such UN resolution, General Assembly Resolution 65/277, "Political Declaration on HIV and AIDS: Intensifying our Efforts to Eliminate HIV and AIDS," of 10 June 2011 did little to undo such circumvention. It did, however, highlight the centrality of the state in the ongoing response to the epidemic. Paragraph 2 sights the sovereign rights of the state in the response, and paragraph 33 places the onus on that response with the state. While paragraph 15 encourages international cooperation, and paragraphs 54 and 55 likewise alert states to their ability to invoke flexibilities in accessing medications, South Africa's experience (outlined in detail in chapters 5 and 6) and a litany of contemporary examples beyond illustrate the inherent difficulties in venturing into a challenge to the existing economic and particularly intellectual property regimes. However, paragraphs 71 and 72 do offer some direction for such a challenge, although their recommendations to states and

---

15   UNGA 2006 Resolution 60/262, "Political Declaration on HIV/AIDS, paragraph 28.

16   Ibid., paragraph 25.

17   Ibid., paragraph 42.

18   Ibid., paragraph 43.

19   Ibid.

international organizations are for voluntary participation:[20] still, the very presence of those paragraphs can be attributed to the myriad changes afoot in the allocation and assumption of responsibility and accountability for HIV response especially shortly before, during and after the 2008 global financial crisis. This trajectory, as described below in terms of the international and domestic repercussions on South Africa's HIV response, crystallizes the view of the GAP.

4.2.1 The United States' Commitment

It is useful to take a closer look at the influence of the United States Government, the largest global donor to HIV/AIDS, and its response to the pandemic under former Presidents Clinton and George W. Bush as well as President Obama. While each contributed to the fight against the disease, their responses differ in important ways, especially in how they interact with and impact those of the South African governments.

While Clinton, unlike former US President Reagan and former South African President Mandela, did address the pandemic, he has done much more since leaving office than he did while serving. Former President Bush, whose impetus to respond to HIV/AIDS resulted PEPFAR, the largest anti-AIDS program in the world, received much credit for this initiative. Many of the conditions associated with it, including policy prescriptions and donor dependency, riled South African President Mbeki, arguably contributing to his dragging his heeds on the South African response to the epidemic. Current US President Obama, who came to office pledging further support for HIV/AIDS, is actually phasing out much of PEPFAR's funding in favor of a more holistic approach to health contained in his Global Health Initiative (GHI)[21] with both positive and negative implications for the fight against the pandemic. The consequences of each of these initiatives and phases, particularly vis-à-vis South Africa's concerns for its domestic sovereignty and sovereign statehood are significant.

4.2.1.1 Clinton and HIV/AIDS
Despite a declared commitment to fighting HIV/AIDS, albeit facing a hostile Republican-dominated Congress, during Clinton's first term, US worldwide funding for the epidemic stagnated, never rising above US$141 million per annum.[22] This increased to US$540 million per year during his second term: paltry sums compared to those later committed under President Bush. In the interim,

---

20   UNAIDS 2011. General Assembly Resolution 65/277, "Political Declaration on HIV and AIDS: Intensifying our Efforts to Eliminate HIV and AIDS" (10 June).

21   GHI is, however, imperiled by the stalemate in the US Congress.

22   See Dugger, C.W. 2006. "Clinton makes up for lost time in battling AIDS." *The New York Times* (29 August). For comparison, see also Stolberg, S.G. 2009. "Obama Seeks a Global Health Plan Broader Than Bush's AIDS Effort." *The New York Times* (6 May); "Obama expands health agenda, but not funding." 2009. *PlusNews* (8 May).

Clinton was instrumental in protecting US pharmaceutical companies against South Africa's 1997 bid to access ARVs.[23]

Upon leaving office, however, Clinton seemed to change his tune. The former President established the William J. Clinton Foundation under whose auspices he negotiated "steep cuts in the price of AIDS medicines through deals with drug companies that cover more than 400,000 patients in dozens of countries" as of 2006.[24] South Africa was among the targeted beneficiary countries; the Clinton initiative clearly illustrating the kind of interference that South Africa, notably then President Mbeki, was determined to avoid.

Arguing that his relationship with political leaders, Mbeki foremost among them, enabled him to advocate for HIV/AIDS intervention, Clinton tried to capitalize upon Mbeki's press-lynching for his lack of action against the epidemic. In 2003, ignoring the role he played in thwarting Mbeki's 1997 attempt to address the disease in the TRIPS case, Clinton said to the South African President, "you know, I really want to help you, and as you know, I may be the only one of those involved in this work who's never been publicly critical of you," "but this is something you have to do."[25] In response, Mbeki invited the Clinton Foundation to "help the country write a comprehensive treatment plan."[26] That plan included provisions through which South Africa could

> Avail itself of some [US] $1.5billion in the form of export-import loans, at commercial interest rates, to buy American drugs at market prices. In addition, by May 2001, five of the world's biggest pharmaceutical companies had agreed to enter talks with African nations on reduced prices, provided the countries concerned agreed to health action plans being drawn up by McKinsey, a leading business consultancy![27]

The lop-sided benefits entailed therein—in favor of the US pharmaceutical companies and consultancy and weighed against the South African Government—were blatant. However, South Africa's negotiating ability was deemed negligible, expected as it was to accept the offer. This left South Africa with two choices: to acquiesce to the externally imposed terms of the offer, or to reject it. Either decision would limit South Africa's domestic ability to respond to the epidemic; tarnish its credibility on international markets, and in the HIV/AIDS industry arena; and hamper its attempts to address criticisms of its approach:

---

23   This case, often alluded to, will be explored and analyzed in detail in Chapter 6.

24   Dugger, C.W. 2006. "Clinton makes up for lost time in battling AIDS." *The New York Times* (29 August).

25   Ibid.

26   Ibid.

27   Gumede, W. 2005. *Thabo Mbeki and the Battle for the Soul of the ANC.* Cape Town: Zebra Publishers: 157.

criticisms that would inspire further interventions against HIV/AIDS that circumvent the government. South Africa rejected the Clinton Foundation offer.

4.2.1.2 Bush and HIV/AIDS

In January 2003 US President Bush launched the PEPFAR, which arguably changed everything in the HIV/AIDS arena. With an initial five-year budget for 2003–2008 of US$15 billion dollars, renewed in 2008 for the ensuing five years to the tune of US$48 billion, PEPFAR's resources and its scope of influence far outweighs those of any other organizations and programs. This has both positive and negative consequences.

Though PEPFAR has undoubtedly contributed significantly to the scale-up in treatment access around the world, particularly in sub-Saharan Africa, it has also wrought additional destruction. Given its sheer size, PEPFAR overwhelms—psychologically and practically in terms of absorption and implementation capacity—and overpowers. It also deliberately circumvents and thereby circumscribes state ability to respond to its epidemic as it deems fit. As an American aid official competing for a US Government contract to deliver antiretroviral drugs in Africa pointedly said, "we're going to grab every trained health-care worker we can get our hands on."[28] This mentality, as well as its implementation, contributes not to the support and strengthening of the sovereign state's ability to enact its responsibility to respond, but to its weakening—without an accounting.

Furthermore, the initial PEPFAR legislation, much like the original Clinton Foundation offer to South Africa, required that all of the ARVs purchased with from its funds be for those approved by the US Food and Drug Administration (FDA), regardless of whether these, patented or generic, had already been accepted by the World Health Organization (WHO). Waiting for FDA approval implied that US manufactured drugs are being favored over, for instance, Indian produced generics, and delays access to ARVs, thwarting the HIV/AIDS response.

Additional pertinent criticisms and shortcomings include: shoddy statistics, which count "not only those assisted through site-specific support of treatment centers, but also those supported by PEPFAR through contributions to national, regional or local 'system strengthening' [including such activities as staff training, laboratory support, logistics, and curriculum development]."[29] Other issues include almost arbitrary scaling-up without attendant attention to care and capacity. For instance, in Soweto, the conglomerate of townships to the south west

---

28   PEPFAR, as well as other global foundations such as the Clinton, mentioned above, and the Gates foundations, also routinely "poach" healthcare personnel from the public sector, paying them higher salaries; undermining general healthcare and imperiling the sustainability of the response to HIV/AIDS if and when such external actors and their associated funding depart. See also Epstein, H. 2007. *The Invisible Cure: Africa, The West, and the Fight Against AIDS*. New York: Farrar, Straus and Giroux: 267.

29   See www.pepfar.gov [accessed 1 July 2012].

of Johannesburg, the NGO Hope Worldwide (Hope) received an US$8 million PEPFAR grant in 2004 to provide care for 165,000 orphans. Since it lacked access to that many orphans,[30] Hope offered Sizanani, a local organization providing meals and care to over 300 children in Soweto a Memorandum of Understanding (MOU). Sizanani had, at the time, been up and running for three years, supported solely by the founder's salary and some meager donations: but it was tactical, and as a result, not designed to be sustainable over the long-term.[31] In the MOU, Hope proposed to provide a review of Sizanani's HIV/AIDS-related needs and responses, to develop and strengthen a local working group on HIV/AIDS, and to develop HIV/OVC [Orphans and Vulnerable Children] strategies, by developing community competency. The MOU would have allowed Hope to count the orphans in Sizinani's care among its statistics to meet the quotas required for the PEPFAR grant. Sizanani declined to sign the MOU.

Around the same time, at least seven of Hope's own counselors quit because "the pressure from PEPFAR to produce numbers made their work all but impossible."[32] In a statement foreshadowing Ambassador Rasool's quoted in the introduction,

> You cannot give quality counseling anymore because PEPFAR has counseling quotas. If you have to do one thousand people by the end of the month [and PEPFAR requires a monthly report to Congress on the number of people it has helped every month], you end up not doing good counseling. It compromises people's dignity. ... All the time we were thinking 'I have to fill this form because PEPFAR is coming![33]

In addition to the statistical pressure and the associated compromised care and capacity, the original PEPFAR legislation also earmarked one-third of the money for abstinence programs, and prohibited any funds from going to organizations that promoted or distributed condoms or contraceptives or offered abortions.[34] It also contained a provision to enable students educated in the United States to relieve their medical school debts by working for a year in AIDS-affected regions in sub-Saharan Africa, without, however, a complementary requirement for training locals: in essence exacerbating the capacity shortage and GAP on the ground.

---

30   A term which is problematic in Africa and in the HIV/AIDS arena: first of all, most orphans have family and many are cared for in still-existing albeit strained family situations; secondly, orphan is generally used when either one parent or both have died—no distinction is consistently made between half- and full-orphans.

31   Epstein, H. 2007. *The Invisible Cure: Africa, The West, and the Fight Against AIDS*. New York: Farrar, Straus and Giroux: 221.

32   Ibid.

33   Ibid.

34   See, for example, Epstein, H. 2007. *The Invisible Cure: Africa, The West, and the Fight Against AIDS*. New York: Farrar, Straus and Giroux.

All of these costs and caveats to South Africa, the epicenter of the HIV/ AIDS pandemic and struggling as a newly sovereign state, are captured in Okey Nwanyanwu's noting that "26 percent of PEPFAR funding never leaves the US, while nearly 80 percent of it benefits the United States"[35] overall (through procurement, technical expertise, strategic support, etc.) as opposed to the recipient countries. In other words, faced with a crisis, in this case the HIV/AIDS epidemic, the recipient South Africa was beholden to financial interests of the US, which were, in turn, accountable to US taxpayers.

The Congressional renewal of the PEPFAR legislation at the end of 2008 amended some of these controversial provisions. The abstinence earmark is gone. The new legislation facilitates the procurement and provision of generic ARVs, and includes provisions to increase coordination of this process in particular with other global organizations such as the Global Fund and the World Health Organization. It has also removed the loan benefit for US students. Yet the mark PEPFAR made under Bush and continues to make is indelible. In this environment characterized by local and global pressure to expand its response to the epidemic and yet beset by fickle funding, South Africa had little choice but to accept PEPFAR and its attendant circumscription of the country's domestic sovereignty by its policy stipulations prepared in Washington, DC and by PEPFAR's field staff consisting of representatives of numerous US international agencies and accountable to US taxpayers, and by the inherent dependency contingent upon its financing—the very dependency that the South African response to HIV/AIDS sought to avoid.

4.2.1.3 Obama and HIV/AIDS

Current US President Obama has taken a different approach to HIV/AIDS than either former Presidents Clinton or Bush. Clinton focused on pharmaceuticals and treatment, arguably attributable to the fact that he was in office at the advent of ARVs. Bush inaugurated PEPFAR, his most significant international humanitarian effort, which included funding for programs geared toward prevention, treatment and care. Obama is widening the focus further, turning his attention to global health more broadly, to maternal and child health as well as to neglected, easily treatable diseases, in particular. These goals are outlined in the GHI[36] as well as in the 2010 National Security Strategy, albeit a bit vaguely.[37]

It appears that the GHI would pare down the funding previously allocated to HIV/AIDS, and would treat it as one health threat among many. Though the pandemic does infect and affect millions of people across the world, primarily in

---

35   Okey Nwanyanwu, former director of the Centers for Disease Control (CDC) for sub-Saharan Africa, quoted in Pretoria, South Africa, 2005; currently CDC country director in Abuja, Nigeria.

36   The success of GHI is, however, in considerable doubt, due to the stalemate between the Republicans and the Democrats in the US Congress, particularly in the Senate.

37   National Security Strategy. 2010. Available at http://www.whitehouse.gov/sites/ default/files/rss_viewer/national_security_strategy.pdf [accessed: 1 July 2012].

sub-Saharan Africa as this analysis makes clear, pneumonia and diarrhea pose an arguably more dire threat to survival for millions more. One consequence of this revised commitment to global health—and security—is the flat-lining of PEPFAR funding at 2009 levels. As a result, HIV-positive people, notably in sub-Sahara, are being turned away from treatment; this detracts from incentives for behavior change and predicates resurgence in incidence accompanied also by the threat of drug-resistant strains of HIV.

The shift contained in GHI thus poignantly illustrates the risks and liabilities of the current treatment-based approach to the HIV/AIDS response, emphasizing its reliance on external funding and associated compromise of the national sovereign ability to guarantee the responsibility to respond.

While the bilateral US contributions to the fight against HIV/AIDS are comparatively enormous and have received the most international attention, three multi-lateral efforts are worth mentioning. These are the Global Fund to Fight AIDS, Tuberculosis and Malaria, UNAIDS, and the World Bank's MAP. They are complemented by a plethora of other public and private foundations, organizations, forums, and coordinating committees, each of which, as for instance the Clinton Foundation and PEPFAR, has its own rules and regulations, policies, and stipulations for addressing and responding to the epidemic. In the heavily populated HIV/AIDS arena, this maelstrom of approaches to addressing the epidemic creates a perfect storm in which South Africa also seeks to navigate its own road of responsibility and accountability.

4.2.2 The Global Fund

The Global Fund, launched in 2001 by then United Nations Secretary-General Kofi Annan, is not so much an organization as a mechanism. It operates as a funding vehicle to attract, collect and distribute international donations on the part of national governments in the fight against AIDS, tuberculosis and malaria. It manages its funding rounds through local Country Coordinating Mechanisms (CCM) that intended consist of local activists as well as governmental representatives, and which to prepare applications for Global Fund financing. In practice, the CCM is often staffed by Global Fund technocrats who draft the country plan. As such, it is subject to not necessarily national priorities as intended, but to the preferences of local-global alliances, and especially its state and non-state donors.

The Global Fund conducts periodic funding application rounds which proceed according to strict, prescribed protocols. These do not necessarily occur in equal intervals, as they are contingent upon the flow of donations, which sometimes results in overlap, lack of spending, or gaps in project support. For instance, in 2001, the Global Fund only spent 17 percent of what it received. As of August 2008 the Global Fund had committed US$11.3 billion in 136 countries to support aggressive interventions against all three diseases. How much of this committed money has actually been dispersed, however, is uncertain—but is certainly less than has been promised.[38]

The dependency of the Global Fund on its donors in turn magnifies the dependencies of recipient countries, including South Africa on these same funding sources. As alluded to previously and will be noted in the following chapter, under dubious and controversial conditions, former South African Minister of Health Manto Tshabalala-Msimang held up a Global Fund grant to hard-hit KwaZulu-Natal. Over and above the political machinations, the episode highlights South Africa's concern over its dependence upon external policies and funding. This concern has proven justified in the aftermath of the 2010–2011 embezzlement crises which led to the cancellation of Round 11 grants, leaving dependent countries dry. It also emphasizes the GAP: nothing held the Global Fund to account in each affected state in such a way as to ensure the response to HIV/AIDS it had been delivering.

4.2.3 UNAIDS

UNAIDS is the oldest of the international multi-lateral organizations dedicated to fighting HIV/AIDS. It is worth noting that its founding in 1996 coincided with the advent of ARVs on the international market. It is also the only UN agency dedicated to one particular, albeit multi-faceted, problem, save that of the more recently founded UN Women. Though UNAIDS has its own Secretariat, it comprises cosponsors which include the UN High Commissioner for Refugees (UNHCR), the UN International Children's Emergency Fund (UNICEF), the World Food Program (WFP), the UN Development Program (UNDP), the UN Population Fund (UNFPA), the UN Office on Drugs and Crime (UNODC), the International Labor Organization (ILO), UN Educational, Scientific, and Cultural Organization (UNESCO), the World Health Organization (WHO), and the World Bank. As a consequence, rather similarly to the Global Fund, UNAIDS is dependent upon its internal donors, as well as external donors to the UN at large, for its financing. This amalgam of co-sponsors participates in UNAIDS Program Coordinating Boards and Theme Groups at the local country level, influencing policy with the impetus on the global agenda, as opposed to that of the state. Likewise, implementation is fragmented, making it even harder for the state to exercise oversight with responsibility and accountability.

Despite the precariousness of such international funding flows, the Global Fund and UNAIDS have stepped up and expanded their efforts since their respective inceptions. These efforts are not insured against shifting donor funding application

---

38   See Bernstein, M. and Sessions, M. 2007. "A Trickle or a Flood: Commitments and Disbursements for HIV/AIDS from the Global Fund, PEPFAR, and the World Bank's Multi-Country AIDS Program (MAP)." Washington, DC: Center for Global Development HIV/AIDS Monitor (5 March) for further details outlining differences between allocations of donor funds and actual receipt.

and dispersing schedules or amounts, procedural delays, donor fatigue, or actual progress against the epidemic. These are also not devoid of duplication or even counter-productive interventions promoted by the different donors with divergent initiatives such as PEPFAR or the Gates Foundation. Finally, these efforts and those implementing them are not accountable to the recipients of their committed and dispersed funding largess, and only, if at all, to the sources of their funding.

The result can be a bewildering array of attempts to allay the HIV/AIDS crisis, accompanied by behemoth bureaucracies with questionable practical applicability. For example, in July 2007, the already considerable UN presence in South Africa established a Joint UN Team on AIDS. Though by that time the South African Government had announced the launch of its second public-sector antiretroviral roll-out as part of a comprehensive anti-AIDS strategy, this UN initiative appeared to take the reins on both local and global AIDS response. This occurred despite the fact that the UN's own HIV/AIDS strategy, substantially unaltered since 1996, has failed to produce measurable inroads against the epidemic and its unabated spread.

As the new Joint UN Team on AIDS prepares to assume its role, a number of developments leading up to that transition highlight the impact of global influence in South Africa's national and local HIV/AIDS sphere. Indeed, the erstwhile UN Theme Group, now Joint UN Team on AIDS participate in the government-led Donor Coordination Forum on HIV/AIDS, whose continuation, under the auspices of UNAIDS, would seem to render both the Theme Group and the Joint UN Team redundant.

First, the previously-existing UN Theme Group on HIV/AIDS supported the South African National AIDS Council in developing a US$103 million proposal for the Global Fund Round 6 in 2006. It remains unclear to what extent the South African Government and civil society were involved in the conception of the proposal, when the process was conceived, coordinated, and approved. It also begs the question of who will control and be held accountable for the proposal's implementation.

Second, using Program Acceleration Funds for 2003, UNAIDS oversaw a review of South Africa's 2000–2005 National Strategic Plan prior to the successful Global Fund proposal as well as to the launch of South Africa's second national antiretroviral roll-out. The funds paid for a national consultation process with civil society partners, and, in order to document the outcomes and recommendations of that consultation, also for a full-time consultant to the Department of Health. This arrangement guaranteed UNAIDS a central role not only in conducting the consultative review, but also in conceptualizing South Africa's latest strategic plan. In so doing, it could ensure that the new plan would be in accordance with the norms and standards set out by UNAIDS and the Global Fund, even if these were not necessarily the most optimal and conducive to responding to the epidemic in South Africa.

Third and similarly, UNAIDS allotted Program Acceleration Funds for 2005 to support Statistics South Africa and the Department of Health to generate high-quality HIV data. This resulted in a convergence of data and reflected in UNAIDS global AIDS epidemic update of 2006. It was billed as a "major success." However, as highlighted in previous chapters, UNAIDS had to revise its own statistics related to the global pandemic downward by 16 percent in 2007. Though mostly attributable to better estimates available in India, most recently the Demographic Information Bureau at the Development Bank of Southern Africa released more reliable data on HIV/AIDS in South Africa as well; data that diverge from those of UNAIDS.

Fourth and finally, Program Acceleration Funds for 2006–2007 and broader UNAIDS support flowed into two sets of HIV prevention programs. The first of these involved programs to promote safer and healthier sexual behavior through life-skills education. The second targeted best practice initiatives for HIV workplace programs. As noted above, both of these initiatives are part of HIV prevention and response policies that have been in place for the better part of a generation and have yet to show substantiated results.[39] Regarding the first, life-skills are unlikely to succeed without supplementary initiatives which create an incentive for their exercise, including food security, education and vocational-training and the realistic prospect of employment. The latter, first trumpeted by Professor Sher and colleagues in 1986, and implemented in various degrees by individual companies such as AngloGroup and then Daimler(Chrysler), have yet to be broadly applied.[40]

These are worth noting because the recommendations and requirements of the HIV/AIDS response as conceived primarily by external state and non-state actors remain the guiding principles of the fight against the epidemic. Their influence and agenda is also reflected in international political prioritization of HIV/AIDS. As such, they preview the context in which the South Africa Government continues to form its response to HIV/AIDS and to enact its domestic sovereignty including its responsibility to respond. In particular, the current shifts are characterized by prominent actors and agenda-setters such as the US presidents and the UN Security

---

39   Helen Epstein posits that the United Nations' HIV/AIDS programs prevail not necessarily because they are practical or work, but because the UN philosophy does not suffer alternatives. Citing Uganda, as will be shown in more depth and detail in Chapter Seven, she points out that "Africans had fought this epidemic on their own through frankness and common sense, compassion for the afflicted, and shifts in sexual norms and attitudes surrounding sexual relationships and the rights of women," and adds that such simple components of success "were the last thing(s) UN bureaucrats would have wanted to hear. It meant that fighting AIDS would require an approach with which they were quite unfamiliar, and for this their existing expertise might not be paramount." "The UN's expertise lay in formulating short-, medium-, and long-term plans; setting up national AIDS committees in African countries; and developing surveillance networks, laboratories, and other health-related technologies," precisely what it brought to South Africa anew in 2007, regardless of previous progress, or of the government's own initiatives, or more importantly, of concrete indicators of success.

40   Such initiatives will be discussed in more detail under the recommendations offered in Chapter 8.

Council, as well as market investors and non-governmental organizations, and local-global networks of special interest groups, all of which wield influence, especially regarding the response to HIV/AIDS. Working in tandem, these bypass the domestic sovereignty of national governments, as seen in HIV/AIDS agenda-setting and interventions.

Caught in between, adapting to the shifts but attempting to assert its independence, South Africa is arguably wedged between domestic priorities and international dictates. Its domestic sovereignty and associated *effective* responsibility and accountability curtailed as a result, the government, and thus the state nonetheless remains ultimately and legally responsible and accountable for the protection and the welfare of its citizens—including those infected and affected by the HIV/AIDS epidemic.

4.3 The National Scene

Having assumed sovereign rights and corresponding responsibilities at its democratic transition in 1994, successive democratic governments worked to act upon these. Policy reflected these priorities, paying special heed to economic fundamentals, and working to enact and maintain especially macroeconomic stability. In particular, Mbeki was intent on avoiding being beholden to external actors. Already in July 1989, writing for ANC leader Oliver Tambo, Mbeki stated that "unless Africa comes in with a solution, with a plan, it might be marginalized, and forced in the end to participate in plans—no doubt in good faith—by others."[41]

> Mbeki was determined to prove to the mandarins of global capitalism that Africans could play them at their own game, and compete within a modern, global economy, without becoming indebted to them. Weaned on Marxist theory and raised by a movement that believed it could shape the destiny of its people, he was never entirely comfortable with the underpinnings of GEAR, as is evidenced by the way he did not promote structural reform, such as privatization, as vigorously as he might have. But—the son of struggling black traders—he was determined to survive independently of white creditors or paymasters. He would do anything to avoid hocking the shop.[42]

At the same time, Mbeki realized that "the democratic state would be faced with an immediate problem [of] how to manage [South Africa's] wealth" and that if the "ANC did not have [or acquire] the resources to run a modern economy," "the consequence would be "counter-revolution."[43] Consequently, Mbeki foresaw that

---

41   Gevisser, M. 2007. *Thabo Mbeki: The Dream Deferred.* Jeppestown: Jonathan Ball Publishers (Pty) Ltd: 547.

42   Ibid., 694.

43   Ibid., 540.

"it's not about what will happen on day one of liberation, [...] it's about what we should do now, to guarantee that when we have won power we don't lose the revolution because we are not prepared to govern":[44] and governing entails promoting "an array of concerns and serving multiple constituencies. To do any good in office, you have to be in office."[45] Hence Mbeki's political calculation: as part of arguably the mantra of the post-revolution, explicitly on display in the balancing act between HIV/AIDS response with competing post-revolution power plays (e.g. in RDP/GEAR and BEE/BBBEE, for example).

4.3.1 Market Constraints: National Ramifications and Response

Before and then during the transition to democracy, South Africa faced constraints by international capital it attempted to attract and strictures it aimed to overcome. The apartheid era government drove the South African state into debt by waging wars in South-West Africa (now Namibia) and Angola externally and by imposing draconian security measures internally, which led to international outcries.[46] The latter resulted in international reactions, which took two forms: proposals for "constructive engagement" and boycotts; with diametrically opposed consequences for South Africa's economy.

Constructive engagement, championed by Chet Crocker, advocated the gradual end of apartheid by propelling the economic integration of the black majority. Proponents argued that such integration would erode South Africa's repressive political system while shoring up the country's economic survival. Yet this argument lost out to the firebrand approach of Randall Robinson of TransAfrica, who appealed for an economic boycott against apartheid-ruled South Africa.

> The Reagan Administration could not hold the line [of a gradual shift in the situation in South Africa as advocated by Crocker] in the face of a bipartisan assault in Congress and sanctions became the order of the day. [They] had a direct and immediate impact, and certainly led to the freeing of Mandela by De Klerk and the subsequent collapse of apartheid.[47]

While popular, the boycott crippled the economy and possibly hastened the end of the apartheid regime—while undermining the sustainability of the country's economic base, especially as international companies and capital fled the pariah state.

In order to lure the lost capital back into the country and to establish its solvency in international capital markets, the governments of Presidents Mandela

---

44   Ibid., 539.

45   Bruni, F. 2012. "Why Obama Isn't Saying 'I Do' to Same-Sex Marriage," *The New York Times* (8 May).

46   Personal correspondence with Ambassador Barkley, 11 February 2008.

47   Ibid.

and Mbeki proceeded to pursue programs of strict fiscal discipline. This economic stance was also influenced by the presidents and their democratic governments: (a) desire to be less dependent upon national capital, as this could obviously leave;[48] (b) perceived need to ensure against dependence upon international financial institutions;[49] and (c) the political and economic compromise between the old and new regime that prioritized the interests of existing and potential creditors.[50] However, while the governments' intentions and associated priorities—of economic independence—were clear and justifiable, the accompanying fiscal measures had the adverse effect of "hampering a new government's ability to address its most pressing needs,"[51] notably those of the burgeoning HIV/AIDS epidemic.

Addressing those "most pressing needs," those listed by Mandela quoted above and associated with the "freedom from want, freedom from hunger, freedom from deprivation" would have required radical reconstruction and development of the South African economy, to reverse hundreds of years of oppression culminating in the institutionalized oppression of the apartheid state especially from 1948 until 1994. While the Mandela government briefly flirted with the Reconstruction and Development Program (RDP) which proposed such a restructuring, it eventually traded this approach for the more market-friendly GEAR strategy. Nonetheless,

> The investment promised by businessmen and foreign countries if the ANC eschewed nationalization did not materialize. Industrialists demanded yet more concessions, claiming they were still not convinced of the government's commitment to a market-friendly economy. They wanted more assurances, a signal or a guarantee that the SACP and COSATU could not still force nationalization on the country. A new economic strategy focused entirely on growth would be a good starting point, the moguls suggested.[52]

---

48   The independence of the South African Reserve Bank, and its strict capital controls, however, makes this much more difficult in the democratic era—but conversely, also works against attracting foreign business and capital into the country.

49   Here, the primacy of independence and of the country's control of its domestic sovereignty comes to the fore—though South Africa repaid its international debt and accepted and IMF loan, and currently in the context of its HIV/AIDS response receives PEPFAR money, the emphasis is against such dependency.

50   This compromise resulted in the repayment of debt, with an unstated declaration not to end up in the same position of dependency again. Personal correspondence with Ambassador Barkley, 11 February 2008.

51   Personal correspondence with Ambassador Barkley, 11 February 2008.

52   Gumede, W. 2005. *Thabo Mbeki and the Battle for the Soul of the ANC.* Cape Town: Zebra Publishers: 85.

GEAR was adopted against the background of the precipitous decline of the South African exchange rate in 1996.[53] At the time Mandela acknowledged that "we are aware that the investor will not invest unless the security of that investment is assured. The rates of economic growth we seek cannot be achieved without important inflows of foreign capital. We are determined to create the necessary climate that the foreign investor will find attractive."[54] As such, GEAR further "stressed the need for market-led growth, fiscal and monetary discipline, and investor confidence."[55] Its prescriptions focused on the stability of the macroeconomic situation, in order to deal with "the realities of an unmanageable budget deficit, high interest rates and weak local and foreign investor confidence" through "greater industrial competitiveness, a tighter fiscal stance, moderation in wage increases, accelerated public investment, efficient service delivery and a major expansion of private investment" in addition to "an exchange rate policy consistent with improved international competitiveness."[56] Mandela even went so far as to justify the new economic gear as a means "to ensure stability and secure the support of groups that had the potential to destabilize the country," and then deputy president Mbeki endorsed GEAR out of the opinion "that the markets still doubted that the ANC was really committed to economic prudence."[57] Mbeki explicitly said that GEAR was to "tune its policies to international markets and investors" in order to try to secure support, financial and otherwise, for that transition. Furthermore, he acquiesced that "South Africa had no choice but to play by the rules of the global economy,"[58] in the hope that investor confidence would attract sustaining capital for the growth of the South African economy and to the benefit of the country's socio-economic and political stability. In short, GEAR was meant to counteract skepticism and garner confidence in the fledgling democracy and transitional state—and to shore up confidence in and the ability to deliver upon the "moral-political obligation and the constitutional imperatives"

---

53   1996 marks dual, conflicting, focuses: On the one hand, South Africa implemented GEAR, loosening its exchange controls and tightening its fiscal policy, weakening its control over its domestic policies, and on the other hand, the advent of ARVs increased the demand for such domestic control to protect South Africa's citizens and to enact the state's sovereign responsibilities. See also Biersteker, T.J. 1992. "The 'Triumph' of Neoclassical Economics in the Developing World: Policy Convergence and Bases of Governance in the International Economic Order." In *Governance without Government: Order and Change in World Politics* (ed.) Rosenau, J. and Czempiel, E.-O. Cambridge: Cambridge University Press: 108.

54   Gumede, W. 2005. *Thabo Mbeki and the Battle for the Soul of the ANC.* Cape Town: Zebra Publishers: 70.

55   Terreblanche, S. 2002. *A History of Inequality in South Africa 1652–2002.* Pietermaritzburg: University of Natal Press: 115.

56   Gumede, W. 2005. *Thabo Mbeki and the Battle for the Soul of the ANC.* Cape Town: Zebra Publishers: 88.

57   Ibid., 62.

58   Ibid., 91.

of the legacy of the liberation struggle and of Nelson Mandela's initial vision for the country.[59]

Yet in effect, GEAR resulted in the jettisoning of

> The Freedom Charter [which inspired Mandela's speech]—the social program of the ANC from the 1950s [on which the RDP was largely based]—was effectively scrapped, as a condition of the ANC entering government.[60] The agreement of the new government to relocation out of the country of its central industrial/financial nucleus, the Anglo-American/DeBeers complex,[61] was massive proof of the relative weakness of the government. It has not been able to deliver on its social program, in any substantial way.[62]

However, as of 2010, GEAR has produced neither the promised growth nor redistribution. Does the status of South Africa then confirm the perception that it is impossible, "in practice, for African states or governments to be tolerant both of the demands of global capital and to the exigencies of their own nationals?"[63]

That question and the answers to it will be further explored in the following chapters. In light of this perverse consequence, despite the governments best efforts to the contrary, "the best way of interpreting Mbeki's 'African Renaissance' is as a nationalist alternative to the loss of his previous ideology,"[64] of the available independence of South Africa from such imposed international constraints—accepted both voluntarily and with persuasion, which served to circumscribed the country's domestic sovereignty and to undercut its ability to respond with responsibility and accountability to the challenges confronting it.

Nonetheless, despite serious set-backs—a second exchange rate crisis in 2002, which devalued South African exports without causing them to increase in magnitude, and the end of the Multi-Fiber Agreement in 2005, which saw the loss of many jobs in the textile sector—South Africa has seen growth averaging 6 percent in the formal economy since 2004 (though it has since slowed in the wake of the 2008 global financial crisis). It has also had some success in attracting FDI. In 2006, the country even ran a budget surplus of 0.6 percent, and in 2007,

---

59   Booysen, S. 2001. "Transitions and trends in policymaking in democratic South Africa." *Journal of Public Administration*, 36(2): 125–144.

60   See the aforementioned compromise.

61   See the above notes on the fleeing of international companies and capital, and their lack of return, also due to the stringent capital requirements imposed by the South African Reserve Bank.

62   Trewhela, P., Sampson, A. and Gordimer, N. 2006. "Looking Back Six Years—to Mbeki." *New York Review of Books* (10 August).

63   Nyamnjoh, F.B. 2002. "Globalizations, Boundaries, and Livelihoods: Perspectives on Africa." *Philosophia Africana*, 6(2): 6.

64   Trewhela, P., Sampson, A. and Gordimer, N. 2006. "Looking Back Six Years—to Mbeki." *New York Review of Books* (10 August).

the IMF praised then President Mbeki and Finance Minister Trevor Manuel for their handling of South Africa's macro-economy.

Then in early 2008, growth began to slow, inflation to climb above 10 percent, and official unemployment to stagnate at 26 percent; unofficial figures pin it at above 40 percent. President Zuma's 2010/11 budget allocations are growing, much of the additions aimed at HIV/AIDS. Yet some of the allocated funding externally based, throwing doubt on South Africa's economic principles and independence. Its pending dependency illustrates how South Africa continues to struggle to achieve its goals of growth, employment, and redistribution, and finds itself stuck between the "often intractable rules of the global economy" and "populist and redistributive rules."[65] Its local-global conflict is not unique and is indeed reflected in other policy problems. The ramifications for the response to HIV/AIDS loom large.

In the meantime, South Africa's democratic governments largely let HIV/AIDS fade into the background preferring to focus on supposedly "bigger," "longer-term" priorities such as integrating the informal and formal economies, and generating GDP growth as a means of tackling inequality. The actions of local-global alliances that filled a void in HIV/AIDS response emerged in the ensuing policy vacuum, waging the counter-revolution Mbeki sought to avoid. In doing so, they went one step farther than implied by the boomerang pattern, not only advocating, but enacting policy. As a result, they arguably decreased the salience of the state,[66] even as their very presence rendered the state—as the residual bastion of the responsibility and accountability to respond—indispensable.

4.3.2 Domestic Constraints: Rights' Demands and Responsibility Dues

As indicated above, the new government of South Africa assumed office in 1994 under the rubric of a revised Constitution. Significantly, that new Constitution enshrined both the individual rights of all of the country's citizens and the associated responsibilities accorded and assumed by the state. Though inaugural efforts to address the HIV/AIDS epidemic pre-date this transition, the new Constitution recreated the domestic political context in which further interventions would and could take place.

Though clearly imparted on paper, rendering the rights and enacting the responsibilities entailed in the South African Constitution proved more complicated. Rights and realities clashed, as did priorities in policy and feasibility under the conditions of national and international forums. While the Constitution's

---

65   Booysen, S. 2001. "Transitions and trends in policymaking in democratic South Africa." *Journal of Public Administration*, 36(2): 125–144.

66   Brühl, T. and Rittberger, V. 2001. "From International to Global Governance: Actors, Collective Decision-making, and the United Nations in the Twenty-First Century." In *Global Governance and the United Nations System* (ed.) Rittberger, V. Tokyo: United Nations University Press: 2.

Bill of Rights[67] guaranteed each and every of the rights in it—education, health, housing, and water, among others—simultaneously and immediately, securing them in reality has been an arduous and seemingly interminable process. For all those that have gained houses and piped-water, for example, the waiting lists of those still without grow. The same is true for the availability of and access to healthcare concerning HIV/AIDS.

The most important rights enshrined in South Africa's Bill of Rights as they pertain to this analysis of the relationship South Africa's response to its HIV/AIDS epidemic and its exercise of sovereign statehood are the *freedom and security of the person*, the rights to *healthcare, food, water and social security*, and the right to welfare, particularly economic welfare.

In South Africa's Bill of Rights the right to the *freedom and security of the person* includes the rights to bodily and psychological integrity.[68] These are paramount rights which constitute the highest order of prioritization in domestic sovereignty, and as such are inextricably linked to the notion of the sovereign state's responsibility to respond. In the case of HIV/AIDS, where the survival of infected persons is contingent upon access to ARVs, which is in turn predicated on state (financial) dependence upon external funding sources, which are not ultimately responsible or accountable to the rights being addressed, domestic sovereignty is by definition compromised and circumscribed. In an example of the power inequality at play, in a case that will be explored in detail in chapter six, when the South African Government attempted to invoke provisions of the TRIPS legislation of the World Trade Organization to secure ARVs, US Vice President Al Gore threatened sanctions against the country,[69] openly invoking the limited statehood inherent in the relationship between domestic sovereignty and global rule-making, without concomitant responsibility and accountability. Indeed, instead of assuming a responsibility to respond where the national government had its hands tied (by TRIPS), the international community in effect contributed to the erosion of such effective protection on the part of the state.

The responsibility to ensure the rights to *health care, food, water and social security*[70] fall under the remit of sovereign statehood. The state is held to account for their realization. As recounted above, the governments of the democratic South African dispensation have made significant process on these counts, notably access to water. Yet amidst the slow pace of provision, especially of housing, as well as

---

67   This Bill of Rights is a cornerstone of democracy in South Africa. It enshrines the rights of all people in our country and affirms the democratic values of human dignity, equality and freedom. See South African Constitutional Assembly 1996. "Constitution of the Republic of South Africa," Act 108 of 1996 (8 May): 7(1).

68   South African Constitutional Assembly 1996. "Constitution of the Republic of South Africa," 12(2).

69   More on this in the analysis in Chapter 6.

70   South African Constitutional Assembly 1996. "Constitution of the Republic of South Africa," 27(1).

persistently high unemployment (explored in more detail below), impatience and dissatisfaction are mounting. For example, in June 2007, South Africa's public service, mostly teachers, hospital workers, and some government functionaries such as court orderlies and stenographers, staged a nation-wide strike that spanned more than two weeks. Demand for a 12 percent, then 10 percent wage increase went unmatched by government offers of six percent and then 6.5 percent.[71] When compromise appeared elusive, the government responded by firing thousands of striking nurses "arguing that they violated a constitutional ban on strikes by essential workers" and "deployed army medical workers in public hospitals."[72] Then in September 2007, municipal strikes over the lack or mismanagement of services took place in 53 percent of municipalities.[73] Neither of these actions served to inspire public confidence, or to shore up capacity.

The same skepticism and even consternation has met South African Government responses to unemployment, which, like the HIV/AIDS epidemic, constitutes a multidimensional and increasingly inter-generational crisis. Employment is an issue of welfare, which also falls under the rubric of domestic sovereignty by virtue of the stipulation that state has the duty to enable and protect the welfare of its citizens. Yet unemployment in South Africa is between 25 and 40 percent of the population. The government has banked on stimulating the economy as a panacea. Yet its commitment to macroeconomic stability brought to bear with fiscal discipline, renders rectifying this situation arduous. For instance, as of 2008, government expenditure was slated to reach 27.5 percent of GDP in 2007/08, with revenue at 28.1 percent, which is on par with high-income countries' revenue average of 28.4 percent of GDP.[74] Yet this has not resulted in increased job creation or employment. In addition, the South African rand loss two percent of its value from January to the 20 February 2008 released of the budget. Interest rates were set at 11 percent to curb inflation with an aim towards encouraging investment. Despite this, US$3.8 billion departed the country in the same time period.[75] This same economic malaise also affected the government's response to HIV/AIDS.

In the case of HIV/AIDS, despite repeated roll-outs of ARVs, these have proven neither a magic bullet against the epidemic, nor promoted a sense—or reality—of security vis-à-vis a sustainable government commitment amidst an assumption of responsibility. In other words, though in rolling out ARVs, the government assumes responsibility to continue to provide these—as a matter of life-and-death for recipient patients and as an effectual right to health as guaranteed by

---

71   Wines, M. "South Africa Strike Foreshadows Political Contest." *The New York Times* (13 June).

72   Ibid.

73   Personal correspondence with Fanyana Shiburi, 7 September 2007.

74   Laubscher, J. 2008. "Polokwane, ANC and the Budget." *Fin24* (12 February).

75   Jacobson, C. 2008. "SA Energy Crisis Sends Rand Tumbling." *The Mail and Guardian* (20 February).

the South African Constitution—the associated economic strictures renders this guarantee precarious.

Though "anti-AIDS measures are in all the business plans of all government departments,"

> For the moment HIV and AIDS has all but disappeared from public attention. Newspapers like the Sunday Times run an on-going 'We all know someone' page, encouraging people to go for tests and relating individual stories. The only two other recent stories concern a dancer who was sent back from Alaska when his HIV-positive status became known and the high school article. Nothing active from government.[76]

As such, as of 2010, notwithstanding a new expansion of the government's HIV/AIDS campaign, including a broader ARV program, the sustainability of South Africa's HIV/AIDS response overall is in question: dependent as it is on global funding shortfalls and impending trade-related intellectual property challenges and dearth of new ARVs under development. This situation, in its broader incarnation not unique to South Africa, portends crises in domestic sovereignty as rights. This is particularly the case with those rights being met by responsibility tasks taken on by an assortment of unregulated state and non-state actors, which bear no ultimate accountability. That remains within the realm of sovereign statehood, however limited.

Thus, as the South African Government struggles to assume and enact its responsibilities, in both theory and practice, for the rights guaranteed its citizens through the Constitution's Bill of Rights, it faces numerous challenges. It is constrained by competing internal priorities and conflicts of interest as well as by feasibility. It is further constricted by its image focus and strained confidence, and by the rules imposed upon it by external actors. The influence of and interactions with the latter in turn alternatively spur its domestic capacity but in the final reckoning impinge upon South Africa's sovereign statehood. This begs the questions: What is South Africa able to do? What does it try to do, particularly in the HIV/AIDS arena? What roles does the governmental leadership take on, and how does this play out, with particular reference to HIV/AIDS?

4.4 Leadership: Responsibility and Accountability

Leadership is crucial for an effective response to HIV/AIDS.[77] Indeed, leadership is important for governance as such, especially in a transitional situation as is

---

76   Personal correspondence with Ambassador Thomas Wheeler, 22 January 2008.

77   See Fourie, P. (forthcoming) "AIDS Policy-making in Contemporary South Africa." In Zondi, S. and Le Pere, G. (eds) *Strategic Responses to HIV/AIDS in Southern Africa.* Johannesburg: IGD; Nattrass, N. 2004. *The Moral Economy of HIV/*

still the case in South Africa. Political leaders should embody the assumption of responsibility and accountability associated with their legitimacy: "If South Africans cease believing in the dream that was promised with freedom, and see it as a dream forever deferred, civil disobedience will grow and become the only form of political expression."[78] Though this understated threat of counter-revolution is not always necessary, it is present in South Africa, as shown above, and should be a spur for action against HIV/AIDS.

A trained economist renowned for his intellectual prowess, the former President Mbeki "understood that in the era of "intensifying global interwovenness," leadership is guided by "continental and global strategic visions" and its exercise depends "on ever deeper integration into the world economy."[79] In the case of South Africa, a middle-income country and a regional hegemon, its leadership tends to assume it possesses the power to negotiate its place in the international political-economic arena and it has the ability to dictate its own development. However, being in essence subordinated to those very same global demands, matched locally, and merged into local-global alliances, divests that same leadership and of some of its tactical ability to implement its responsibilities to respond. Indeed, "the lines were drawn for ten years of conflict that would focus international attention on South Africa and obloquy on President Mbeki, a conflict between, on the one side, people with AIDS and their idealistic sympathizers, and, on the other, politicians determined to rectify centuries of racial injustice."[80] Consequently, South Africa finds itself wedged between local and global pressures in its governance, particularly with regard to the high-octane issue of HIV/AIDS. Regardless of the immediate outcome, the state also remains ultimately responsible and accountable for whatever response is forthcoming.

Political contexts, politics, and political leaders themselves, across the board, those in the HIV/AIDS arena are not exempt to these pressures. Seeing the agenda, determining what is even possible to conceive of as a policy issue,[81] these leaders make decisions; they proffer and appropriate funding; they oversee (or stymie)

AIDS. Cambridge: Cambridge University Press; Nattrass, N. 2007. "Now in fiction: the president on AIDS." *The Mail and Guardian* (23 July).

78 Taljaard, R. 2007. "If Those in Power Do Not Listen Nor Care, They Are Failing the Constitution." *Cape Argus* (2 August).

79 Patrick Bond, quoted in Alexander, N. 2002. *An Ordinary Country: Issues in the Transition from Apartheid to Democracy in South Africa.* Piertermaritzburg: University of Natal Press: 141.

80 Iliffe, J. 2006. *A History: The African AIDS Epidemic.* Athens, Ohio: Ohio University Press: 73.

81 Calland, R. 2006. *Anatomy of South Africa: Who Holds the Power?* Cape Town: Zebra Press. See also Herbst, J. 2000. *States and Power in Africa.* Princeton, New Jersey: Princeton University Press: 31. "There is nothing exotic about African politics. Rather, as elsewhere, political outcomes are the result of human agency [actor-oriented analysis offered by Krasner, too: particular actors in particular context] interacting with powerful geographic and historical forces. And, as is the case in other parts of the world, the viability

implementation; they evaluate feedback, and decide how to proceed, or not. This last point is particularly important in election-driven political systems, as it impacts the continuation or termination of a previous policy. This is especially relevant (again) in the current funding climate which threatens the sustainability of South Africa's ARV roll-out. The HIV/AIDS policy arena in and around South Africa is crowded, both locally and globally; so it is worth mentioning a few key players to make sense of the scene and to be able to delve into further analysis of the state's response to the epidemic.

4.4.1 Leadership and HIV/AIDS

Taking into account the role of South Africa's leaders' self-perception and that of its stance toward HIV/AIDS, as well as the impact thereof on the ensuing response to the epidemic, the following leaders emerge as the most relevant to this analysis: former Presidents Mandela and Mbeki, who have been mentioned, as well as current President Zuma; the late former Minister of Health Manto Tshabalala-Msimang; former Minister of Health Nozizwe Madlala-Routledge, and her successor as Minister of Health Aaron Motsoaledi; as well as the Treatment Action Campaign (TAC) and MSF; and various business leaders.

At this stage two things are important to note: first of all, an invisible tie seems to linkformer President Mandela, former President Mbeki and current President Zuma: an arch of an idea, the idea of sovereign statehood, primarily in the domestic realm, and independence. Mandela, generally remembered as the great conciliator, was also keen to assert South Africa's newfound freedom and independence, going so far as even to toy with nationalization, and neglecting HIV/AIDS as a hindrance to his political aspiration and aims. Mbeki, as will be explored below as well, likewise and with much vitriol, ignored the severity of HIV/AIDS and subordinated it to his prioritization of South Africa's domestic sovereignty and in a broader incarnation of the African Renaissance. Zuma, though comparable to Mandela in striking a concessionary tone and seemingly reversing Mbeki's belligerent stance against HIV/AIDS with renewed and expanded antiretroviral roll-outs, actually sustains the former presidents' preoccupation with independence and sovereign statehood.[82] Despite South Africa's increased dependence upon donor funding to facilitate its newest ARV roll-out, Zuma is arguing for the country's donor independence and resurgence in its domestic sovereignty.

Second, the actors listed above have played crucial roles in defining the policy arena and the practice associated with HIV/AIDS in South Africa. Their actions, or inactions, have been consequential of the trajectory of South Africa's response to its HIV/AIDS epidemic. Consequently, they constitute guiding elements

---

of African states depends on leaders successfully meeting the challenges posed by their particular environment."

82   Council on Foreign Relations 2009. Global Health Update (23 December).

influencing how South Africa has acted on its sovereignty and its ultimate responsibility to respond.

4.4.2 Leadership and Denial

The track record of leadership in particular on HIV/AIDS in South Africa is paved with potholes. It is mired in personal beliefs and comfort levels—or lack thereof—in discussing the sex-fueled epidemic, and implicated in projections of power. It is characterized by twists and turns, progression and digression. Yet there is one core component in the South Africa scene, a person part of the country's HIV/AIDS response before and during his presidency: former President Thabo Mbeki. He was there at the beginning, and almost through the (bitter) end of the response to the epidemic. Any comprehensive review and analysis of South Africa's response to HIV/AIDS has to include him in its focus.

Though Professor Sher met with Nelson Mandela in 1994, Mandela remained publicly silent on HIV/AIDS. He would not speak out until a decade later, when he, followed by the Sisulu family and Chief Buthelezi, acknowledged the toll taken by the epidemic on their own families. Mandela announced the death of his son, Makgatho; Buthelezi the death of both a daughter and a son.

In the meantime, the torch passed to first deputy and then President Mbeki. He spoke out relatively early and eloquently, addressing the reality and the devastation of the virus. On 9 October 1998, when Mbeki launched the Partnership against AIDS, he said in his inaugural statement:

> HIV/AIDS is among us. It is real. It is spreading. We can only win against HIV/AIDS if we join hands to save our nation. For too long we have closed our eyes as a nation, hoping the truth was not so real. For many years, we have allowed the HI-virus to spread, and at a rate in our country which is one of the fastest in the world. Every single day a further 1,500 people in South Africa get infected. To date, more than 3 million people have been infected.[83]

Eerily, this incidence rate remains the same today. Bluntly stating the facts, Mbeki asserted the far-reaching implications of the impending destruction—and he, as the head of the state—assumed responsibility:

> By allowing it to spread, we face the danger that half of our youth will not reach adulthood. Their education will be wasted. The economy will shrink. There will be a large number of sick people whom the healthy will not be able to maintain. Our dreams as a people will be shattered.[84]

---

83   Mbeki, T. 1998. "Address by Deputy President Thabo Mbeki: Declaration of Partnership against AIDS" (9 October), available at http://www.anc.org.za/ancdocs/history/mbeki/ [accessed: 20 July 2009].

84   Ibid.

Then something happened. Within a year, with his election as president, when he convened the controversial Presidential Advisory Panel,[85] Mbeki had turned from this apparent acceptance to an irate insistence that HIV/AIDS did not have, could not have, a place in the new, independent South Africa.

The dramatic turn seems to be a reactionary response to the perception and practice of limited domestic sovereignty, a loss of sovereign statehood; and an affront to Africa and the African Renaissance.[86] Addressing the Advisory Panel,

---

85   Despite the controversy that is arouses, it is useful to see the influence of kgotla and indaba in the convening of Mbeki's Advisory Panel. Kgotla-style leadership involves absorbing, taking everything in, and then making a decision, always in compromise, where "everybody recognizes everybody's else's interests." Ndaba refers to the tradition of African elders debating together and emerging with one united position: a style often attributed to the ANC's closed-door politicking. Indaba brought traditional leaders together for "days, weeks, or even longer" until "a consensus was reached": upper most was consensus. Amidst the stigma, the misunderstanding, the contested roles of Western medical doctors and medicines and of sangomas and other traditional healers, debating and determining a consensus position might have been a tangible, important, and effective element of the fight against HIV/AIDS.

86   Mbeki's skepticism of antiretrovirals, while misguided, does have traceable roots in history and in contemporary skepticism concerning some Western medicine in Africa. Three examples illustrate this. First, "in the 1930s, for instance, the anthropologist Ellen Hellman and the psychiatrist Wulf Sachs conducted an extended period of fieldwork in Rooiyard, a shantytown in Doornfontein, Johannesburg. During the time they spent there, rumors swept through the shantytown, which soon proved to be true, that is had been targeted for demolition. Sachs had asked several Rooiyard residents whether he could take their blood and test it for syphilis. He promised to provide medication for those who tested positive:" due to the demolition, residents received not treatment, and correlated the testing of "contaminated blood," with the demolition itself. See Steinberg, J. 2008. *Sizwe's Test: A Young Man's Journey through Africa's AIDS Epidemic*. New York: Simon & Schuster: 149. Second, more generally, "Across colonial Africa, medicine was always understood as a vital ingredient in white political power. The needle that penetrates African skin to extract or inject substances into African blood has never been a neutral technology; it is an image that has always been hungry for meaning ... Between the 1920s and the 1940s, for instance, it was widely believed throughout central and eastern Africa that whites and their agents killed Africans in order to steal their blood," which whites purportedly needed to stay alive in Africa. See Steinberg, J. 2008. *Sizwe's Test: A Young Man's Journey through Africa's AIDS Epidemic*. New York: Simon & Schuster: 150. Third, "in November 1918, when the Spanish Influenza was felling the young and the healthy, and people spoke of the long needle of the white man coming to inject more harm, Pondoland had just commemorated the 24th anniversary of its formal annexation. Its people were under few illusions that their relationship with colonial power could amount to much more than mutual plunder. There is thus not much mystery in the fact that a little-known white technology was greeted with extreme caution." See Steinberg, J. 2008. *Sizwe's Test: A Young Man's Journey through Africa's AIDS Epidemic*. New York: Simon & Schuster: 151. Given also contemporary drug trials, some of which are conducted in Africa under conditions that would not be permissible in Western countries whose pharmaceutical companies produce and profit from the ensuing

and its scientifically dubious composition, Mbeki cited the research published in the *South African Medical Journal*, which revealed that the first incidence of HIV reported in sub-Saharan and South Africa was in 1985—in (white) homosexuals who, along with intravenous drug users and hemophiliacs, who both then and now constitute the main high-risk groups for HIV/AIDS in the US and Europe. Why is the situation in (South) Africa so different?

Mbeki quoted from the 1999 World Health Organization report which estimated that of 5.6 million people living with HIV worldwide, an almost inexplicable 3.8 million of these were in sub-Saharan Africa. Though the region housed less than 10 percent of the world's population, it had the highest HIV-related mortality rates: 85 percent of the global total, representing 2.2 million people. "We are talking about people—it is not death of animal stock or something like that, but people. Millions and millions of people."[87] "Why here, why us, why now?"[88]

In his address to the Advisory Panel, President Mbeki attempted to answer his own questions—and to assume responsibility for an appropriate response to the epidemic:

> What we [know is that there is a virus, HIV. The virus causes AIDS. AIDS causes death and there's no vaccine against AIDS. So once you are HIV positive, you are going to develop AIDS, and you are bound to die. We responded with that part of the response the Minister was talking about—public awareness campaigns, encouraging safe sex, use of condoms, all of those things.[89]

Then he hit upon an incongruence; that while the epidemic met with an unprecedented public health response, other diseases, ever-present and perhaps associated with HIV/AIDS, did not. At this point, Mbeki did not take responsibility—personally or as the head of state—but hid behind the notion of "one," anyone, and instead of thrusting HIV/AIDS into the limelight *alongside* additional (health) issues, he attempted to throw it out altogether—arguably part of what would become his mangled but deliberate political calculation in addressing, by not, HIV/AIDS.

---

drugs, this caution is warranted. In light of this, that "Mbeki read calls for universal AIDS treatment as an attack on South Africa's sovereignty and as harmful to its people" should not be surprising. See Steinberg, J. 2008. *Sizwe's Test: A Young Man's Journey through Africa's AIDS Epidemic*. New York: Simon & Schuster: 152.

87   Mbeki, T. 2000. "Remarks at the first meeting of the Presidential Advisory Panel on AIDS" (6 May), available at http://www.anc.org.za/ancdocs/history/mbeki/ [accessed: 1 July 2012].

88   Steinberg, J. 2008. *Sizwe's Test: A Young Man's Journey through Africa's AIDS Epidemic*. New York: Simon & Schuster: 6.

89   Mbeki, T. 2000. "Remarks at the first meeting of the Presidential Advisory Panel on AIDS" (6 May), available at http://www.anc.org.za/ancdocs/history/mbeki/ [accessed: 1 July 2012].

> One noted that we had never said anything in all of this public awareness
> campaign, that people need to practice safe sex and use condoms in order to
> stop the other sexually transmitted diseases—syphilis, gonorrhea and so on—as
> though these did not really matter. What mattered was this virus.[90]

This viewpoint offered two important opt-outs to former President Mbeki: first,
to deny that the HIV/AIDS be treated as special case, and second, to subsume it
under his preferred priorities, notably the promotion of the African Renaissance
and the protection of South Africa's sovereign statehood. It also had profound
policy implications for the HIV/AIDS response in South Africa, influencing
what was acceptable to place on the agenda, what it was then possible to decide
upon, and what was possible to implement. This political and policy progression
also interacted with South Africa's interpretation and exercise of its domestic
sovereignty, as will be discussed in the next chapter.

The shift in Mbeki's thinking on HIV/AIDS, his folding it into his conception
and promotion of the African Renaissance and South Africa's concomitant
leadership role therein, becomes poignantly clear throughout the following year—
2000. That October, Mbeki, jettisoning the intellectual juxtaposition of HIV/AIDS
and poverty, of past and present, resorted instead to cognitive dissonance and to
simple blame.

> If one agreed that HIV causes AIDS, it followed that that treatment lay with
> drugs manufactured by Western corporations. The pharmaceutical companies
> therefore needed people to believe that HIV and AIDS were linked, in order
> to peddle their products. One drug company, which he did not name, had
> confessed, he said, that it had spent vast amounts of money on the search for an
> AIDS vaccine, but had abandoned the effort after failing to isolate the virus. This
> fact remained hidden from the public, Mbeki claimed, because the company's
> share price would plummet if the truth were told.[91]

----

90   Mbeki, T. 2000. "Remarks at the first meeting of the Presidential Advisory Panel
on AIDS" (6 May), available at http://www.anc.org.za/ancdocs/history/mbeki/ [accessed: 1
July 2012]. In this context of preferential AIDS awareness and treatment, Mbeki asks why
of all diseases, HIV/AIDS is singled out: is it because it is so much more epidemic than
other, endemic diseases? Is it because it can be cast as an African disease? Is it because
special-interests, such as pharmaceutical groups, have less profit to gain from pursuing and
selling treatments against these?

91   Gumede, W. 2005. *Thabo Mbeki and the Battle for the Soul of the ANC.* Cape
Town: Zebra Publishers: 167. It is important to note that the isolation of the HI-virus is
and remains a complicated process, though it has been done. Additionally, it must also
be stated that no effective vaccine has yet been developed, and that the mutations in the
virus itself make this an ongoing challenge. The challenges themselves do not render the
attempts futile. Indeed, the existing and evolving drugs against HIV have been proven to
reduce viral load and to prolong the lives and their quality in those who consistently and
correctly take them.

In this context of preferential AIDS awareness and treatment, Mbeki asks why of all diseases, HIV/AIDS is singled out: is it because it is so much more epidemic than other, endemic diseases? Is it because it can be cast as an African disease? Is it because special-interests, such as pharmaceutical groups, have less profit to gain from pursuing and selling treatments against these? By asking these questions in this way, Mbeki opened the floodgates to false information. He seemed to espouse a denialist stance, though he couched his argument in the vestiges of historic victories over oppression and insisted upon the inviolability of sovereignty.

Yet denial is a shirking of responsibility. AIDS-denialists assert that HIV is harmless, and that any interventions against it are harmful and in the case of ARVs, toxic and deadly. Abetted to this position is the accompanying alternative argument that as denialist [David] Rasnick asserts "the link between AIDS and socio-economic status is truly the underlying basis of AIDS in Africa."[92] As has been discussed above and elsewhere,[93] HIV/AIDS in (South) Africa is undoubtedly aided and abetted by poverty—but this is not a cause-and-effect relationship.

Two additional caveats with regard to denialism and HIV/AIDS are worth noting here. First, with regard to diet, foods such as lemon, garlic, olive oil, African potato, and beetroot[94]—are, especially in the case of beetroot, expensive, and in the case of African potato extract, actually shown to reduce CD4 counts and cause bone-marrow suppression in HIV-positive people, possibly hastening their death as opposed to supporting their life. Likewise, garlic eaten in conjunction with a drug regimen including Saquinavir (a protease inhibitor) reduces the blood levels of that drug and thereby its antiretroviral efficiency, compromising treatment.[95] Second, Rath's vitamins, in addition to being more expensive than first-line ARV treatment, are prescribed in extremely high doses, themselves causing toxicity. Finally, it should also be noted that those needing treatment who receive it in the very late stages of AIDS are unlikely to recover and thus more likely to die. This has nothing to do with any ARV toxicity erroneously asserted, but with the body's inability to rally even with the onslaught of medications.

Mbeki's denialism, related as it was to his ardent attempts to vouchsafe South Africa's domestic sovereignty, had the opposite effect. As the former president appeared to renege on the state's responsibility to respond, seeking an unattainable consensus, he faced challenges, both locally as well as from external actors. The alliances in advocacy and action that these created, and the interventions that they

---

92   Nattrass, N. 2007. *Mortal Combat: AIDS Denialism and the Struggle for Antiretrovirals in South Africa*. Scottsville: University of KwaZulu-Natal Press: 48.

93   See also Poku, N. and Whiteside, A. (ed.) 2004. *The Political Economy of HIV and AIDS*. Aldershot: Ashgate; and Nattrass, N. 2007. *Mortal Combat: AIDS Denialism and the Struggle for Antiretrovirals in South Africa*. Scottsville: University of KwaZulu-Natal Press.

94   As recommended by former Minister of Health Manto Tshabalala-Msimang.

95   Nattrass, N. 2007. *Mortal Combat: AIDS Denialism and the Struggle for Antiretrovirals in South Africa*. Scottsville: University of KwaZulu-Natal Press: 143.

implemented, served to undermine the domestic sovereignty he tried to strengthen, notably in the HIV/AIDS arena.

Mbeki repeatedly highlighted the need for a holistic approach to attaining the host of rights and responsibilities guaranteed in the democratic South Africa. In the meantime, when the South African Government's bid to challenge the controversial implementation of TRIPS failed under pressure from international pharmaceutical companies backed by foreign governments failed,[96] the local NGO TAC took the government to court for failing to provide the drugs. In the aftermath, Mbeki explained his refusal to declare a national emergency to access ARVs by saying, "declaring a national emergency for the simple reason of accessing any drugs, sends a signal that tends to narrow the response to AIDS to the issue of one particular drug,[97] a position consistent with his holistic prioritization.

More so even than a fight around the South African response to the HIV/AIDS epidemic, Mbeki's position, and its consequences, reveals a "political battle whose contours extended beyond the mere detail of AIDS policy and into the broader arena of state-civil-society relations." Mbeki "was locked into a conflict over the nature of state power itself," a battle over who had the right to address the epidemic, a fight pitting state and non-state actors against one another—though ostensibly striving towards the same goal, the defeat of HIV/AIDS.[98] He was right to address the epidemic as a struggle between state and non-state actors.[99]

That tension is also the result of the unresolved power and policy prioritization dispute inherited from the transition from the apartheid era to democracy. For instance, the leadership and cadre of the TAC had also, to a large extent, been fellow activists against apartheid. TAC's challenge to the then-president's approach to the HIV/AIDS epidemic came to symbolize, in perception and in practice, the counter-revolution Mbeki sought to combat and quell.

> For some in the Treatment Action Campaign who remember what the struggle for liberation represented, our government's response to HIV/AIDS fills us with anger. It is after all this government that should free us of the legacy of Apartheid by dealing with the HIV epidemic, the lack of access to health care and education, poverty and unemployment. So, when it fails to provide the necessary leadership

---

96   According to dependency theory analysis, pharmaceutical companies, as transnational companies (TNCs) can "expect help from 'their own' government, which may broaden the campaign by calling on other external and internal allies, and using the additional instruments of retaliation at its disposal which range from cutting off aid to trade embargoes or even war." *Dependency Theory: A Critical Reassessment*. London: Frances Pinter (Publishers) Ltd, 1981: 137. This was clearly seen in former US Vice President Gore's threatened sanctions against South Africa in response to that country's challenge to pharmaceutical patents.

97   Nattrass, N. 2007. *Mortal Combat: AIDS Denialism and the Struggle for Antiretrovirals in South Africa*. Scottsville: University of KwaZulu-Natal Press: 63.

98   Ibid., 83.

99   Ibid.

despite numerous opportunities to make much needed treatment available, we are compelled to question it.[100]

As such, Mbeki responded to the TAC, but also to the HIV/AIDS epidemic in South Africa more broadly, by striving vehemently to shore up the state's domestic sovereignty.

Yet he lacked the power to corral the external state and non-state actors to his decision-making. This intransience on both "sides," without a framework to define the responsibility and accountability of each, drove a wider wedge between them. Neither could do without the other; but the lines of authority blurred and the delegation of responsibility and accountability obscured lead not to mutual strength but to the GAP.

4.5 HIV/AIDS and State Sovereignty

Mbeki then took his battle abroad to try and trump up solidarity on behalf of the sovereignty of his state, while much of the more vocal global advocates were appealing for only a response to the HIV/AIDS epidemic. On 14 December 2000, in an address at Brazil's Bahia University, Mbeki appealed to the African Diaspora and invoked the African Renaissance, saying

> Together we [Africans] are faced with the challenge of defeating the political and economic conditions that, as we speak, condemn the majority of our fellow humans, particularly in poor countries, to the conditions similar to the ones on the Slave Ship. We have to fight this state of existence where people live as though they are 'prisoned in the bars of a single jail,' where our people seem to be 'delirious' from malaria, TB, AIDS and many preventable and curable diseases.[101]

Ostensibly asserting and claiming responsibility, he continued. "nobody can do it for us. Only ourselves—we who know the debilitating effects of the pangs of hunger—should marshal our energies, harness our resources and use our comparative advantage strategically for our own development. This is what the African Renaissance seeks to achieve."[102] Ironically, if his aim was to shore up South Africa's domestic sovereignty—by forging a path of independence from pharmaceutical companies—he actually contributed to undermining it. Already in his remarks to the Presidential Advisory Panel, Mbeki admitted that by stalling initiatives to stay the spread of the epidemic might be seen as betraying people; but

---

100   Ibid., 117.

101   Mbeki, T. 2000. "Address at the University of the State of Bahia, Brazil" (14 December), available at http://www.anc.org.za/ancdocs/history/mbeki/ [accessed: 1 July 2012].

102   Ibid.

he also indicated that not to question the reality of HIV/AIDS and the role of local and global actors in the spread of and response to it would likewise be betrayal:[103]

However, by focusing on the African Renaissance and stalling responses to the epidemic, Mbeki effectually opened the floodgates not only to criticism, but also to the formation of local-global alliances, including those spearheaded by the TAC. Interestingly, Mbeki understood this dynamic.

> The impact of HIV/AIDS on the population, the economy, and the very fabric of our society undermines not only development, but poses a serious threat to our security and life as we know it. ... And South Africa's negotiation of its choices will impact and be impacted not only by its internal dynamics, but also by 'regional and global forces.'[104]

These "regional and global forces," the context, leadership, and alliances outlined above, circumvented the government in responding to the HIV/AIDS epidemic and consequently threatened its domestic sovereignty by compromising the state's authority and its ability to enact its responsibilities to respond.

4.6 Conclusion

As has been illustrated, South Africa faced and faces a number of demands in the sphere of its international and national areas. This is especially true at the outset, and ongoing, phase of its transition to democracy. Addressing HIV/AIDS is one priority among many. Though intertwined with associated rights and responsibilities as spelled out in the South Africa Constitution, HIV/AIDS has not always—or ever—been the over-arching political priority of either the government or of the majority of South Africa's citizens. Nonetheless, the very nature of the epidemic and of its interrelationship with those attendant rights and responsibilities laid out in South Africa's Bill of Rights, and yet dependent on international conditions, make addressing it vital with respect to the country's exercise of its domestic sovereignty and responsibility to respond. The next chapter will present an integrated case study of South Africa's responsibility to respond to HIV/AIDS through the lens of its compromised sovereign statehood.

---

103   Gumede, W. 2005. *Thabo Mbeki and the Battle for the Soul of the ANC*. Cape Town: Zebra Publishers.

104   Barnett, T. 2006. "A Long-Wave Event. HIV/AIDS, Politics, Governance and 'Security'." *International Affairs HIV/AIDS*, Special Issue, 82(2): 311.

Chapter 5

Policy Polemics I:
Apartheid's Demise to HIV/AIDS' Rise

The previous chapter laid out the international and domestic frameworks within which South Africa negotiates its response to the HIV/AIDS epidemic, taking into account internal and external factors of influence that link and differentiate the governments of Mandela through Mbeki to Zuma. The emphasis on sovereign statehood—as a means to assert and demand independence that is in effect not to be had; but nonetheless as a right to determine the contents of the responsibility to respond—threads its way through all. It will be explored and analyzed in detail here.

The South African Government's response—from agenda-setting and identifying the problem through to the feedback loop—is primarily understood in policy terms. Yet it is a far from straightforward response. Instead, South Africa's policy process to respond to HIV/AIDS follows a rather circuitous route, at times appearing to abandon the initiative, and repeatedly circling back unto itself. It contends with crises in confidence and leadership, is interrupted and influenced by South Africa's democratic transition, as well as by local demands and global rule-making.[1]

The majority of analyses of South Africa's reaction to HIV/AIDS contain a threefold assumption: that the country and the government should have registered the extent of the problem posed by the epidemic; that it should have acknowledged this; and that it should have acted in a particular way to address the epidemic. As South Africa has not responded to the HIV/AIDS epidemic according to these strategic prescriptions; consequently, its response has largely been labeled a failure.

Contrasting this, this analysis will offer a threefold refute to that set of assumptions. By dissecting the three phases in which the South African Government and the South African state responded to its HIV/AIDS epidemic, covered in this and the following chapter, taking into account the accompanying international and domestic circumstances and conditions, it will illustrate not the state's failure per se, but its continuous contention with its responsibility to respond. Finally, it will tease out the theoretical and practical lessons that can be learned from this reading of the South African case through the lens of the Governance Accountability Problem, the GAP.

---

1   See "Theories and Models for Analyzing Public Policy." In *Improving Public Policy* (eds) 2000. Cloete, F. and Wissink, H. Pretoria: Van Schaik.

The three phases it identifies are between ca. 1981–1998, during which the state acknowledged the problem, but *chose*, based on the context and conditions of its domestic sovereignty, to prioritize the transition to democracy over this insipient threat to its birth; between ca. 1998–2003, during which it was forced to content with responding to HIV/AIDS according to prescriptions foisted upon it; between c. 2003–2013, which manifests the continued struggle of the state to respond, even as the external actors once so energized, lose interest, and with it, cease their tasks.

The road South Africa chose to travel is riddled with controversy. The verdict of its "failure," moreover, is generally and simplistically attributed to a lack of a political will. Without exonerating its short-comings and failures, this analysis aims to illustrate South Africa's response to the epidemic and their pattern from a slightly different perspective. Emphasizing the country's negotiation of domestic priorities and those of external state and non-state actors and entities exerted in and on the national response in the HIV/AIDS arena, it will reveal a pattern of reaction that sheds light on the rules-of-the-game and the role that especially domestic and global contexts, actors and actions played in the HIV/AIDS response. In doing so, it offers a more nuanced conclusion than has been typical: arguing that South Africa, bound by a local-global alliance of external, state and non-state actors actions, finds itself thrust out of the line of power and yet vested with ultimate responsibility for the country's HIV/AIDS response.

Perhaps South Africa could have, and should have, responded to the epidemic with a full-scale ARV roll-out imminently after the arrival of ARVs on the market in 1996. Doing so would have granted the wishes of many of the local-global alliances putting pressure on the state to enact its responsibility to respond in a particular way. Indeed, it would have gone a ways towards delivering upon the second tenet of sovereignty—the protection and provision of welfare—for South Africa's HIV/AIDS infected populace. However, doing so, like failing to do so, caught South Africa in a catch-22.

Promulgating an ARV roll-out then would have tied the South African state to the agenda and policy-making of non-state actors. This would have, as indeed it did in 2003, rendered it, and more importantly its ability to act upon its responsibility to respond, to HIV/AIDS but also further afield, dependent upon forces outside of its control. The South African Government was not prepared to enter into such a bargain.

Therefore, the battle between these contradictory "coulds" and "should" also, as analyzed, here, resulted neither in failure nor in success, but in an uninspiring truce with some noteworthy insights and implications. This chapter evaluates the ensuing implications for its domestic sovereignty, and in particular it's associated responsibility to respond to HIV/AIDS—with lessons beyond.

5.1 Phase One (c. 1981–1998)

The beginning of the HIV/AIDS epidemic was inauspicious. It emerged in the midst of what would turn out to be the last decade of the apartheid regime's rule. As freedom for the majority of South Africans emerged, HIV/AIDS and death hovered on the horizon.

Despite warnings of the impending epidemic, many were not heeded. Consequently, the epidemic spread, with these warning first silently and then more loudly, drowning out other voices in reaction. Today it seems undisputed that HIV/AIDS is a serious problem in South Africa. Yet the way there has been long and winding, and disputes still rage over its severity, and especially, over the plausible and possible responses to its ravages.

5.1.1 Inauspicious Beginnings: A Slow-striding Death Sentence

The first symptoms associated with the disease were those of pneumonia and Kaposi's sarcoma, a rare cancer. Both surfaced, seemingly exclusively, in young, homosexual men. In lieu of another explanation, HIV/AIDS was immediately, and viciously, portrayed and politicized as what US President Ronald Reagan publicly called the "gay plague." The year was 1982. Significantly, at the same time US President Reagan removed South Africa from the list of pariah states and inaugurated the process of "constructive engagement," a development that possibly diminished the sense of immediacy in South Africa's response to the disease as it embarked on a course dedicated first to economic development with the notion of supporting its sovereign responsibility to respond on a comprehensive basis.

Shortly thereafter in 1983 US scientist Robert Gallo of the National Institutes of Health and French scientist Luc Montangier of the Institute de Pasteur vied for the honor of being the first to identify what became the human immunodeficiency virus,[2] tests to detect the virus and eventually treatments against it would follow. In the meantime, steadily, but slowly, the first soft steps of awareness of HIV would become louder, and sound as footfalls of alarm that fell in a soundproof room.

5.1.2 Identifying the Problem: Sounding the Alarm

Professor Sher stood at the forefront of the research and recognition of the spread of HIV/AIDS in South Africa. After attending the first AIDS Conference in Atlanta, Georgia, USA in 1984, he visited Robert Gallo's laboratory at the National Institutes of Health (NIH). There he received several vials of cultured HIV to take back to South Africa, where he would study them and soon be able to

---

2   A point of interest: Susser, I. 2009. *AIDS, Sex, and Culture: Global Politics and Survival in Southern Africa*. West Sussex, UK: Wiley-Blackwell, notes that it was actually a woman in Montangier's lab who "discovered" HIV.

test whether it was present in the patients he was treating with symptoms similar to those observed in the US.

Towards the end of 1985, Abbott Laboratories in the US released its antibody test, the so-called ELISA (Enzyme-Linked Immunosorbent Assay), which replaced Dr Lyon's fluorescent antibody test in detecting HIV in South Africa. This would later be supplemented by the Western Blot test for added accuracy.

Professor Sher and his colleagues went right to work, testing the 250 blood samples drawn from homosexual men in Johannesburg in 1983. The result revealed the silent presence of the virus in the early 1980s, showing that "between 10 and 11 percent of this group had been HIV-positive. At the time, South Africa's HIV prevalence rate in the general population was estimated at 0.02 percent." Though this, and at the time most of the prevalence rates for sub-Saharan Africa fell far below the epidemic threshold of 1 percent prevalence, the rate nonetheless illustrated the presence of the virus and its potential increase. That increase has been borne out in reality: HIV breached the one percent threshold in southern Africa in the early 1990s, 10 years after initial awareness and alarm over the virus.

5.2 Internal but Non-state Agenda-setting and Implementation

Despite the prejudices and preoccupations of politicians, by 1987 scientists in South Africa were taking not only a lead in research but also in response. In October, Professor Sher, along with colleagues Professors Prozotsky and Metz and Dr de Wet Ras opened the AIDS Center at the South African Institute for Medical Research (SAIMR).[3] Funded with roughly half a million rand courtesy of SAIMR, South African Breweries and the South African Chamber of Mines, the AIDS Center was the first of its kind. It focused on education and created a "train the trainer" program, which was subsequently replicated across the country, off-shoots of which can be found in the reputed peer educator programs of public and private, state and non-state, organizations to this day.[4] Significantly, the Center's operations, from the outset through its closing, foreshadow the tactical and implicit assumption of essential state responsibility by non-state actors in

---

3   Notes from Professor Ruben Sher, acquired March 2005.

4   Notwithstanding its laudable attempts to promote awareness and to stem the tide of the HIV epidemic, the AIDS Center operated on a number of false pre-conceived and perpetuated social-political notions. Notably, its educational initiatives misconceived and underestimated the extent of the epidemic for South Africa, in particular its effect on the heterosexual population. This is largely due to the fact that "the educational information came from the United States; mainly from homosexual pamphlets and those agencies which were beginning to produce pamphlets, [like] NIH," a crisis situation and response wholly different from that which South Africa was beginning to face. Chapter 8 offers more discussion on prevention.

responding to HIV/AIDS. The South African state, still governed by the apartheid regime, did nothing.

The AIDS Center contributed to actions and reactions to HIV/AIDS in South Africa, particularly before the entry into the market of viable treatment options. In 1987 the first anti-AIDS drug, later to be known collectively as ARVs, emerged in the US and then entered the global market. This first drug, known as AZT, originally a chemotherapy drug developed in the 1960s, offered new hope for life amidst what was rapidly becoming an onslaught of death.

5.3 External Conditions: Death Rattle of Apartheid Replaced with Death Knell of AIDS

The arrival of AZT and its promise of life for those who could access it coincided with the slow death of apartheid at the hands of a long resisted but ultimately triumphant freedom. It was a pyrrhic reemergence, as the resurrected South Africa, sovereign and independent, faced the ashes of the HIV/AIDS onslaught.

In its neighborhood, South Africa faced "international pressures as well as the ongoing war in Angola and all along the border."[5] Further afield, the country was the object in a fight over extending of loans to the ruling regime. The US loan policy promulgated under President Reagan diverged in the end from "constructive engagement," and contributed significantly to the debt that the fledgling democracy would soon inherit, increasing South Africa's dependence upon foreign capital and investments during the transition. Combined with boycotts against the apartheid regime, which "had a direct and immediate impact,"[6] these external pressures helped lead to the freeing of Mandela by De Klerk and the subsequent collapse of apartheid. At the same time, "the impact of an international/American policy that had as its purpose the ending of apartheid in fact had the result of hampering a new government's ability to address its most pressing needs."[7] This was because the newly emerging democratic South Africa inherited an essentially bankrupt state with little money and means to deliver upon the rights guaranteed in the new Constitution, including those to health and by association, to the fight against HIV/AIDS.

5.4 The Internal/External Influence on Initiation and Agenda-setting

As outlined in the previous chapters, South Africa's response to its HIV/AIDS epidemic has taken place amidst existing and evolving rules-of-the-game set by the political-economic structures and strictures of markets and policy-makers at

---

5   Personal correspondence with Ambassador Richard Barkley, 11 February 2008.
6   Ibid.
7   Ibid.

the local, national and global levels. These have had and continue to have bearing on South Africa's own policy space, its self-perception, and its practical room to maneuver, particularly with regard to its ability to deliver upon its sovereign responsibility to respond to the rights of its citizens, notably with regard to its HIV/AIDS epidemic.

The tension between rights as enshrined in the Constitution and the responsibility of the South African Government to guarantee them amidst local and global pressures to pursue particular priorities—economic, political, issue-specific—influences and characterizes South Africa's policy arena since the inception of its democracy. One outcome was GEAR, which aimed to steer South Africa away from dependence upon international financial institutions and investor capital, and towards sovereign control of the country's economic sphere: a laudable impossibility. GEAR constitutes one backdrop to South Africa's political agenda, embodying as it does the primacy of economic independence and a focus on independence. It is also buffeted by BEE, formally introduced in 2004, and expanded to BBBEE legislation stipulating shares of black ownership in South Africa's businesses. These measures constitute not so much an employment initiative as an answer to the sunset clauses that protect government bureaucrats from termination due to the governance transition, and as an attempt to implement redress through the reallocation of economic ownership. However, on the domestic front, these have not yielded the economic redistribution envisioned. Similarly, neither has GEAR drawn the international investment it aimed to capture. Both attempts however, encapsulate projects by the South African Government to tackle its domestic and international challenges—to put to rest doubts about its competence, to deliver upon its responsibilities and accountability—head-on. In addition to these, a few other influences presented here are worth paying attention to, with a special focus on how they interacted to shape South Africa's perception and practice of its sovereign responsibility to respond, especially as related to HIV/AIDS.

5.5 Political-economic Hurdles and HIV at the Dawn of Democracy

Viewed in retrospect by Finance Minister Trevor Manuel, who worked with Mbeki for over a decade before, during, and after South Africa's transition to democracy,

> My purpose has always been to remain sovereign. We saw 10 years of remarkable change in Zimbabwe on borrowed money. Then came 1991 and the first structural adjustment loans fell due. It coincided with my appointment as head of the ANC's department of economic policy. It became a challenge to take

decisions to stay out of the clutches of other decision-makers; not to land at the door of the IMF.[8]

In other words, Manuel meant for South Africa to be independent, to be able to determine its own policy course, to set its priorities and follow its prescriptions—even though, as evidenced, such complete control is not possible in an ever-more intertwined world.

Nonetheless, by striving towards such an instance, this stance arguably—and ironically—led to prioritizations and policy prescriptions that restricted South Africa's political-economic position and power, limiting its power to influence and negotiate, and stymied the ability to enact its responsibility to respond; first, because the country tried to set itself apart, and later, because it tried, arguably too late, to (re-)enter the fold despite shifting rules-of-the-game as seen in the aftermath of the 2007–2008 global financial crisis. "That they are so determined to be sovereign is perhaps understandable considering the length and cost of the anti-Apartheid battle. Ironically, they stress sovereignty at about the exact time that the global economy is beginning to demand incremental changes to the very concept."[9] South Africa embarked on its course to assuage the fears and attract the funds of investors, and to respond to the rights of its freed populace, while at the same time attempting to insulate itself from the associated strings attached. This is especially evident in its early HIV/AIDS response, when the government refused to countenance ARVs, the prescriptive response to the epidemic proffered by the local-global alliances around the state. South Africa chafed against its ensuing dependency upon external funding, while at the same time seeking unstipulated financial support. It strove to be both credit-worthy and not to need credit at all: an irreconcilable set of priorities that would reappear in the government's circuitous HIV/AIDS response.

Nonetheless, the South African Government incurred significant strain in trying to secure is state sovereignty and to enact its sovereign statehood. Towards these ends, the South African Government assumed the debt burden of its predecessor, rendered the Reserve Bank independent,[10] signed the General Agreement on Tariffs and Trade (GATT), later the WTO,[11] and promulgated GEAR, all the while banking on the benefits of such economic discipline to spur growth and development, including as a buffer against the ravages of the HIV/AIDS epidemic.

Explaining the necessity of the strategy's adoption, then Deputy President Mbeki stated, as quoted in detail above, that the South African Government would exert its power to reassure potential investors of the soundness a decision to put

---

8   Manuel, T. 2007. "Polokwane Briefing: Not in My Father's House." *The Mail and Guardian* (13 December).

9   Personal correspondence with Ambassador Barkley, 13 February 2008.

10   Personal correspondence with Professor Patrick Bond, 22 January 2008.

11   Ibid.

their money into the country.[12] All of the actions that state took towards this end were designed to showcase South Africa's independent capabilities in managing its economy with the purpose of attracting FDI, and with the ultimate aim of securing its sovereign capacity to respond on the back of macroeconomic growth and stability.

But the odds shifted against the enterprise.

It is difficult to underestimate both the pressure placed on South Africa to orient its political-economy towards internationally lauded neo-liberal market principles, or to understate the survivalist imperative that made accepting such principles in policy a priority. The new democracy was essentially bankrupt. In the run-up to the 1994 elections, 20.4 billion rand fled the country. In addition, the South African Reserve Bank's forward exchange rate policies resulted in outstanding payments of US$16 billion, which risked default. South Africa also faced the repayment of an IMF loan. Many or perhaps even most of these monies might have been deemed "odious debt," on which the new government could have righteously defaulted or requested forgiveness. Yet in the interest of accruing the above-mentioned investor confidence and open credit lines, South Africa's young democracy chose to honor these debts. As a consequence, South Africa's ability to prioritize and implement social-political imperatives was constricted. Despite its aspirations of internal independence from especially economic dependence, domestic sovereignty concedes some of this independence. Yet the tension remains. As such, Manuel's emphasis on South Africa's independence in its domestic economic policy is arguably the most important, perhaps the determining priority of South Africa's democratic transition. It became the central element steering the country's course, as is starkly on display in South Africa's struggle to balance broad domestic demands and international dictates, including its responsibility to respond to its HIV/AIDS epidemic. GEAR embodied the compromise: lassoing South Africa's independence to its domestic sovereign control while acceding to the demands of the global financial and monetary markets.

GEAR derived from and decreed a host of changes in South Africa's political-economic sphere. These restricted choices in the country's policies. Rejecting nationalization in order to attract and retain capital investment, in January 1995 the new government introduced the process of privatization, supporting it with financial liberalization in the "form of [partial] exchange control abolition in March 1995."[13] Taking heed of the capital flight which contributed to the devaluing of the peso in Mexico around the same time, South Africa also raised "interest rates to a record high, where they have remained ever since."[14] Incongruent with these strict measures, the value of the South African rand has fluctuated throughout the

---

12   Gumede, W. 2005. *Thabo Mbeki and the Battle for the Soul of the ANC.* Cape Town: Zebra Publishers: 62.

13   Personal correspondence with Professor Patrick Bond, 22 January 2008.

14   Ibid.

ensuing decade, and exchange controls, though loosened, remain in place. In the meantime, the South African Government has stuck to its tight fiscal script.

> The South African government chose the [...] most conservative option, with the goal of eventually placing sovereignty in the hands of all of the citizenry. But in doing so it surrendered the only effective means of enabling the rest of society to actualize their rights, for without redistribution they remain in a condition in which they are lacking the resources to do so. The hope is that the process of 'transformation through austerity' would, 'in the end,' generate sufficient growth to eliminate any distributional constraint.[15]

The theory postulated that domestic sovereign control, so long sought by the majority of the population, would render the South African Government economically and fiscally able to determine and act upon its policy priorities. However just as the end of the apartheid era did not automatically end South Africa's decline, neither could these lofty aims be magically conjured by the fiscal discipline imposed at democracy's inauguration.

Indeed, despite this calculation, capital inflows, especially of foreign direct investment, have not been forthcoming as predicated, nor have the promised rewards of growth-enabled redistribution. In fact, in some cases, it has been worse: for example, AngloAmerican of the Anglo Group, founded in South Africa and which had its primary stock exchange listing in Johannesburg, moved it to London in 1998; a lost vote of confidence in South Africa. Thus despite its efforts, South Africa could not guarantee its successful control of its context and circumstances. Instead, by attempting to, it helped construct its political-economic strait-jacket.

The consequences of South Africa's compliance with the shifting rules-of-the-game and the impacts of these on the country's quest for independence and control are made evident in two prescient examples relevant to the HIV/AIDS response: the promulgation of TRIPS, and the volatility of exchange rates. First, South Africa constricted its options by acquiescing to the new rules. Second, shifts it could not control imposed limits in turn. Indeed, both policies stymied the new democratic governments' ability to secure sufficient economic funds for their programs, including those for HIV/AIDS.[16]

Promulgated in 1994, TRIPS was to be adopted progressively by all World Trade Organization members. All developed economies had a year to ensure that their patent laws conformed with TRIPS prescriptions; all developing and transitional economies had five years; and all least developed economies initially 11, later extended to 21 years, or to 2016. Brought to the WTO by a group of enterprising pharmaceutical companies led by Pfizer, TRIPS not only imposed

---

15   Hamilton, L. and Viegi, N. "The Nation's Debt and the Birth of the New South Africa," work in progress (September 2007), *Cambridge Journal of Economics* (February 2009 revised submission).

16   Personal correspondence with Ambassador Richard Barkley, 11 February 2008.

protections on intellectual property rights, including in arts and science, ensuring global conformity and promoting trade, but also regulated access to medicines, including to ARVs. Its stipulations impact not only patented, but even generic versions of drugs. Though TRIPS allows for some exemptions from its strict patent rules in the event of a declared "national emergency," making limited allowances for the use of voluntary or compulsory licensing or of parallel imports, these are severely restricted. By signing the agreement, a criterion of coveted membership in the WTO, which South Africa joined 1 January 1995, the country limited its own options in its response to its HIV/AIDS epidemic[17] even while it facilitated its entry into global trade. This apparent trade-off again highlights South Africa's balancing act between the independence of its domestic sovereignty and its nonetheless associated dependence upon external actors and in this case apparatus, upon which its ability to enact its responsibility to respond hinges.

Likewise, volatile exchange rates impact South Africa's economic independence and response to its HIV/AIDS epidemic. Cases in point are the devaluation of the South African rand in 1996 and again in the midst of the Asian financial crisis of 1997; and the attacks on the US Embassies in Nairobi, Kenya and Dar e Salaam, Tanzania in 1998. The value of the rand plummeted by 15.17 percent against the US dollar in the aftermath of the two sets of events. These simultaneous security and economic crises contributed to financial volatility on the international markets, and rendered especially investment into emerging markets less attractive.

So, South Africa faced on the one hand, the self-imposed restrictions on its independence, and externally applied circumscriptions as well. These dual—local-global—strictures on South Africa's independence, and more importantly on its ability to apply its responsibility to respond are starkly evident in the HIV/AIDS arena. It is here, amidst this tension, heightened by the daily fact of people dying, that South Africa consistently prioritized adherence to capital market mantras with the notion that stability, once achieved, and only then, would provide an independent basis for an HIV/AIDS response. In the interim, South Africa concluded that the exorbitant price of ARVs excluded the possibility of offering them in the public sphere. The large-scale purchase of the drugs would have undermined South Africa's ability to pursue the GEAR goals of "economic austerity and financial prudence."[18] In addition to the wholesale costs of ARVs, Thenjiwe Mtintso, then assistant secretary general of the ANC also pointed out that "making anti-retroviral drugs available is only one side of the story; the state will have to take responsibility for all the costs of AIDS-infected individuals."[19] Finance Minister Trevor Manuel bluntly asserted that claims of the effectiveness of ARVs were a lot of "voodoo," and that purchasing them for a dying set of people was a waste of limited resources. Such prejudices, grounded in a dream—deferred—would

---

17   More on TRIPS below.

18   Gumede, W. 2005. *Thabo Mbeki and the Battle for the Soul of the ANC.* Cape Town: Zebra Publishers: 162.

19   Ibid.

plague South Africa's response to its HIV/AIDS epidemic long before it would reverse course and attempt to make good on its sovereign responsibility to respond.

5.6 Option Consideration, Decision-making, Policy Publication, Resource Allocation; and Return to Agenda-setting

This delay ensued despite ample evidence of the necessity and early ability of the state to respond with responsibility to the rights of its populace. On 16 April 1988, the *South African Medical Journal* published a special article by the AIDS Advisory Group based at the AIDS Center at SAIMR entitled "Strategic plan for containment of AIDS in South Africa." Armed with the available knowledge and resources, the strategy advocated prevention, treatment and care. For an interim period after the introduction of ARV medications prevention would be neglected, but it would make a come-back as part of a three-pronged intervention combination which continues to inform the current counter-measures against HIV/AIDS. In 1989, the AIDS Center held its first meeting with *sangomas*, traditional healers, from throughout South Africa. In recognition of their socio-cultural power and influence, by the mid-2000s, *sangomas* would be legally recognized and their methods re-integrated into HIV/AIDS treatment and care.

Professor Sher once again stood at the forefront of this initiative to respond to HIV and to integrate *sangomas* as well as other traditional leaders in South Africa in the effort. In 1991, he had met with Mangosutho G. Buthelezi, Zulu Chieftain. At the time, Buthelezi headed the non-independent black Bantustan, or designated homeland, of KwaZulu under the apartheid regime from 1972 until South African independence in 1994.[20]

> At this meeting, at which I was very warmly received, we discussed the gravity of the AIDS situation in the region. I later learnt that as a result of this discussion the government donated R60,000 towards drama and music as a means of education as they both appeal to the African people. At the time I was convinced of the importance of involving political leaders in the fight against HIV/AIDS.[21]

Contrary to initial hopes, however, the road to public acknowledgement and practical action against the HIV/AIDS epidemic would be long and littered with obstacles. These included distrust between, among others, the incile Buthelezi,

---

20   Buthelezi also founded and led the Inkatha Freedom Party (IFP), the leading political rival to the African National Congress, which had its party seat in the KwaZulu town of Ulundi. It is difficult to understate the influence of Buthelezi particularly among Zulus, the majority black African population in South Africa, and beyond, politically and socio-culturally. As such, Sher's approaching him with regard to HIV/AIDS promised far-reaching implications.

21   Notes and interview with Professor Ruben Sher, 8 March 2005.

who had worked with the apartheid regime, and returning exiles; a distrust at times mirrored and magnified between the ANC and the IFP and their respective supporters.[22] Such domestic political tensions are par for the course, and in the case of HIV/AIDS, reflected and refracted again at the international and global level, as more and more actors, and local-global alliances became involved in the response to South Africa's particular epidemic. So while South Africa cautiously catapulted itself into a democratic era, the battle against HIV/AIDS remained bogged down on all sides of the political, not merely medical, partisanships and patronage.

In 1992, South Africa's political leadership acknowledged HIV/AIDS. It also launched NACOSA, which had a mandate to develop a national strategy on HIV/AIDS. The strategy closely resembled that proposed in the 1988 *South African Medical Journal* article. Yet the strategy profiled in the *South African Medical Journal* was side-swiped in the waning days of apartheid, and that of NACOSA was side-lined by the competing priorities at the inauguration of democracy. Attesting to this, on 31 March 1993, the new democratic government closed the AIDS Center. It cited lack of funds as the official cause of the closure:[23] arguably an issue of understanding, prioritization and feasibility. This opened the floodgates for international advocacy and activism, to try, via the boomerang approach, or direct intervention, to cajole and coerce South Africa into responding to and assuming its responsibility to respond vis-à-vis HIV/AIDS in a particular manner.

Closing the AIDS Center and therein severing ties to this initiative forged during the apartheid era did nothing if not ignore and stand by to the continued spread of HIV/AIDS in South Africa. Indeed, the virus flaunted its new freedom, bringing to bear the dire prediction made by Chris Hani about the severity of the epidemic resulting in "untold damage and suffering by the end of the century."[24] Yet closing the Center seemed to close the door on the necessity to consider the problem; but it tried perhaps to hide it from public view until evidence of HIV/AIDS was strewn across the country.

5.7 Phase Two (c. 1998–2003)

In what would prove an already belated attempt to turn the tide of HIV's spread in South Africa, the government, the South African state, necessarily refocused its attention from the longer to the immediate term. Doing so it also shifted its primary focus from delivering upon all of the rights of all South Africans, to meeting its responsibilities to some of the most vulnerable of the moment, namely those infected with and those affected by, HIV/AIDS. The timing coincided almost

---

22   See also comments on inciles/exiles in Chapter 2.
23   Notes and interview with Professor Ruben Sher, 8 March 2005.
24   Nattrass, N. 2007. *Mortal Combat: AIDS Denialism and the Struggle for Antiretrovirals in South Africa*. Scottsville: University of KwaZulu-Natal Press: 39.

perfectly with the global attention aligned to health, which, in the count-down to the turn of the twenty-first century, proclaimed:

> Governments have a responsibility for the health of their people which can be fulfilled only by the provision of adequate health and social measures. A main social target of governments, international organizations and the whole world community in the coming decades should be the attainment by all peoples of the world by the year 2000 of a level of health that will permit them to lead a socially and economically productive life.[25]

This sentiment has been borne since -though not yet reliably implemented. Against in March 2013, Richard Horton, editor of British health journal, *The Lancet*, argued "the purpose of government is to uphold the dignity of its people,"[26] and added that

> The capability to make free choices about who you want to be and what you want to do partly depends on innate abilities, which in turn depend on a host of prenatal influences, such as maternal health and nutrition. Freedom to make independent choices also depends on the abilities we each possess as children and adults, which in their turn depend on our health, among other determinants. Finally, our freedoms depend on the political, economic, and social environment we experience. These three categories of influence shape our capabilities, of which health is one essential kind. They are essential requirements for a life lived with dignity.

The facilitation of such a life lived with dignity is a core conceptual component of the relationship between individual rights and state responsibility to provide for an enabling environment.

> It shows why health ought to be a core political concern. It allows us to incorporate disability, not only preventable mortality, as a central priority of the health system. It invites us to consider the political structures needed to deliver health as a capability, not merely as health, and how we might hold those political structures accountable for their promise to deliver capability as an outcome.

As such, Horton, no doubt also inspired by Amartya Sen's seminal work, *Development as Freedom*, again highlights the relationship between individual rights and state responsibilities to enable citizens to attain, enjoy and act upon their rights.

---

25 From the Declaration of Alma-Ata, paragraph V.

26 Horton, R. 2013. "Why governments should take health more seriously." *The Lancet*, 381(9871) (23 March).

Of course, fulfilling this right, in other words meeting this obligation, requires a state to possess the "necessary means for individuals to access health care." But whether that means that the state has to provide healthcare beyond access, and to what extent it is obligated to provide it, remains unclear. For example, a state could allow its citizens to access healthcare through external state and non-state actors, a possibility that became a reality in the HIV/AIDS response in South Africa, and elsewhere, with significant consequences for and to the state's authority over and ability to guarantee sustained healthcare access and provision: the right to health and its provision exists without a "corresponding duty" on the part of external state and non-state actors, to "refrain from impairing a state's responsibility to satisfy" those health obligations. In other words, as of this writing, no mechanism exists to ensure that such external state and non-state actors continually provide healthcare access and provision as part and parcel of a sovereign "package" of human security—and no provision is made for such sovereign responsibility to be definitively shared with or transferred to (with the possibility of being revoked and reclaimed) to another actor. Therefore, the state remains in theory if not in perfect practice, the ultimate harbinger of an individual's human security, and thus also the guarantor of healthcare access and provision. As a result, "in this case, the right to access reasonably priced generic drugs because no individual should die for lack of readily available treatment—which would seem to derive from the right to health—did not trump the commercial rights of pharmaceutical companies."[27] Yet the state faced clear and vocal censure for failing to its obligations, as poorly articulated and applicable as they were. So the South African Government would have to pay full-price for hundreds of thousands to millions of doses of medicines, and risk paying even more if the currency devaluated.

When all was said the done and the dust settled the erstwhile adversaries came to an agreement. In 2001, the pharmaceutical consortium dropped the case in exchange for a South African concession to purchase their on-patent drugs and to refrain from pursuing parallel imports. Since the ensuing government purchase tenders locked the South African Government into paying high prices even as these began to fall, thanks to pressure from Brazil, as well as generics, mostly from India, entering the market, it can be concluded that the settlement favored the pharmaceutical companies and less so South Africa and its HIV-infected population in particular. Far more people might have been able to access ARV medications had the full TRIPS provisions been applied, and had the two elements of the principle provision of the right to health been implemented; namely, that the South African state act on its responsibility to provide access to and provision of the means to the right to health in a sustainable and guaranteed fashion, including by naming the HIV/AIDS epidemic as a national emergency, and that external state and non-state actors, including pharmaceutical companies and their host and home states (at least) "refrain from impairing a state's responsibility to satisfy" those health obligations. Neither one of those scenarios came to pass.

---

27   Davies, S.E. 2010. *Global Politics of Health*. Cambridge: Polity Press.

On the one hand, the South African Government, bound by its Constitution enshrining the right to health, and as a signatory to the ICESCR, committed itself to fulfilling its responsibilities to the right to health for all of its citizens. On the other hand, in order to meet those obligations, particularly to those HIV-infected, it needed to rely on the implementation of provisions of the TRIPS agreement, as well as the cooperation of external state and non-state actors on a reliable basis so as to meet its sovereign responsibilities for the intermediate and long-term delivery of human security. Neither was forthcoming.

5.7.1 Political-economy of Decision-making: The Role of Drugs

Despite such early recognition of the presence and potential of the epidemic inspired initial political attention, it spurred little sustainable response. Already in 1994, the newly appointed South African Cabinet endorsed the first national strategy against HIV/AIDS. It highlighted and emphasized three pillars of response:

1. Prevent HIV transmission
2. Reduce the personal and social impacts of HIV infection
3. Mobilize and unify provincial, international and local resources.

Successive strategies against the epidemic would, with the addition of treatment provision under the second point, continue to mirror this initial outline. However, none of the subsequent national plans, of 2000–2005, the 2003 operational strategy, or of 2007–2011 would conjure much confidence or succor much success in forestalling or fighting the epidemic. Nonetheless, other progressive steps do mark the interim.

The most significant was that posed by the advent of ARVs. ARVs, especially when administered in combinations of so-called "cocktails," so-called HAART changed the course of HIV. While not a cure for the virus, the drugs play a key role in slowing disease progression from HIV-infection to full-blown AIDS. In some instances, HIV has been transformed into a chronic disease, manageable with a life-time of treatment regimens, which must be continually adjusted to avoid and respond to viral resistance to the medications. This reality mostly applies to the disease management of HIV-infected individuals with access to ARVs in developed economies. For the majority of South Africans, it remains out of reach.

Two things explain this: complications in access to ARVs, coupled with but also separate from their exorbitant, though in some cases falling, prices. As such, ARVs constitute a double-edged sword: on the one side, touting the promise of life; on the other side, tantalizingly out of reach, portending death. HIV/AIDS is and remains an epidemic of life and death, in terms of the virus itself and in terms of aiding or abetting interventions against it.

As elucidated in the previous chapter, most ARVs were developed by private Western pharmaceutical companies, some with additional public financial support. The ensuing patents belong exclusively to the pharmaceuticals, with the result that drug prices remain out of reach to a majority of poor and middle-income countries and their populaces. The most prominent companies include: Abbott Laboratories (USA), Boehringer Ingelheim (Germany), Bristol-Myers Squibb (USA), GlaxoSmithKline (UK), Merck Shape and Dome (USA), Pfizer (USA), and Roche (Switzerland). They are responsible for most first- and second-line ARVs. Given their international and often multi-national pedigree, and their accompanying political and economic clout, their impact extends far beyond the medicines they produce.

Hence the fights.

It is worth noting that one instigator for the TRIPS conflict in South Africa was the country's passage, on 23 November 1997, of the amended Medicines and Related Substances Control Act. Article 15C of the Act explicitly stated that the national government had the power to determine that the "rights with regard to any medicine under a patent granted in the Republic" may actually not apply to medicines "put onto the market by the owner of the medicine, or with his or her consent,"[28] even if such action contravened the Patents Act of 1978, Act No. 57 of 1978, and presumably also TRIPS, which only makes provisions for the breaking and circumventing of patents in cases of declared national emergency. As such, South Africa could be accused of flaunting international regulations and overstepping the boundaries of intellectual property law, TRIPS Article 39.3; except that as an arguably developing and transitional economy it ought to have been exempt from TRIPS until at least 2000 (and in the event, the country's first national roll-out of ARVs was only promulgated in November 2003 and initiated in April 2004). In its eagerness to join the WTO as a full-fledged member as soon as possible, however, and to dispel any notion of itself as a developing or under-developed state, the South African Government acceded to TRIPS at the first possible opportunity, in 1995. Despite the Medicines and Related Substances Act, South Africa had little way out of the TRIPS requirements.

Its response to HIV/AIDS stalled.

Much as South Africa strove to keep its HIV/AIDS policy a domestic concern under its own control, its laggard response fueled the epidemic on the one hand and created a lesion: a schism between state and external state and non-state responsibility and accountability. Into its wake stepped local-global alliances that operated under and over and around it, and thus under and over and around the South African state.

---

28   "Medicines and Related Substances Control Act 101 of 1965 after amendment by the Medicines and Related Substances Control Amendment Act (Act 90 of 1997)," available at http://www.pharmcouncil.co.za/documents/ACT%2090%20OF%201997.pdf [accessed: 1 July 2012].

5.7.2 In Brief: A Deeper Insight into Pharmaceutical Fights

As introduced in some detail above, South Africa has had a stormy relationship with pharmaceutical companies in particular pertaining to medicines to treat HIV/AIDS. Even over and above this fight, as has been shown, when it comes to patented pharmaceutical drugs and generic medicines used to treat and prevent HIV/AIDS, a number of factors compete in what has become a contentious fight between intellectual property and public health. First at issue are branded antiretroviral drugs. These are more often than not profitably protected by patents owned by pharmaceutical companies. However, the initial development of a significant number of these drugs proceeded through infusions of public funds, via for instance the National Institutes of Health (NIH) in Bethesda, Maryland, USA. Although the NIH retains the legal right, by virtue of its fund infusion, to render products to whose production it contributed public, it has thus far failed to do so.

The second issue concerns generic drugs. For one thing, their legality is contested. Though any drug can be produced legally and generically once a patent expires, a number of stumbling blocks have been put in the way of this process, particularly in the HIV/AIDS arena. The validity of extended and new patents for merely incremental changes, referred to as "ever-greening" to drug formulations constitutes one fight. There are at present, in 2012, at least two relevant battles[29] being fought over this particular issue before Indian courts, with far-reaching consequences for intellectual property and access to generic medications. The contest over the authority of TRIPS and its application—as seen in the cases of South Africa, Brazil, and Thailand—is another. Finally, the ways and means of legal innovation, for instance of India's creation of the three-in-one generic-based antiretroviral pill, forms a further fight. This is at present being addressed by patent pools, in an effort set up through the United Nations system.[30]

These two sets of issues constitute the core of the dispute that pits pharmaceutical innovation and intellectual property against public health. There are, despite the dismal-appearing odds at resolving these and coming to a compromise. With regard to the first issue, pharmaceutical companies can authorize generics through so-called 'voluntary licenses.' These protect intellectual property to a greater extent than do compulsory licenses, and also secure the patent-holder a larger profit. Indeed, this has even occurred. Boehringer Ingelheim authorized South African generic company, Aspen Pharmacare, to produce its antiretroviral blockbuster, Nevirapine, used in numerous antiretroviral cocktails and especially importantly in the prevention of mother-to-child-transmission. With regard to the second issue, where voluntary licenses fail, compulsory licensing remains an option, though this

---

29   The more prominent one is being brought by Novartis for Glivec a drug used to treat two rare cancers, see Hermann, R.M. 2012. "Novartis before India's Supreme Court: What's Really at Stake?" *Intellectual Property Watch* (2 March).

30   More on this in the recommendations in Chapter 8.

step requires greater cooperation from the World Trade Organization and national governments to ensure it is accepted and enforceable.

Illustrating these issues is the particular fight concerning two antiretroviral drugs, Norvir and Kaletra, both produced by Abbot Laboratories. Abbott initially received funding for the development of what became Norvir through the National Institutes of Health (NIH). As mentioned above, NIH could have invoked its legal right to allow the production of generic versions of Norvir prior to the expiry of its patent. In May 2004, NIH held a public hearing to debate this option. A research scientist responsible for much of Norvir's initial development testified that Abbott was unlikely to have funded that early research without the US$3.5 million 1998 grant. Abbott countered that it spent US$300 million of its own money conducting clinical trials prior to Norvir's market approval. NIH ruled against authorizing the breaking of the patent.[31]

In the meantime, in 2003, Abbott initiated a contentious marketing strategy designed to reduce the use of Norvir and to replace it with the more expensive Kaletra. At the time, Abbott controlled 35 percent of the global protease inhibitor market, the class to which both Norvir and Kaletra belong, with global sales totaling US$400 billion. Simultaneously, the company faced competition from two new protease inhibitors: Bristol-Myers Squibb Co.'s Reyataz, which was as effective as Kaletra and had the added benefits on cholesterol levels and required fewer pills a day, and GlaxoSmithKline PLC's new drug.

Striving to maintain and maximize its profits, Abbott conceived three strategies. All revolved around Norvir. It is vital to note that Norvir was not approved for use alone, but was only allowed in combination with additional ARVs, mostly due to its side-effects. Nonetheless, Abbott considered removing Norvir from the US market, "selling the medicine only in a liquid formulation that one executive admitted tasted like vomit," discouraging the drug's use in combinations, claiming that "it [Abbott] needed Norvir pills for a humanitarian effort in Africa."[32] An Abbott spokeswoman later contended that "the company never seriously considered pulling Norvir from the global market or withdrawing the pill version in the US."[33] The last option involved raising the price of Norvir.

The last strategy carried the day. Abbott quintupled the price of Norvir, and justified it stating that Norvir had been previously under-valued, and posting a cost-comparison chart on its Norvir website. This chart showed "that Norvir remained cheaper than other protease inhibitors," but implied therein that it could be taken alone. This move was dishonest on two counts. First, it revalued Norvir without taking into any account the public investment made by NIH, thereby inhibiting as opposed to facilitating access to the drug. Second, the cost-comparison chart was

31   Carreyrou, J. 2007. "Inside Abbott's Tactics to Protect AIDS Drug." *The Wall Street Journal* (3 January).
32   Ibid.
33   Ibid.

blatantly misleading. In June 2004, the US Food and Drug Administration (FDA) ordered Abbott to remove it.[34]

Nonetheless Abbott achieved its aim. Over the next two years, sales of Kaletra in the US rose 10 percent, a rise largely attributable to the astronomic cost increase of antiretroviral regimens that included Norvir. For instance, these increased, on average, from annual costs of US$2,504 to US$11,187 for a Reyataz/Norvir combination, and by another US$5,000 or more in regimens hat included more than one daily dose of Norvir. As a result, Kaletra became the cheaper option, priced at about US$7,000.

Though the company exempted some US federal medical assistance programs such as Medicare and Medicaid, from Norvir's price increase, this restriction did not apply to foreign countries attempting to access ARVs. This has two important consequences. First, it appeared that a company could arbitrarily raise the price of an antiretroviral drug at any time, to any price. Second, just as Abbott raised the price of Norvir South Africa announced its 2003 Operation Plan which inaugurated its public sector roll-out of antiretroviral drugs. The drug tender approved by the plan locked the government into paying the same prices for the ensuing four years. The quintupled price rise for Norvir thus constituted far-reaching fiscal consequences for South Africa's roll-out, both in 2003 and later, influencing as it did perceptions around access to drugs, and the intentions of the patent-holding companies.

In this context, it is also worth mentioning that PEPFAR was getting off the ground at the same time. The largest share of its drug tender was awarded to Abbott, at US market prices.

On a final note, though South Africa acquiesced to not invoking the TRIPS agreement after 2001, Brazil and Thailand made no such promises. The latter two countries both broke the patent on Kaletra. Abbott responded with an offer of a 55 percent price cut. Yet even this price reduction was hardly enough. At US$1,000 for Kaletra, per patient, per year, the drug remained out of reach for poor and even middle-income countries.[35] This continued to be a spark that fueled flames of a fight between middle-income and wealthier countries backing their pharmaceutical companies over the cost, and worth of—at times millions of—human lives.

This fight, this battle, at heart constituted a power struggle between states and both other states, at times backing their pharmaceutical companies' interests, as well as unaccountable global actors and entities, notably the non-state actors and advocates pleading for a certain response to HIV/AIDS. The multi-faceted struggle begs the question: who holds the power? Who determines, who decides how to respond to such a crisis? Who dictates who may live and who must die? Who is responsible? Who is accountable?

---

34   Ibid.

35   Harrison, V. 2007. "Abbot to Lower Price of HIV Drug." *Pharmaceutical Business Review Online* (11 April).

*5.7.3 The Role and Impact of Pharmaceutical Drugs for
HIV/AIDS in South Africa*

Though drugs, and the fights over them, are far from the only factors in HIV/AIDS treatment—other components include overall health infrastructure, accessibility of healthcare, treatment of opportunistic infections, adequate nutrition and food security, and receptiveness and responsiveness to treatment including the ongoing struggle against stigma—they constitute and represent a real lifeline. Indeed, attesting to this, in the wake of the 1998–2001 court case in South Africa, outlined above, the pace of initiatives for drug access rapidly accelerated. These were spurred in particular by local-global alliances of advocates and activists, as well as by business initiatives both individually and through supply chains, and by the peer pressure of the United Nation's International Labor Organization's Program (ILO) on HIV/AIDS and the world of work, and outfits such as the New York based GBC, founded by former US Ambassador Richard Holbrooke, who also helped to bring the issue of HIV/AIDS before the UN Security Council.

These were also enabled by the development of generic ARVs. The entry of these drugs onto international markets promised to transform HIV/AIDS from a debilitating disease ending in swift death to a chronic, manageable illness, and not only for those well enough and wealthy enough to afford patented medications. Foremost among these were the innovations by Indian manufacturers not yet bound by the TRIPS accord,[36] which combined different active ingredient formulas, otherwise patented by competing companies, into one pill. So in February 2001, Indian generic manufacturer Cipla offered a combination pill for first-line antiretroviral treatment to the market for US$350 per patient per year, a marked contrast to the thousands of dollars which patented HIV/AIDS treatment cost. The availability of generics was also underscored by the passage at the World Trade Organization's ministerial conference at Doha, of a waiver stating the intellectual property should not take precedence over public health, seemingly paving the way for more generic manufacturing and importation.[37]

Acknowledging the trend towards prioritizing public health over absolute patent rights, pharmaceutical companies joined in the furor of facilitating access to antiretroviral drugs, notably by establishing local-to-global partnerships. For

---

36   All countries were exempted from applying these provisions to drugs invented before 1995, which could be copied and manufactured as generics. Those drugs invented after 1995 which were under patent could be coped via compulsory licensing especially in the case of national emergency, though this continued to be contested. The timetable to introduce TRIPS-compliant legislation varied from one year for the developed, Western countries, to up to 20 years (extended to 2016) for the least developed countries.

37   Article paragraphs 31f and 31h of TRIPS. For more information, see also Wogart, Jan Peter, Gilberto Calcagnotto, Wolfgang Hein, and Christian von Soest. 2008. "AIDS, Access to Medicines, and the Different Roles of the Brazilian and South African Governments in Global Health Governance." GIGA.

instance, GlaxoSmithKline (GSK) granted South African generics' manufacturer, Aspen Pharmacare, a voluntary license under which the latter could produce GSK's antiretroviral drugs AZT, 3TC, and Combivir. GSK exempted Aspen Pharmacare from paying royalties to GSK with the proviso that Aspen donate 30 percent of its net sales too one or more non-governmental organization fighting HIV/AIDS in South Africa. This development undoubtedly boosted GSK's public image as the concept of 'corporate social responsibility' (CSR) came into vogue, and also promoted the burgeoning local-to-global alliances around HIV/AIDS.

The most significant of such alliance involves South Africa's local TAC. Inspired in part by the anti-apartheid struggle in which many of its leaders were active as well as by American AIDS activists such as ACT-UP, TAC joined with MSF of France in what would prove a powerful such alliance focused primarily on the provision of antiretroviral drugs.

In April 2000, TAC and MSF teamed up to launch HAART at three public clinics in the informal settlement of Khayalitsha, on the outskirts of Cape Town. In January 2002, three members of the TAC traveled to Brazil, where Mbeki had given his Bahia address quoted from above, and returned with generic antiretroviral drugs for use in Khayalitsha. This action contravened laws against the import of medications by individuals and put the South African Government in an awkward position regarding its 2001 pledge not to pursue parallel imports. Yet the move was immensely popular, if not practical. It is also illustrative of the applied pressure of local-to-global alliances particularly on state structures.

The alliance has two key consequences. First, it illustrates the possibility of providing complex treatment in a resource-poor setting. It also showcases one effect of local-global cooperation, which appears to assume some of the traditional tasks of national government, without, however, taking on the responsibility and accountability that ultimately rests with the sovereign state. As a result, the control sphere of the government becomes yet more circumscribed. Second, the alliance evidences the evolution of a local movement to one that "worked within global structures of governance and assistance."[38] In the short-term it provided HAART treatment to a limited number of patients and shamed the South African Government into implementing a more comprehensive response to the epidemic. Yet over the longer-term, it compromises the government's control of its decision-making regarding HIV/AIDS intervention as the alliance does not assume responsibility and accountability for a sustained HAART program which the South African state must ultimately carry.

Then-President Mbeki reacted badly to this move; possibly trying to play by the established rules of the global market game, at the cost of lives of his domestic constituency. So seemingly incongruently, instead of embracing and acting upon the evidence clearly established, and still pursuing his focus on poverty and domestic sovereignty, President Mbeki lashed out at the insinuation that Africans were

---

38   De Waal, A. 2006. *AIDS and Power: Why There is No Political Crisis—Yet.* London & New York: Zed Books: 9.

uniquely predisposed to acquire and transmit HIV. In the fall of 2002, in an email written largely by former ANC Youth League head Peter Mokaba, to members of his cabinet, Mbeki had reiterated his accusation that Western pharmaceutical companies stood to profit from the spreading epidemic.[39] These companies did profit, though only after it was established that Africans could access medicines; but, as evidenced above, business was also at the forefront of ensuring that its employees had such access.

Desperate to prove that South Africa was an exception in a world that routinely condemned black governments to failure, and also a success in turning a revolutionary movement into managed governance, Mbeki and his allies dismissed the criticism of the president's questioning the link between HIV/AIDS and asserting the toxicity of antiretroviral drugs and refusing to make them publicly available, as racist and refused to admit they had erred. Mbeki warned the ANC would not be cowed by "racists hankering for an apartheid past" or those who "wanted to see a black government fail to prove their own beliefs that blacks cannot govern efficiently."[40] Dlamini-Zuma, once one of the most vocal advocates warning of the HIV and AIDS crisis and calling for interventions, spewed vitriol on the Democratic Alliance (DA), saying "if they had their way, we would all die of AIDS."[41] In sum, however, it is Mbeki who doubtlessly infused skepticism and injected confusion regarding the epidemic back into an already contentiously debated arena and in doing so served to undermine efforts to address HIV/AIDS. As such, his words might be regarded as reflecting frustration of being constrained by uncontrollable externalities of disease and impossible financial demands. That loss of control is most obvious in the interaction between the government and the pharmaceutical industry. Without generic medications which the South African Government foreswore to pursue after the loss of the 2001 TRIPS' trial, or external funding, which it would accept, South Africa could not meet its responsibility to respond. That bind infuriated Mbeki. It epitomized his lack of control over necessary interventions to provide for and protect the South African populace, and showed the limits of South Africa's domestic sovereignty. The pharmaceutical arena thus became the—repeated—target of Mbeki's ire. His anger, however, did nothing to enable Mbeki or his government to assume integrated tactical and ultimate responsibility and accountability for responding to South Africa's HIV/AIDS epidemic.

Making matters worse, the Minister of Health, Manto Tshabalala-Msimang, allegedly blocked a Global Fund grant intended for HIV/AIDS response in South Africa's hardest-hit province of KwaZulu-Natal. She cited procedural irregularities in her decision, but reinforced the public perception of inequality: like that incurred after the revelation of ANC parliamentarians receiving ARVs

---

39   Gumede, W. 2005. *Thabo Mbeki and the Battle for the Soul of the ANC.* Cape Town: Zebra Publishers: 163.

40   Ibid. 155.

41   Ibid.

while these were denied the public, KwaZulu-Natal, a poor, majority Zulu province, was denied HIV/AIDS funding by a Xhosa-dominated leadership.

Reacting to this and to similarly thwarted efforts to roll-out antiretroviral treatment across South Africa, the TAC took the Minister of Health to court for murder, and threatened to charge her with genocide. Though the government's actions and inactions fall short of exhibiting concrete evidence of killing or wanting to kill HIV-infected citizens of South Africa, and therefore for invoking R2P, the neglect of the needs of those is a failure of the state to protect human and especially health rights: a failure of its responsibility to respond.[42]

Despite this furor, it is worth noting that TAC's ideology and tactics stem from the anti-apartheid struggle, as noted in the previous chapter. As such, TAC and its leaders were and are integral products of and players in the shaping of South Africa's democracy. "TAC uses some of the same language of people's struggle, because that is South Africa's language of politics," and

> TAC has no agenda of overthrowing the government or denying its legitimacy. Many remain as members of the ANC. Not only do they have personal friends and comrades within the party and government, but they are very sympathetic to many of the policies of the Mbeki government. It is their government and constitution; they are still proud of both.[43]

As TAC has been the most vocal local voice against the actions of the South African Government on HIV/AIDS, its criticisms cut deeply through history into the present. TAC and Mbeki were on the same side, only it seems impossible to see amidst the lines drawn in the sand. Together though, TAC and the government would find a way to cross the rubicon of AIDS response and at the same time safeguard the state and its ability to assume its responsibility to respond.

Indeed, South Africa was busy re-writing its patent laws and challenging TRIPS. The government launched an Annual HIV/AIDS and STD [sexually transmitted diseases] Review. While the former action appeared to stall South Africa's response to the HIV/AIDS epidemic, the latter acknowledged the crisis and set out to find a solution. Seemingly incongruent to each other, both actually were closely related.

In particular, both initiatives confront the issue of financing. South Africa's challenge to TRIPS centered on the cost of providing ARVs to its populace,

---

42   See Lisk, F. 2009. *Global Institutions and the HIV/AIDS Epidemic*. New York: Routledge Global Institutions: 73: "It was in the context of its WHO/GPA's global AIDS strategy of 1987 that universal human rights were linked with the protection and needs of PLWHA. This was the first time that a public health strategy had been framed in human rights terms and anchored in international law and, by implication, made governments ultimately responsible for the health and well-being of their populations."

43   De Waal, A. 2006. *AIDS and Power: Why There is No Political Crisis—Yet*. London & New York: Zed Books: 37.

and the Annual Review addressed the same challenge. In it the government advocated ensuring adequate funding at national and provincial levels within the healthcare environment to ensure delivery; and recommended an agreed-upon resource standard for all provinces to directly place financial resources into HIV/AIDS. Though sound recommendations, notably for integrating HIV/AIDS measures into the existing healthcare environment, implementing these remains a central problem in South Africa's response to the epidemic.

Putting the challenge into perspective, the Review also noted that the South African government's health funding appropriation per person, per year in 1999/2000 prices amounted to 10 rand.[44] This effectively excluded the ability to fund ARVs.[45]

ARVs, once they were part of possible HIV/AIDS response, remained and dominated the agenda to address the epidemic, both locally and globally. On the one hand, ARVs' inherent promise of longer life instead of the immediacy of death for infected individuals was predicated upon their provision. On the other hand, the South African government's commitment to its democracy became, for the special population segment that was infected and affected by HIV/AIDS and vocal about it, synonymous with ARVs as well. So as the South African Government confronted the high prices and the problems of access to the drugs, amidst competing domestic and international demands, it found itself held hostage, locally and globally, and by correspondingly local-global alliances, to surmounting these.

While the South African Government vacillated on how to meet these competing demands, both its and others, notably non-state and external, responses against the epidemic accumulated. This pattern would eventually lead to a perceived and a practical impotence of the government, which would contribute to compromising its ability to act upon its sovereign responsibilities including its responsibility to respond. Thus instead of merely bowing to the pressure brought to bear by advocacy organizations, as proposed by the boomerang theory, similar organizations would actually do the work expected of the government, shifting the tactical but not the ultimate responsibility entailed therein.

---

44   The South African Department of Health 2000. "HIV/AIDS/STD Strategic Plan for South Africa, 2000–2005" (February): 29.

45   Perhaps in an effort to offer an alternative, in 1997 the South African government supported a purported "African cure" to HIV/AIDS. This "African cure," Virodene, later proved to be a toxic substance, but the battle over its admission and administration reached Parliament and pitted advocates of Western and traditional or indigenous medicines against each other. It would take nearly another decade for these two opposing groups to cooperate, in some of the ways which Professor Sher advocated at the beginning of the epidemic. In the meantime, the Virodene scandal seemed to eclipse much of the South African government's efforts to fight the HIV/AIDS epidemic.

5.8 (Forcing) Decision-making

Despite its priority-setting of the independent exercise of its domestic sovereignty, South Africa could not wait until that realization was perfected to decide upon a course of action against HIV/AIDS. It had already tested the patience of an increasingly vocal activist sector in South Africa, and lost. Those activists, the TAC foremost among them, were forging alliances with international donors and NGOs, networks that were addressing HIV/AIDS outside of government control. The result served paradoxically to the intent of South Africa's policy priorities, to undermine the state's domestic sovereignty as opposed to shoring it up.

The South African Government moved to make decisions[46] to respond to HIV/AIDS and to take control of that response. In doing so, it confronted plagues over its (self-) perception and its practice of sovereign statehood. While not completely abandoning the obfuscation that characterized Mbeki's questioning of the link between HIV/AIDS, the government clarified its stance on the relationship between the epidemic and poverty, and its aspired-to role in changing the global "rules of the game," and embarked on a practical response to the impact of the disease.

5.8.1 Perception and Practice

In the meantime, the South African Government formally acknowledged the severity of the spreading HIV/AIDS epidemic and launched some stratagems to address it. On behalf of President Mandela, who, despite his early meeting with Professor Sher, remained silent on the issue of HIV throughout his presidency, Deputy President Mbeki announced the inauguration of the "Partnership against AIDS" on 9 October 1998, excerpts of which were quoted above. Mbeki expressed recognition of the present and potential threat posed by a spreading HIV/AIDS epidemic. However, the Partnership has yet to produce any tangible results. Measures to address the crisis remained mired in the debate between an immediate medical response and the economic priorities of the democracy. The fact that the two were and are increasingly intertwined would complicate attempts to separate them in initiatives against the epidemic and attempts to safeguard the South African economy and it as a base of the provision of comprehensive security and welfare.

Illustrating this, also in October 1999 South African Minister of Health, Manto Tshabalala-Msimang rejected the Medical Control Council's (MCC) approval of the first antiretroviral medication. Highlighting safety issues, the Minister cited

---

46   See also Czempiel, E.-O. 1992. "Governance and democratization." In *Governance without Government: Order and Change in World Politics* (eds) Rosenau, J. and Czempiel, E.-O. Cambridge: Cambridge University Press: 258; on decision-making as a definitive function of a sovereign state, notably according to the function of a "rule," and thus of acting according to "rules of the game," as applied to sovereign states and impacting their domestic—as opposed to their Wesphalian—sovereignty.

lack of a satisfactory review process as her explanation.[47] While dismissing the evidence collected by the MCC, in November 1999, the Minster commissioned the Cochrane Center, an international healthcare NGO that "reviews clinical trials on new drugs and has branches all over the world, to research the risk of anti-retrovirals, especially AZT."[48] The move sent a message of distrust in the South African MCC versus that of an international NGO, seemingly undermining the country's own credibility.

This reaction to the initial tension in turn instigated what would evolve into a series of reactionary responses. In an alternating pattern, on the one hand, the South African government would dismiss indigenous knowledge in the fight against the disease. On the other hand, it would question Western science, its efficacy, and its motives in pushing its medicines to treat HIV/AIDS, especially in Africa. All the while, pressure to respond to the epidemic and to maintain a functioning macro-economy would increase. As the epidemic intensified and the government took spurious action against it, Mbeki would return to the separate and integrated themes of epidemic and economy, but the government's rhetorical and practical responses were no match for the virulence of the virus.

Still the speeches soared—with validity. On World AIDS Day, 1 December 1999, President Mbeki spelled out the specific threats of HIV/AIDS for the South African economy. He iterated deep concern for the future of each infected and affected individual's survival, and also for the survival of the state of South Africa, saying

> Every day a child suffers and has to learn to fend for him or herself when a parent dies as a result of this disease. Every day, when someone, who is infected, dies, we lose a lifetime of skills and experiences; we suffer a blow to our economy that we have only just begun to rebuild.[49]

He added a call to all South Africans to cooperate with each other locally and with the global community to educate, and to work together to protect and preserve individuals and economic investments threatened by HIV/AIDS across the board. He cited in particular, agriculture, mining, factories, schools, hospitals, and government. Mbeki noted further that "there can be no talk of an African renaissance, if AIDS is at the door of our continent."[50] Yet later, Mbeki would renege on this stance, striving to 'rescue' South Africa and its renaissance, even as HIV/AIDS already crossed the threshold of the continent and country.

That reality did prompt responses more than mere rhetoric. In contravention to a Ministry of Health prohibition on the provision of Nevirapine, an antiretroviral

47   Gumede, W. 2005. *Thabo Mbeki and the Battle for the Soul of the ANC*. Cape Town: Zebra Publishers: 160.

48   Ibid.

49   Mbeki, T. 1999. "Address on World AIDS Day" (1 December). Available at http://www.anc.org.za/ancdocs/history/mbeki/ [accessed: 1 July 2012].

50   Ibid.

instrumental in preventing mother-to-child-transmission (MTCT) when given just before, at and after birth, the Premier of KwaZulu-Natal, Dr LPHM Mtshali, announced he would accept pharmaceutical giant Boehringer Ingelheim's offer of the antiretroviral Nevirapine for free, and would roll-out PMTCT in the province. Nearly five years after the acknowledgement of the crisis of HIV/AIDS in the 1997 Annual Review, hastened by the lack of subsequent practical action, he said

> We had to act, and may God forgive us for waiting so long. We shall not wait one day longer, nor allow any space for further excuse, delaying tactic or preposterous theory which may get in the way of saving our children … For me this is a matter of principle and common decency. I have turned upside-down the scientific facts to find a reason which can justify the failure to act and ameliorate the suffering and reduce the death of so many of our children, [and] I have found one. The undisputed facts before me are that there are sound scientific bases on which Nevirapine is recommended, which include that it is effective in reducing the number of HIV/AIDS infected babies born to HIV-positive mothers. It is cost-effective in that it is more expensive not to treat [and have to treat sick persons later] and it is safe. There to me is where the issue stops.[51]

The Premier's statement marks a significant shift in the political perception and prioritization of the response to HIV/AIDS. Up until this point South Africa's presidents—Mandela and Mbeki—set the tone and charted the course: of silence, of deferral. This desperate cry, from a leader at the relatively lower echelons of government but at the frontlines of the response to HIV/AIDS, yields an echo. It also signaled a broader shift.

Shortly after the KwaZulu-Natal premier's initiative, additional provinces including Gauteng, the Eastern Cape and Limpopo, likewise made Nevirapine available to prevent mother-to-child-transmission followed suit. The battle over Nevirapine illustrates South Africa's sense of being beleaguered between its sovereign responsibility to respond and the dependence implied in order to achieve this goal. Yet the debate over the provision of drugs, especially in light of the newest (2013) WHO recommendations to provide ART to all infected persons regardless of CD4 count, is ongoing.

5.8.2 Practice as Policy Implementation

Notwithstanding the internal struggle over whether to confront the swelling HIV/AIDS epidemic, South Africa did continue to seek ways to answer the 'how' of response to counter the crisis. In January 2000 the South African Government launched the South African National AIDS Council (SANAC). Meant as an umbrella organization for all of South Africa's AIDS initiatives, it lacked sufficient

---

51   Nattrass, N. 2007. *Mortal Combat: AIDS Denialism and the Struggle for Antiretrovirals in South Africa*. Scottsville: University of KwaZulu-Natal Press: 100.

streamlining to function, encompassing so many bureaucracies as to become unmanageable. It includes 16 government ministries, 18 government departments, the parliamentary committees on health, as well as 17 civil society sectors,[52] numbering at least 51 participants.

SANAC is not alone in its role as an overarching AIDS coordinating body. Included among the myriad of other coordinating and oversight organizations are: the South African Cabinet, which has decision-making authority over HIV and AIDS policies; the Inter-Ministerial Committee on AIDS (IMC), chaired by the Deputy President and composed of the Ministers of Health, Social Development, Education, Agriculture and Land Affairs, Mining, Public Service and Administration; and the Policy Committee of the National Health Council (NHC), which assembles the Minister, Deputy Minister, Director General and all Deputy Director Generals of Health, all provincial health MECs (members of the executive council) and their Heads of Department. In addition, HIV/AIDS policy is organized domestically by the Social Sector Cluster, which brings together all government departments; a national Interdepartmental HIV/AIDS Committee; and individual HIV/AIDS Units in all government departments. Finally, there are also a slew of so-called "Additional Implementing Agencies," which refer mainly to provincial, district and local authorities and which are oftentimes augmented by local and global community service and non-governmental organizations addressing HIV/AIDS.

A zigzag line of ostensibly hierarchical policy-making runs through this assortment of ministries, departments, organizations, and civil society, non-state actor, representatives. Yet nowhere does it clarify exactly who does what and who is responsible and accountable for that doing:

The Cabinet regularly delegates HIV/AIDS discussion to the IMC, while retaining its decision-making authority. This stymies the process of policy analysis through implementation. Similarly, the other assorted institutional entities as well as individual players involved can continuously devolve and redistribute responsibility. Accountability becomes a casualty of this revolving process. The result has been prevaricating HIV/AIDS policy and practice.

Beyond HIV/AIDS, this pattern points to another broad theme. It is indicative of the prevailing and wide-ranging contest over prioritization, assumption of responsibility and alignment with accountability. It is a question of power and authority within the country: political and economic, exiles and inciles; and externally, with pressure applied by state and non-state alliances. Within these strictures, the country is attempting to align its policy prescriptions with its practical capabilities and capacities and its aspirations, while also taking into account local and global demands upon it. This leads to inconsistent policies and applications, which interact and are aptly illustrated in the case of HIV/AIDS. Moreover, the

---

52   South African National Department of Health website, www.doh.gov.za [accessed: 1 July 2012].

scope and assumption of responsibility and accountability become entangled, both locally and globally, with no clear delineation of authority. The result is the GAP.

5.9 Conclusion

At the end of these first two phases of South Africa's response to its HIV/AIDS epidemic, two conclusions can be drawn. First, the coincidence of the end of the apartheid era with the dawn of democracy in South Africa colluded to do irreparable damage to any response to the burgeoning epidemic. International as well as national priorities were far from the insipient epidemic. When the former focused on the issue, the latter remained by turns preoccupied and insistent on an alternative course. Second, the overriding demand of external actors on a particular response to the epidemic served to emasculate the South African response, both politically and tactically, while neglecting to establish an 'in the event of' framework that would secure sustainable responsibility and accountability. Seizing on this GAP, and as national and international conditions shifted, so, too, did the political course, in a third phase. It also saw the South African state (re)claim some of its circumvented sovereignty and control over its responsibility to respond.

Chapter 6
Policy Polemics II:
Rising to the Challenge of HIV/AIDS

The existence of the GAP, whose emergence is illustrated in the previous chapter, becomes clearer in the final phase of the analysis of South Africa's HIV/AIDS response presented here. This is because in the years from 2003 through 2013, the focus of this chapter, the South African Government assumed not only responsibility but also accountability in its response to the HIV/AIDS epidemic. In doing so, South Africa ceased to deny the reality of the GAP or to exonerate its roles, and instead sought to confront and to bridge it in both word and deed; spelling out what the country could afford and allocating amassed domestic funding to fit a locally designed response, as opposed to allowing ad hoc interventions sourced with outside support. This shift parallels a broader change in global (aid) policy, towards "country ownership," which, as in the case of South Africa, is and can be possible where and when a country rises to the occasion of its responsibility and demand, credibly and capably, that the accountability dispersed by the GAP rest ultimately with it.

In the run-up to this new phase, the GAP yawned wide. Reflecting it, a dual set of external influences on South Africa's prioritization and response to HIV/AIDS arrived in conjunction with TRIPS-Plus in 2000. It tipped the balance in response to HIV/AIDS towards a more immediate medical and away from an alternative, preventative and holistic approach. The benefit of the immediate medical approach lay in the long-term gains reaped from a large up-front investment in treatment and care to contain current human and economic costs, and to forestall further infections; its drawback in the precariousness of the initial balance-of-payments, (in)terminable dependence upon external sources of finance and inputs, including drugs, and the incalculable rates of infection and resistance, the latter raising the costs of further future treatment and care. At the same time, this tipping point would provide an impetus for the South African Government to grab the reigns of its response, especially to ensure the validity of its ultimate accountability. The timing was (still) not of the country's choosing, but the time was ripe nonetheless.

Starting with TRIPS-Plus and the game changer it represented: the TRIPS-Plus laws' breadth exceeds the protection of intellectual property rights entailed in the original TRIPS agreements. They are usually introduced into bilateral trade agreements in return for greater investment, particularly by the United States. An executive order signed by President Clinton also in 2000 and endorsed by President Bush in 2001 exempted southern Africa. However, parallel to that exemption, the

Bush Administration pursued a free-trade agenda with Southern Africa, which affected access to ARVs.

Following upon its introduction and adoption, whatever else the intended consequences, the TRIPS-Plus policies spurred local-to-global alliances. These notably benefit select interest groups which pursue their aims within the conditions created by such foreign and similar international legislation successfully. The ensuing alliances play a pivotal role in contributing to circumscribing the South African Government's attempt to keep control over its domestic sovereignty while also exercising its ability to act according to norms of its sovereign accountability to responsibility to respond—though the government's at times reactionary response has also abetted this process.[1]

A number of notable international developments indicate the emergence of the above local-global alliances. In July 2000 at the 13th International AIDS Conference, activists staged a march demanding access to treatment. The same month, the United Nations General Assembly convened the first-ever special session on a disease, focusing on HIV/AIDS. In the session's wake, the United Nations Security Council passed Resolution 1308, which designated HIV/AIDS a "threat to international peace and security,"[2] raising both awareness of the epidemic and the stakes in addressing or neglecting it.

Later that same year, on 18 September 2000, the United Nations General Assembly adopted the Millennium Development Goals (MDGs). Each goal is accompanied by a series of explicit targets. The sixth goal pertains to HIV/AIDS and articulates the aim to "combat HIV/AIDS, malaria, and other diseases,"[3] and according to 6A, to "have halted by 2015 and begun to reverse the spread of HIV/AIDS."[4] A bit of time remains before the judgments over the achievement of this goal fall.

In the meantime, the United Nations and especially the Security Council's recognition of HIV/AIDS as being more than merely a health issue, contributed to greater understanding and appreciation of the role of health and disease as threats not only to individual lives, but broadly to peace-keeping, social cohesion,

---

1   The circumscribing of the responsibility and authority associated with sovereignty is not solely attributable to intervening internal social and external forces. However, these internal social and external forces and influences, and the reactions they inspire, such as the former South African Minister of Health Manto Tshabalala-Msimang's attempts to thwart access to anti-retroviral therapy and to establish herself as the final authority on medicines' approval (see also Kapp, C. 2008. "New hope for health in South Africa." *The Lancet*, 372, 1207–1208) do contribute to curbed state sovereignty.

2   Initially, the United Nations Security Council considered HIV/AIDS as a particular threat to peacekeeping operations. This perception was, however, likely slightly overblown, but the general concern over the influence of HIV/AIDS on peace, security, and stability remains a central tenet of assessments of the epidemic regionally and globally.

3   United Nations 2000. Millennium Development Goals, Goal 6 "Combat HIV/AIDS, Maleria and other diseases." United Nations.

4   Ibid.

economic growth and development, and political stability. As a result, the above-listed events and associated promises heralded a new era of AIDS-awareness and set the stage for concerted action.

6.1 Phase Three (c. 2003–2013): Carryover and Continuation

Global voices joined the fray to facilitate drug access and to put pressure on the South African Government. In addition to the Global Fund to Fight AIDS, Tuberculosis and Malaria, as well as initiatives of the World Bank and UNAIDS, in January 2003 US President George W. Bush launched PEPFAR. The funds were to be dispersed in the original 15 focus countries including South Africa, as well as in a total of nearly 100 others. Though some finance is directed through the Global Fund, PEPFAR's multilateral coordination is unmatched by its bilateral emphasis.

Most significant is PEPFAR's financial contribution to the fight against the HIV/AIDS epidemic: it is by far the largest donor program in the world. This has two major consequences in the case of South Africa. On the one hand it alleviates some of the financial burden of the South African Government's response to HIV/AIDS. On the other hand, in doing so and creating a parallel response structure tied to an external source, PEPFAR largely bypasses that same South African government, supplanting some sovereign control. Applications and approvals of PEPFAR-funded projects are processed by the US Embassy and managed by US representatives, relieving the South African Government of some of its capacity as well as funding constraints, but without assuming accountability to the South African government or its citizenry and recipients of PEPFAR aid. Instead PEPFAR remains answerable to the US Government and US taxpayers.[5]

PEPFAR, with all of its potential and problems, reignites the contest over access to antiretroviral drugs. In its initial inception, PEPFAR stipulated the almost exclusive purchase of patented antiretroviral drugs. This reinforced the monopoly of many of the pharmaceutical companies active in the development of HIV/AIDS drugs and broadly expanded their market reach. These include: Abbott Laboratories, Boehringer Ingelheim, Bristol-Myers Squibb, GlaxoSmithKline, Merck Sharp and Dome, Novartis, Pfizer and Roche. PEPFAR did later endorse the use of some select generic ARVs, notably those produced by Aspen Pharmacare of South Africa and Cipla in India.[6]

As is evidenced, the antiretroviral market is dominated by a very limited number of brand-name and even fewer generic companies. In addition, PEPFAR requires USFDA approval of all of drugs purchased with its funding, even in

---

5   Despite the renewal of PEPFAR in 2008, intended to continue into the nearer and even foreseeable future, the program is subject to annual Congressional review and budgetary allocation. It remains to be seen whether this program, amongst many others, will survive the financial crisis and turmoil of 2008/2009 and beyond.

6   See charts on HIV/AIDS pharmaceuticals below.

cases where the WHO has already authorized the use of particular drugs. This hampers procurement and timely access to these vital treatments while increasing their expense. Consequently, options for treatment are limited and not always predictable, and are further constrained by the especially high prices of second-line treatment. These aspects play prominent roles both in South Africa's budgeting for ongoing, sustainable treatment and in the associated perception and reality of its ability to negotiate and deliver the best possible intervention against HIV/AIDS for its populace.

As such, secondly, this did and does put the South African Government in a precarious position. If it acquiesces to a system of ARV supply as part of a response to HIV/AIDS, it has to accept that it cannot completely control the inputs and outcomes. This situation is characteristic of limited statehood, and includes circumscribed control over shifts in the market involving prices and availability and therefore access to ARVs, while at the same time subordinating itself—the state—to the procurement of these medicines to improve and prolong the lives of its HIV-infected citizens. This circumscribed state sovereignty is further characterized by a lack of state control over the consequences of such a policy on its sustainability and on its domestic sovereignty more broadly, including its ability to and assumption of its responsibility to respond.

This led, third, beyond these realities which threatened to implicate the South African state in reneging on its responsibility to respond, in the state instead reassessing options.

Thus, in April 2003 Hetero, a generic antiretroviral manufacturer following on Cipla's example from two years prior, announced it would offer its medicines for a mere US$201 per patient per year. The offer seemed to underscore the enhanced feasibility of a treatment-oriented HIV/AIDS response. Yet in June the MCC deregistered the Nevirapine as well as numerous first-line treatment regimens. This sparked cries of outrage and demand from within South Africa, and echoed from outside of the country and accelerated the emergence of the local-global alliances evolving and circumventing the South African Government's control over its domestic sovereignty in the HIV/AIDS arena. On 12 August, the Rural Doctors Association of South Africa (RuDASA) appealed to the government for leadership and resources to manage HIV and AIDS in the public sector. On 20 August, HIV/AIDS doctors expressed anger at the MCC's "unacceptably slow" registration of a 600mg dose of the anti-AIDS drug efavirenz, made by Merck. On 14 September, the MCC reaffirmed the safety of Nevirapine. With that Nevirapine decision, the arch that bound AIDS activists from local as well as global arenas converged on the ground in South Africa. Capitalizing on this organizational momentum as well as the rising outrage over stymied access to ARVs amidst awareness of the availability of generics, on 26 September, the Generic Antiretroviral Procurement Project and the TAC Treatment Project asked pharmaceutical giant Boehringer Ingelheim for permission to import generic Nevirapine for use in combination antiretroviral therapy. Disregarding the South African Government's 2001 acquiescence to pharmaceutical demands not to issue compulsory licenses or to engage in parallel imports of antiretroviral drugs, and in the process thereby circumventing the state's sovereign control over its trade and health policies, the two NGOs threatened to take Boehringer Ingelheim to court to issue compulsory licenses if it did not agree. The company quickly relented and granted the Generic Antiretroviral Procurement Project and TAC permission to produce Nevirapine. As the local-global arch converged and assumed tactical tasks in providing for ARVs. Pitted against it, the South African Government appeared little more than a bystander, or worse, a thwarter of HIV/AIDS drug provision. It appeared to have little control over, and therefore limited sovereignty in its responsibility to respond, despite its initial, tentative, steps to (re)assert its sovereignty while also responding to HIV/AIDS.

Consequently, PEPFAR most profoundly illustrates the long-term human security costs of unresolved delineation of responsibility without corresponding accountability. First, it bound the South African state to provide a level of ARV provision which it might or might not be able to guarantee on its own. Second, it introduced the volatility of exchange rate fluctuations into an equation where the state would have to purchase, in rand converted into dollars, the ARVs it required. Finally, this external facilitation of HIV treatment as well as the associated state and budget dependency would implicate the South African Government in meeting citizens' rights' demands over which it maintained questionable ability to act to deliver on a guaranteed basis on that sovereign responsibility and accountability. As has been illustrated and argued here, this guarantee remains with the state.

The very circumscription of domestic sovereignty, particularly of guaranteeing the welfare of its citizens, in this case, of the state's ability to afford treatment of HIV/AIDS, resulted in the local-global outcry and alliances that led to prevention, treatment, and care interventions that have not resolved but rendered 'manageable' this particular pandemic. Second, at the same time, this intervention, offered without the appropriation of the accountability attenuated to sovereignty, at the same, forced South Africa to reassert its sovereignty, its ownership of the response to its HIV/AIDS epidemic because when the funding dried up in the midst of the global financial crisis of 2007–2008, South Africa was left responsible for the rescue without the lifeline.

Already in the interim, however, the South African Government tried to rectify this before such a rescue was necessary.

In October 2003, the South African Cabinet committed the government to providing universal access to HAART through the public sector, allocating initially 296 million rand for ARVs, increased to 300 million rand for 2004/2005, and then for 2005/2006 the total HIV/AIDS budget increased to 4.3 billion rand, nearly a billion rand more than the previous fiscal year allocation. On 19 November, the South African Cabinet approved the Operational Plan for Comprehensive Treatment and Care for HIV/AIDS. Reflecting the previous HIV/AIDS fights, their aftermath, and the political-economic shifts chronicled above, the South African Cabinet attributed the feasibility of the roll-out foremost to:

1. A fall in the price of drugs over the past two years without which this program would have been impossible, including new opportunities to manufacture some of these drugs in South Africa, as well as successful negotiations with pharmaceutical companies.

2. Second, the roll-out was arguably made possible by the availability of and access to: new medicines and international and local experience in managing the utilization of ARVs and other interventions.[7]

3. Thirdly, it referred to an attendant focal point of South Africa's HIV/AIDS response, one which would repeatedly crop up both as a positive and as a negative dimension: growing appreciation of the role of nutrition in enhancing people's health and efficacy of medicines.[8]

4. Fourth, it emphasized the building of a critical mass of health workers and scientists with skills and understanding of the management of HIV/AIDS.[9]

5. Fifth and finally, the Cabinet again cited the availability of fiscal resources to expand social expenditure in general, as a consequence of prudent macro-economic policies pursued by government as a key contributing factor to the ability of the South African government to launch a public sector antiretroviral roll-out at this time.

Each of these points underscores South Africa's focus on independence, both in rendering its policy decision to respond to HIV/AIDS and to effect that decision. As such it is a policy predicated on South Africa's concrete ability to fulfill its responsibility to respond.

It marked another start, but not the finish in South Africa's response to HIV/AIDS.

Belatedly renewing its sense and seizing its ownership of HIV/AIDS response, in the run-up to the first South African AIDS Conference, held in Durban in August 2003, the South African Government formally announced its endorsement of a national treatment plan, including ARVs. Cabinet approved the provisional

---

7 The issue of "other interventions" would later become contested territory, as South Africa's controversial Minister of Health, Manto Tshabalala-Msimang would, to offer a well-ridiculed example, promote garlic, beetroot, lemon, and the African potato as a—dangerous—alternative to ARVs.

8 Nutrition, notably adequate and balanced nutrition, is vital for the uptake, tolerance, and effectiveness of antiretrovirals. As mentioned in the above, however, nutrition should not be seen as a substitute to ARVs.

9 Achieving such a "critical mass" of health workers and scientists with expertise in the field of HIV/AIDS is an ongoing challenge, plagued in particular by the so-called brain drain of health professionals from the public to the private sector, as well as from South Africa internationally, and also by the drainage of health care professionals from other medical fields to HIV/AIDS, leaving these decimated even while HIV/AIDS services expand. Much more can be said on this topic, and will be touched upon in the evaluation and conclusion in chapters seven and eight as related to domestic sovereignty and the state's responsibility to respond.

plan on 8 August, and recalling previous endeavors such as cooperation with the Cochrane Center on AZT, South Africa experts joined hands with the Clinton AIDS Foundation to create the operational plan, which was adopted on 19 November 2003, and launched with a slight delay in April 2004. South Africa finally received yearned-for global accolades.

The roll-out coincided almost exactly with the 2004 elections. These took place on 15 April 2004, and the ANC won 69.68 percent of the vote. This seems to indicate roaring approval of ANC government and governance. Yet the apparent enthusiasm hardly masks the transformative face HIV/AIDS put on the country: the voters' roll indicates that almost 1.5 million of South Africa's 20,674,926 million voters were removed between 1999 and 2003 due to death. The increase in mortality among ages 30–49 clearly indicates the relationship between HIV and that mortality.[10] Thus despite the ANC's resounding 2004 electoral victory, given the surrounding circumstances particularly pertaining to HIV/AIDS, "dwindling trust between government and electorate, hollowing out of the electoral process and of the legislature, demands for AIDS treatment, external influences and long-term demographic and intergenerational breach effects described above could all come together to produce odd and unexpected results."[11] Perhaps aware of the precariousness of its hold on power, the government pushed ahead with its planned roll-out.

However, things did not go especially smoothly. The Operational Plan aimed to have 54,000 people on treatment in the public sector by March 2004. Instead the roll-out only got off the ground that April, and so in March, it had none.[12] The promised funding allocation of 296 million rand allotted for ARVs alone only arrived in August 2004, when the National Treasury announced a 300 million rand allocation to the Department of Health for its comprehensive HIV/AIDS treatment plan for fiscal year 2004/2005. The plan was over a year late. Even by March 2005, the public sector roll-out only met 80 percent of its intended target; that is about 43,000 people. The program was also unable to spend its National Treasury allocation, resulting not only in under-serving treatment, but also in a spending gap. Nonetheless, the National Treasury increased its budget allocation for 2005/2006, aiming to be able to provide for 150,000 people receiving HAART by March 2006, a target that was actually within reach as 111,786 people were enrolled in HAART in the public sector by the end of December 2005. The Treasury budget estimate sufficed for the estimated 150,000 HAART recipients through 2005, but the Operational Plan's goal of treating 453,650 people by March 2006 was far from met. This in turn led to accusations of lack of capacity—a cause of concern in a health system challenged to cope not only with HIV/AIDS,

10   Barnett, T. 2006. "A Long-Wave Event. HIV/AIDS, Politics, Governance and 'Security'." *International Affairs HIV/AIDS*, Special Issue, 82(2): 309.

11   Ibid., 311.

12   See also Nattrass, N. 2007. *Mortal Combat: AIDS Denialism and the Struggle for Antiretrovirals in South Africa*. Scottsville: University of KwaZulu-Natal Press.

but also with additional opportunistic infections, chronic diseases, and other healthcare concerns, notably maternal and child health.

6.2 National Engagement for the Responsibility to Respond

In the interim, the South African Government repeatedly actors it had left untouched in its hands-off, ad hoc approach to the response to the HIV/AIDS epidemic. Now, assuming more effective responsibility to respond, on 16 October 2003, the South African Competition Commission found Boehringer Ingelheim and GlaxoSmithKline in contravention of the Competition Act for abusing their dominant market positions by charging excessive prices on ARVs. Aiding this ruling were shifting international attitudes altering the balance of power, making it possible for South Africa to reassess its position—and to maintain control of its chosen response to HIV/AIDS arguably from here on out.

Thus for example, in January 2005, the five-year transition period allotted to India to adopt TRIPS-compliant legislation protecting intellectual property rights, ended. As a result, while all drugs developed prior to the introduction of TRIPS in 1995 remained patent-free, those produced generically by a local manufacturer able to prove "significant (own) investment" would automatically be granted a production license though required to additionally pay the original developer a "reasonable" royalty, while all drugs developed after 1995 or never manufactured as a generic were subject to intellectual property right provisions. In the latter case, India could also technically issue a compulsory license to produce such drugs. In fact, further facilitating generic provision, Hetero reduced its price to US$168 per person per year.

Further upping the ante on antiretroviral treatment, on 23 October 2004, the Clinton Foundation announced that it made a deal with generic manufacturers Aspen Pharmacare, Cipla, Ranbaxy, and Matrix on the prices of their ARVs. These companies agreed to sell generic versions of triple-drug therapy at a cost of just under US$13 per monthly dose, or US$156 annually. South Africa would make use of some generics, after its initial locked-in tenders expired, but rejected the Clinton Foundation's brokerage. Nonetheless, the ongoing tensions in the response to the epidemic would continue to exist, as the South African Government placed a premium on its ability to decide and to act against HIV/AIDS as independently as possible. As such, it decided to act when the factors listed above aligned. Nonetheless, just as the government could not insulate itself from the expanding epidemic, neither could it pick and choose its response in perpetuity, removed from the continuously emerging local and global alliances to address it.

At the same time though in the background, the South African Department of Health established 199 public health facilities capable of providing HIV/AIDS related services by the end of 2005, including antiretroviral treatment. These facilities were distributed across all of the country's 53 districts and covered at least 62 percent of local municipalities. They seemed to serve their purpose, albeit slowly: by June 2006, more than 175,000 people were receiving HAART across all 53 of South Africa's districts. By the end of 2012, South African had achieved approximately 60 percent treatment coverage of those who qualified (prior to the May 2013 changed guidelines released by the WHO), according to UNAIDS.

Nonetheless, the initial low numbers of people accessing ARVs certainly constituted cause of alarm. While some of South Africa's provinces successfully executed the ARV roll-out, notably the Western Cape, which reached the Operational Plan's rollout target by mid-2004 and exceeded it by 2005 with the early intervention and assistance from MSF, others proved unable to spend the funds allocated to them. Indeed, much of the success of antiretroviral treatment roll-out in the most affected provinces of KwaZulu-Natal and Gauteng, the Eastern and Western Cape, was significantly supported by external funding, followed by the Eastern and Western Cape, accounting for over 53 percent of recipients in the public sector. Nonetheless, Limpopo only reached 12 percent of the target by the end of 2005, and Gauteng, the Northern Cape, and North West Province only reached roughly 50 percent of the target by the end of 2005.[13]

In addition to the difficulty of reaching such targets was the complication inherent in guaranteeing the sustainability and accountability of the intervention. Indeed, during this initial phase of South Africa's national roll-out, a critical cause of concern was that "one of the driving forces for the public sector rollout appears to be external assistance from donors," who are responsible to their financiers, e.g. their home governments, and not held responsible and accountable to their recipients, who are, ultimately, wards of the state. This leads to the "danger that the contribution of donors to the public sector HAART [highly-active anti-retroviral therapy] rollout has taken the pressure off the national Department of Health to ensure that existing, allocated resources from the national Treasury for the rollout are being used effectively and appropriately."[14] A critical consequence of such reallocation of responsibility is its precariousness. The national government retains constitutional responsibility and accountability for the provision of healthcare for its populace. With the roll-out of antiretroviral treatment in the public sector this means the sustainable implementation of such medical intervention. Yet if external actors are acting out this responsibility, their accountability remains in question.

This disconnect can be seen in relief in the UN General Assembly's Political Declaration 60/262, which firmly places the responsibility for responding to the epidemic with states. While welcoming and lauding the participation of external, non-state actors, it makes no provisions for their accountability.

Perhaps recognizing this danger, in March 2007, the South African Government again moved to address HIV/AIDS. After a review commenced and completed in the aftermath of the International AIDS Conference in Toronto, the South African

---

13   Nattrass, N. 2006. "South Africa's 'Roll-Out' of Highly Active Anti-Retroviral Therapy: A Critical Assessment." *JAIDS Journal of Acquired Immune Deficiency Syndromes*, 43(5): 618–623.

14   Ibid.

Government released the HIV/AIDS and STI[15] National Strategic Plan for South Africa, 2007–2011, under the leadership auspices of Deputy President Phumzile Mlambo-Ngcuka. It reiterates the infrastructural achievements in terms of provision of healthcare facilities and clinics, as well as the general priorities of prevention, treatment and care outlined in each successive HIV/AIDS strategy since 1988. In a nod to Mbeki's numerous articulated concerns regarding African ownership of response to HIV/AIDS, also in 2006, the President set up the Presidential Project on African Traditional Medicine as well as the African Pharmaceutical Industry.[16] Yet despite, or even because of, these initiatives, as indicated in the wake of the 2004 and 2009 elections, pressure on the state to adhere to its constitutional imperatives mounted; showcasing the state's ultimate responsibility to respond.

6.3 Resolving the Dilemma of the Responsibility to Respond for State Sovereignty

Though the national government did not endorse it, in January 2004, the Western Cape government expanded its HAART program. By the end of March, 2000 patients had started treatment, relying on an emergency drug procurement mechanism. This put the government, both provincial and national, in the precarious predicament of having decided, de facto, to extend life-saving treatment to people, but without being prepared to guarantee its sustainability: highlighting the GAP. In the end, the government becomes culpable for any death caused by the subsequent denial of such treatment, but without having actually, legally, assumed or delegated responsibility for treatment in the first place. In addition, the expansion of the Western Cape HAART program set a precedent for other provinces. Indeed, on 15 March, Gauteng announced that it would become the second province to provide antiretroviral drugs to its public sector patients starting on 1 April. This created the perception at least of a heartless national government, and accelerated the acrimony of the fight over scarce resource allocation between HIV/AIDS and other policy priorities.

Conceding its compromised position, the government had accepted a grant from the Global Fund in February 2004 to continue its fight against HIV/AIDS. However, the dependence that accepting the Global Fund grant implied pried open the portals of South Africa's jealously guarded domestic sovereignty. The grant relieved some of the state's financial burden vis-à-vis fighting the epidemic, and therein arguably

---

15   Sexually transmitted infections.

16   Before he died in 2007, Professor Ruben Sher had been working on an "Africanization" project, in which medical facilities in particular would be adapted to African culture, including care facilities that would allow for family stays, as well as the provision of traditional food, and cooperation with traditional healers, sangomas, while also administering "Western" medicines and using "Western" medical technology. This will be touched upon again in the recommendations offered in Chapter 8.

also exonerated the government from some of the responsibility of responding to HIV/AIDS. As the national government distanced itself from the HIV/AIDS response it did not control, its responses to the epidemic became increasingly detached while it tried to maintain a modicum of independence and with it, its ability to determine how to deliver upon its responsibilities to respond.

On 8 February 2004, in an address publicized by the South African Broadcasting Corporation, President Mbeki expressed concern over the accuracy of mortality statistics and questioned the ability to determine whether AIDS was as fatal as claimed. On 20 February, the Minister of Health disputed that the government had promised to begin the roll-out by March, and spokesman Sibani Mngadi contended that the ministry was busy checking clinics where drugs would be dispensed, setting up a system to track patients and writing training manuals. Meanwhile, a government report leaked in March 2004 estimated that 100,000 public servants were HI-positive, presenting a very real threat to reliable government administration.[17]

In response, on 10 March, the TAC threatened legal action in the event of government failure to launch HAART. The group gave the Minister of Health until 17 March to respond to a letter demanding the purchase of "an urgent interim supply of ARVs pending the finalisation of the tender process" or face litigation. Just over a week after the TAC deadline, on 25 March, the National Department of Health promised to provide an emergency supply of antiretroviral drugs as an interim measure awaiting the completion of the formal tender process. The contention served to reinforce the perception that the government, in addition to being heartless despite its pledge to respond to HIV/AIDS, was not in control of the process. Indeed, in many senses the government was not in control—due both by its voluntary limiting of its sovereign statehood, and by the involuntarily limiting effects on its sovereign statehood wrought by assumption of responsibilities to respond to HIV/AIDS by local-global alliances active in the arena, as shown above.

6.4 Embracing the Responsibility to Respond

State sovereignty still has a critical role to play in providing, protecting and preserving human security. Yet its ability to act on this proviso is constrained as never before. As Mathews' argues, "more and more frequently today, governments have only the appearance of free choice when they set economic rules,"[18] a truth played out in South Africa's neo-liberal economic policies following the fall of apartheid—and to the distress of the traditionally leftish now ruling African National Congress, and its allies, the Congress of South African Trade Unions

---

17   Gumede, W. 2005. *Thabo Mbeki and the Battle for the Soul of the ANC.* Cape Town: Zebra Publishers: 162.

18   Lisk, F. 2009. *Global Institutions and the HIV/AIDS Epidemic.* New York: Routledge Global Institutions: 73.

(COSATU) and the Communist Party. "Markets are setting de facto rules enforced by their own power"[19]—and often backed by their state governments, as well as in the epic state-financed bailouts of private financial entities in the 2007 crisis and beyond, as taxpayers continue to come to the rescue. "States can flout [such market regulations], but the penalties are severe—loss of vital foreign capital, foreign technology, and domestic jobs,"[20] to say nothing of access to desperately needed medicines, as in the case of HIV/AIDS in South Africa.

Despite the passage of another nearly 10 years, not much has changed in South Africa's HIV/AIDS response, or in the associated unresolved allocation of sovereign responsibility and accountability. There remains a disconnect between the delivery of sovereign protections to ARV-related health and human security and the ultimate guarantee of the sovereign responsibilities and associated accountability. Since 2003, South Africa has consistently broadened and updated its ARV roll-out and HIV/AIDS strategic plans [5] to reflect World Health Organization (WHO) recommendations (though not always with immediate effect, citing the familiar financial and fiscal constraints) and changing landscape of ARV access. Nonetheless, upwards of 10 percent (roughly 5.7 million) South Africans remain infected with HIV, and current medical literature belies an anticipated decline in incidence (new infections). Indeed, the opposite appears to be true. "Currently some four hundred thousand South Africans are newly infected annually—a staggering toll that must be radically reduced lest treatment bankrupt the nation."[21]

In effect, South Africa's worst fears, of external reliance without commensurate accountability, compounded by raised expectations of an unlimited HIV-response, may well be being brought to bear. And the South African state, now as at the outset, bears the ultimate responsibility and accountability for the health and human security of its HIV-infected populace, whether, essentially, it can afford to, or not: a report by Results for Development, quoted in the 10 January 2011 Global Health Update by the Council on Foreign Relations "reckons [that] Pretoria will need to conjure one hundred and two billion dollars over the next twenty years to handle its epidemic."[22] But will it?

Perhaps in cooperation, as the UN General Assembly's Political Declaration on HIV and AIDS 65/277 of 10 June 2011, encourages—but again, does not (cannot) mandate or link to accountability mechanisms.

Ironically, this lesson is now coming into the mainstream, and in 2013, even the US Government, having "bolstered local decision-making, training, and ownership of these efforts [to improve health around the globe], trying to help developing countries follow South Africa's unfolding example of reducing external donor

---

19   Ibid.
20   Ibid.
21   Garrett, L. 2011. "Council on Foreign Relations Global Health Update" (10 January).
22   Ibid.

support and make HIV and other public health efforts locally funded":[23] an outcome directly related to South Africa's HIV/AIDS response trajectory, but attesting to the role of non-state actors in global health—but to their lack of responsibility and accountability. Indeed, "the Gates Foundation is doing extraordinary work, but it operates without accountability or transparency and needs competition. Bill Gates has admitted as much himself in multiple interviews, acknowledging that his efforts wield an uncomfortably large amount of unchallenged power over global health."[24] Thus South Africa's experience highlights not the relative impassiveness of sovereignty, but of its powerful reassertion. It confirms that the global response to HIV/AIDS, scattered among assorted state and non-state actors and interventions, such as global governance in its current rendering, bears no ultimate responsibility and accountability for the health and welfare of citizens, the nation-state indeed does.

President Mbeki's own financial advisors, the same who argued against an antiretroviral roll-out, came to call for just such an action. "Members of his international investment council warned him … that investors found the confusion over the government's approach to the disease unsettling, if not downright frightening."[25] In other words, a consensus began to emerge that engaging against HIV/AIDS—notably with ARVs—would be a better investment in South Africa's economic growth and political stability than not doing so.[26] Finance Minister Trevor Manuel endorsed the new dictum, as did Reserve Bank Governor Tito Mboweni. Manuel even "began dropping hints to the president of the looming economic consequences"[27] of continuing to do nothing. In 2003, Manuel reiterated and expounded upon this, but reemphasized the priorities of independence, saying that

> Economic integration must be managed because it carries the possibility to severely restrict the degree of policy choice that a country has. It is worth reminding ourselves that the degree to which a country's choices are limited, and that country's need for access to capital, are directly proportional. The key variables are first, the financing of the fiscal deficit and second, the dependence on external capital for financing economic expansion.[28]

---

23   Garrett, L. 2012. "Money or Die." *Foreign Affairs* (6 March).

24   Ibid., emphasis added.

25   Gumede, W. 2005. *Thabo Mbeki and the Battle for the Soul of the ANC.* Cape Town: Zebra Publishers: 171.

26   As late at December 2008, however, some voices continued to maintain that in not providing antiretrovirals to those who need them will cull the excess, unemployable, populations of severely-affected countries such as South Africa; personal correspondence with Professor Franklyn Lisk. So far, however, no data support that the untimely deaths of significant portions of the working-age populations in such countries actually has this effect.

27   Gumede, W. 2005. *Thabo Mbeki and the Battle for the Soul of the ANC.* Cape Town: Zebra Publishers: 171.

28   Bond, P. 2004. "From Racial to Class Apartheid: South Africa's Frustrating Decade of Freedom." *Monthly Review* (March).

Although Mbeki's advisors increasingly accepted the necessity of responding to the HIV/AIDS epidemic—and of paying for it—the dictums of fiscal prudence and independence remained influential forces around the ensuing policy choices, which did not necessarily include full-scale HIV/AIDS response as promoted by the emerging alliances of local-global external state and non-state actors. For this, South Africa has been almost unremittingly accused of neglect, a charge that ignores the relevant concern over concomitant responsibility and accountability. This GAP, as seen throughout, is also a legitimate cause for reflection on the most effective responses to the HIV/AIDS epidemic.

Indeed, arguments for the necessity of a more comprehensive HIV/AIDS response, with national and international components though unclear lines of ultimate accountability, mounted in the run-up to the launch of NEPAD, Mbeki's African Renaissance brain-child, in June 2005.[29] NEPAD would, it should be noted, depend on foreign financial support, which would be premised upon sound economic and political fundamentals. These, in a twist, increasingly came to include responses to the incurring decimation caused by HIV/AIDS.

This twist though enabled the South African Government to seize the reigns of both its state sovereignty and its response to HIV/AIDS with its own fists. In July 2002, it established a joint Health-Treasury task team to investigate issues related to the financing of an enhanced response to HIV/AIDS, including provision of antiretroviral treatment.[30] The release in October 2002 emphasized the urgency of such a response: the Department of Health's 13th national HIV sero-prevalence survey, at the time still based on the sero-prevalence of pregnant women attending ante-natal clinics and extrapolated to the entire population, revealed more than 600,000 new infections in 2002.

6.5 Evaluating South Africa's Responsibility to Respond Response

The roll-out initiative came none too soon,. In June 2003 the World Bank published the report, "The Long-Run Economic Costs of AIDS: Theory and Application to South Africa," stating that South Africa faced progressive but eventual economic collapse as a result of HIV/AIDS.[31] This upped the ante on South Africa's actions, spurring both its assertion of responsibility in the name of sovereign statehood and

---

29   Gumede, W. 2005. *Thabo Mbeki and the Battle for the Soul of the ANC.* Cape Town: Zebra Publishers: 171.

30   "Question & Answer: Cabinet's decision on the Operational plan," 19 November 2003.

31   Local experts such as Standard Bank chief Iraj Abedian and the South African Business Coalition dismissed the report as inaccurate and unreliable. Indeed, there are causes for concern in the assembly of HIV prevalence data and its impact upon the economy. Nonetheless, as statistical methods have been improved, such as those used the Development Bank of Southern Africa as shown in Chapter 2, the impact of HIV/AIDS has

especially its struggle to compete for its control of influence and involvement in the HIV/AIDS—and broader political-economic—arena.

South Africa's invigorated response to HIV/AIDS at this juncture received support in the form of two facilitating international trends: increased foreign direct investment (finally), and aid tied to HIV/AIDS as well as falling prices of generic antiretroviral medications. With regard to the latter, US President Bush signed fast-track legislation to enable the US Food and Drug Administration, which must specifically approve the use and thus purchase of all medicines with US money, to give "tentative approval" to essential HIV/AIDS medications, including generics to be used abroad and paid for with PEPFAR monies. This went some way toward alleviating a lag that had stalled access to generic medications since 1996, allowing for the approval of 46 different generic HIV/AIDS medications by June 2007, though the use of generics continued to fall short.

Responding to these new conditions, the South African Department of Health belatedly awarded the tender for antiretroviral procurement first called in March 2004. On 2 March 2005, 16 months after announcing its operational plan, 15 months after Cabinet approved provision of antiretroviral treatment, and 13 months after the tender process commenced, it revealed the winners. Though they included generics, notably those made by Aspen Pharmacare in Cape Town and Cipla Medpro of India, as also arranged with the Clinton Foundation, these were far out-numbered by patented medications, with over half of the entire tender going to Abbot Laboratories and Merck, Sharp and Dome.

The ARVs accessed through the Department of Health's tender, combined with those purchased with funds from the Global Fund, PEPFAR and additional external actors—though not the Clinton Foundation, whose deal-brokerage the Department rejected—rapidly scaled up the numbers of South Africans receiving treatment for HIV. Due in particular to the large sums provided for ARVs from the Global Fund and PEPFAR, this "took the pressure off the South African state to such an extent, that only 51,494 HAART patients needed to be fully covered by the government budget."[32] The Table 6.1 (page 142) illustrates this.

This had a number of consequences. First, it bound the South African state to provide a level of antiretroviral provision which it might or might not be able to guarantee on its own. Second, it introduced the volatility of exchange rate fluctuations into an equation where the state would have to purchase, in rand converted into dollars, the ARVs it required. Finally, this external facilitation of HIV treatment as well as the associated state and budget dependency would implicate the South African government's responsibility to its citizens in an arena over which it maintained questionable ability to act and meet its accountability.

---

become more accurately measurable—and is considerable, especially when accumulated and taken into account over the longer-term.

32   Schulz-Herzenberg, C. 2007. "A Lethal Cocktail: Exploring the Impact of Corruption on HIV/AIDS Prevention and Treatment efforts in South Africa." Institute for Security Studies and Transparency International Zimbabwe.

Table 6.1   Donor amounts received by South Africa, in US dollars

	2004/05	2005/06	2006/07	2007/08	2008/09	2009/10	Total
Global Fund	25.2	17.1	29.2	29.9	26.7	9.2	137.4
KZN	19.0	7.8	11.9	11.9	11.9	–	62.5
NDoH	–	–	4.4	4.0	–	–	8.4
Western Cape	6.2	9.4	12.9	14.0	14.9	9.2	88.5
PEPFAR	89.3	148.2	221.0	–	–	–	458.5
Total	114.4	165.3	250.2	30.0	26.8	9.2	595.9

Note: Schulz-Herzenberg, "A Lethal Cocktail: Exploring the Impact of Corruption on HIV/ AIDS Prevention and Treatment efforts in South Africa. For a breakdown of donor monies received and traced in South Africa for 2004."

In the meantime, the South African Government attempted to keep its promises, allocating resources to fight HIV/AIDS from the National Treasury to the provinces via direct transfers, equitable share grants, conditional grants and special budgetary allocations. Yet as the chart shows, South Africa struggled with managing its budgetary expenditure, a situation which highlights the ongoing capacity constraints existent in the country, with dire consequences for the sustainable and uninterrupted treatment of HIV/AIDS. Indeed, on 13 July 2005, 10 people were shot in Queenstown in the Eastern Cape Province while protesting to gain antiretroviral treatment. Nonetheless, by September 2005, 85,000 people were enrolled for ARV treatment in the public health sector with more than US\$3.4 million allocated for procurement of antiretroviral drugs for the period to the end of 2007.

Further, the question of drug tenders for ARVs has been and continues to be a contentious one. The 2004 delayed tender locked the government into paying prices that by the end of 2007 were nearly double the falling private sector price for first-line drugs such as Nevirapine. The 2007 tender called for competition in the purchase price of 10 drugs and will only run for two years, theoretically expanding treatment options and ensuring against the price lock of the 2004 tender. In addition, "companies will receive preference points for local manufacturing capacity and black ownership, but the largest number of points will be awarded for pricing."[33] Critics however argue that even the two-year time frame is too long, not allowing for the "procurement of new, better or cheaper drugs that may come onto the market."[34] Nonetheless, antiretroviral provision is flowing, albeit repeatedly in fits and starts.

The country reaped initial praise of its efforts with the World Health Organization June 2005 progress report on the expansion of AIDS treatment

---

33   "Question marks over ARV tender." *PlusNews*, 29 February 2008.
34   Ibid.

stating that "South Africa has committed US$1 billion over the next three years to scaling up antiretroviral treatment, by far the largest budget allocation of any low- or middle-income country."[35] Heeding its actions and international acclaim, in August 2005, South Africa joined the WHO Afro Regional Declaration to declare 2006 a year of accelerated HIV prevention.

Few practical results would follow in its wake. Only in 2008 did the outgoing UNAIDS director, Peter Piot, renew the call for prevention focus. But much remained and remains to be done.

6.6 Verdict on South Africa's Responsibility to Respond

Asserting its domestic sovereignty in the HIV/AIDS arenas, South Africa reinserted its sovereign statehood into local and global governance. In late 2000, the South African Government announced the HIV/AIDS/STD Strategic Plan for South Africa for 2000–2005. On 28 January 2001, Mbeki addressed the World Economic Forum in Davos, Switzerland, remarking on the two elements of poverty and power.[36] His remarks frame the ongoing altercation engaging in the immediacy of HIV/AIDS response, and the assertion of domestic sovereignty.

The title of his speech was "Addressing the Backlash against Globalisation, a Southern Perspective of the Problem—Remarks at the World Economic Forum."[37] In it he iterated, forcefully, the constraints challenging the developing world, caught as it is between local conditions and global dictates. Defining globalization as "the integration of national systems of production and finance ... driven by policies of liberalization in trade and finance,"[38] Mbeki addressed a number of key points central to the perspective of the global South. He contended that "the choice for countries of the South is not whether to engage with globalization or not, but how to engage with it."[39] He asserted national governments' responsibility in mitigating the negative impact of globalization, and, in what was clearly a reference to TRIPS, and with prescience with regard to the subsequent failure of the Doha Round of trade agreements, stated

> The first key challenge is the reform of international financial and trading institutions to take on board the concerns of the countries of the South. For example in regards to the WTO there is a need to re-examine their rules

---

35   UNAIDS 2006. Global Epidemic Update 2005: 16.

36   Though he did not explicitly target pharmaceutical companies in this context, Mbeki did highlight the imbalance of power which their influence and interests had represented in his earlier remarks and rebukes which did directly concern them.

37   Thabo Mbeki speech at Davos, 2001, point 5, available at http://www.anc.org.za/ancdocs/history/mbeki/ [accessed: 1 July 2012].

38   Ibid.

39   Ibid.

(governing intellectual property rights, dumping and countervailing measures, subsidies, etc.).[40]

and "there is a need for a renewed commitment to partnership between the international social partners that entails a shared responsibility to eradicate poverty, social exclusion and marginalization. On the part of developing countries this means a commitment to create conditions of peace, stability and good governance."[41] Mbeki's final point emphasized the mutual responsibility of developing and developed countries, and of local and international systems of governance, to coordinate; perhaps offering a prelude to a new form of delegated or shared governance. Up until this point, the South African Government seemed to involuntarily shed some of its sovereign control of its responsibility to respond. In the ensuing void, external actors competed to assume if not responsibility then responsible action. Yet the actions that resulted were implemented without a clear delineation of responsibility or accountability between the ultimately accountable state and the actual deliverers of its sovereign responsibility to respond.

Evidencing this, in August 2001, the South African Government refused to make the antiretroviral Nevirapine available to pregnant women to stem the tide of mother-to-child-transmission (MTCT). Subsequent court orders, first by the Pretoria High Court and then by the South Africa's Constitutional Court required the government to make the medication available at all public health-care facilities in the country. The battles seemed to underscore the government's proclivity against assuming its responsibilities vis-à-vis HIV/AIDS towards its population: a perception made all the more poignant by the revelation during parliamentary questioning in October 2001 that a number of ANC parliamentarians were accessing antiretroviral medications paid for by their state medical aid. This heightened the prevalent perception that "the government could afford to pay for medicine for its own officials and representatives, but such help was too costly for the masses."[42] Throughout the trajectory of HIV/AIDS response in South Africa, financial costs of addressing the epidemic and particularly for providing antiretroviral and accompanying treatment to fight HIV/AIDS have been at the center of the controversy. Indeed, as the Nevirapine contest was playing out between the courts, parliament and activists in South Africa, in the fourth quarter

---

40   Mbeki speech at Davos, 2001, point 8. This statement is particularly relevant in 2008, as the global financial system is under considerable strain if not experiencing outright collapse. While developed countries resort to nationalization, subsidies, and bail-outs, and the developing world is looked toward for support, particularly in terms of investment and consumption, the double-standard in representation and application of the rules of international financial institutions is particularly galling for that same "developing world."

41   Mbeki speech at Davos, 2001, point 14.

42   Gumede, W. 2005. *Thabo Mbeki and the Battle for the Soul of the ANC.* Cape Town: Zebra Publishers: 168.

of 2001, the value of the South African rand plummeted again: by 13.96 percent against the dollar.

Since at the time all ARVs had to be imported, this event, as well as the unpredictable volatility of the rand to come, severely hampered cost projections and the ability of the government to pay for a sustainable antiretroviral program. This constraint would recur. It never really diminishes. Yet the emphasis has shifted, away from avoiding ARV provision, towards offering it.

6.7 Verdict on South Africa's (Limited) Sovereignty

Then on 22 September 2004, President Mbeki delivered another passionate address, this time to the 59th session of the United Nations General Assembly. He focused primarily on the Millennium Declaration and the sweeping set of development goals declared under its auspices and known as the MDGs. In doing so, Mbeki attempted to force attention to the challenge of holistic health and human development, as opposed to the singular crisis of HIV/AIDS.

Poignantly noting that to most of humanity, the attainment of the MDGs is likely to be a "dream deferred," as food insecurity and war constitute their immediate concerns, he pointed out that "depending on where we stand relative to the power equation, we will hold radically different views about what constitutes humanity's most serious threats and challenges, and therefore what must be changed to respond to that perceived reality."[43] Mbeki argued that those furthest removed from the power equation would rank poverty and underdevelopment, "translating into cold statistics about shortened life expectancy, deprivation and want,"[44] among their highest priorities for human development. Yet he acknowledged that because these poor are on the periphery of decision-making in the global arena, they "will have no possibility to persuade this Organization [the UN], mockingly described in the Millennium Declaration as 'the most universal and most representative organization in the world,' to translate what they have concluded into obligatory injunctions ... which all member nations will have to accept and implement."[45] In making this statement, Mbeki addresses the GAP.

Indeed, the challenges in responding to HIV/AIDS only increases. At present, the response to HIV/AIDS is again embattled on the medical side by the steady stream of viral mutations. This will likely always be an issue, and a

---

43   Mbeki, T. 2004. "Address of President Thabo Mbeki at the 59th Session of the United Nations General Assembly." New York (22 September).

44   Ibid.

45   Ibid. Indeed, in the early 2002, US FBI investigators went to South Africa to assess the country's anti-terrorism preparedness. Though the US has done much for South Africa's fight against HIV/AIDS, the pressure to provide and implement anti-terror measures stands in stark contrast to the provision and aid—and more flexible patent legislation—for anti-HIV/AIDS initiatives.

spur for new treatments. Innovation has slowed, and as such, drug pricing, of first-, and particularly second- and third-line ARVs remains a contentious issue. Related challenges include limits, bottlenecks and lack of logistical capacity and staffing, pertaining not only to the number of treating doctors and nurses, but to laboratories and storage, notably under refrigeration. Finally, the aftermath of the global financial crisis is also testing the resolve of the state and of external partners to provide funding for the necessarily ongoing response to HIV/AIDS. Thus both the cost and the challenge of allocating responsibility and accountability in the response to HIV/AIDS continue to mount.

6.8 Lingering Challenges

The lingering challenges remain significant. Roughly 5.7 million South Africans are infected with HIV, and there is currently no evidence that incidence is declining. According to Deputy President Baleka Mbete, speaking at South Africa's 4th AIDS Conference in March 2009, 695,293 South Africans were receiving antiretroviral treatment, which only represented half of those who need it. At that time, SANAC reported that the need for antiretroviral treatment is expanding by half a million people per year. At that rate, South Africa would have had to double the number of people on therapy every year until 2012 to reach all those who need it. This goal has not been reached, despite mounting evidence showing that antiretroviral therapy can lower viral load and thus infectivity,[46] contributing to a reduction in incidence, and costing less in the long-term than treating and caring for HIV/AIDS patients. Theory, however, does not make practice. In fact, the data show a worse scenario unfolding. According to the "best case" scenario as postulated on the report" *Making Progress against AIDS*, an estimated 1.2 million South Africans will have died of HIV and AIDS by 2012.[47] Furthermore, UNAIDS global statistics, which while inexact, highlight a definite trend by which for every two people starting antiretroviral treatment, another five are becoming infected with HIV.[48] A report by Results for Development, quoted in the 10 January 2011 Global Health Update by the Council on Foreign Relations "reckons [that] Pretoria will need to conjure one hundred and two billion dollars over the next twenty years to handle its epidemic. Currently some four hundred thousand South Africans are newly infected annually—a staggering toll that must be radically reduced lest treatment bankrupt the nation."[49] Thus the response to HIV/AIDS remains both a political and economic problem saddled to the state.

---

46   Interview with Professor Ruben Sher, 8 March 2005.
47   "New ideas at 4th national AIDS conference." 2009. *PlusNews* (1 April).
48   See, UNAIDS 2006. AIDS Epidemic Update 2006.
49   Garrett, L. 2011. "Council on Foreign Relations Global Health Update" (10 January).

The continued enormity of the HIV/AIDS health challenge confronting the country was brought to bear by the Medical Research Council's Debbie Bradshaw. In the South African Health Review 2008, published in December 2008 by the Health Systems Trust, she is quoted as saying: "it is clear that the health of the South African population has worsened. South Africa can be considered to have a quadruple burden of disease, including diseases and conditions relating to poverty and under-development, chronic diseases, injuries and HIV and AIDS."[50] This "quadruple burden" poses a threat to the present and the future in South Africa: individually and structurally. Individually, HIV incidence continues to pose a real and present danger to life, as life expectancy has fallen 12 years from that in 1996; and as maternal and child mortality have risen. Structurally, the challenges are reflected in the fact that in 1994 there were 25 doctors per 10,000 people, falling to 24.4 in 2007, that the number of nurses fell from 251 to 110 per 10,000; that in 1989 38 percent of doctors and 79 percent of nurses worked in the public sector, figures which fell to 30 percent and 40 percent respectively, in 2007, and that 40 percent of those nurses are likely to retire in the next five to ten years.[51] In addition, overall, more than a third of public sector positions are vacant, with economic and political consequences: an indication of the hollowing out of the state.

HIV/AIDS remains un-remittent and multi-faceted. The epidemic—and more importantly, its response—is and remains wedged between the priorities set by national demands and international pressures of defeating poverty, of malnutrition and food insecurity, of economic exclusion, and power imbalances, and as such a central, existential threat to individuals in and the state of South Africa. The survival of individuals directly and indirectly affected by HIV/AIDS, their political constituency and representation, their economic contributions, their knowledge transfer, and children, are crucial to a stable and sustainable South Africa. As such, HIV/AIDS is intertwined within the very power imbalances that Mbeki criticizes: in hijacking individual lives with inter-generational effects as well as international attention, HIV has hung itself on the coattails of alliances spanning from national advocates to international actors. Political-economics have played a role, too, as illustrated by the presence of HIV/AIDS on national and international and global agendas, influencing international policy priorities and prescriptions on aid, trade and investment.

The epidemic, as has been seen, is far from receding. In addition to the lives cut short and lost, the orphans left, and the cross-cutting consequences socially, economically, and politically, the challenge of conceiving and implementing an HIV/AIDS response for those infected and those not (yet) infected, remains perhaps the most pertinent. Given this, the most critical component of propounded and paramount importance are antiretroviral medications, and of equal pertinence, access to them.

---

50   Kapp, C. 2009. "Barbara Hogan: South Africa's Minister of Health." *The Lancet*, 373(96600) (24 January): 291.

51   Ibid.

ARVs changed the course of the trajectory of disease for individuals, as well as with their arrival that of the South African state's response to the HIV/AIDS epidemic. Now access to them is in jeopardy. A number of critical factors threatens the necessarily sustainable production and procurement of ARVs: the sourcing of their raw material; their availability per se; real access to them; funding for their innovation and obtainment on the part of both states and individuals; and contending interpretations and applications of international intellectual property right laws. Possible solutions will also be put forth in chapter eight on recommendations.

While at their advent in the mid-1990s it was generally accepted that they would not be made available or accessible to the majority of HIV-infected individuals, notably Africans, who were generally deemed too poor and too logistically incompetent to comply with their complicated regimes,[52] this changed drastically with the inauguration of PEPFAR and the Global Fund, and with the prevalence of generics.[53] These programs, initiated and sustained largely with international funding, greatly increased African access to ARVs.

Crucial to the efficacy of ARVs is consistent access to the drugs by the population that needs them. This stems the progression of the individual's disease and also contributes, as noted above, to reducing incidence at the population level. If the continuous access to ARVs is interrupted, the individual disease rears up—often also mutating, forging resistance to the drugs and thereby making the disease harder to treat in other individuals—facilitating its further spread and increasing the difficulty of responding to it.

Making identifying who qualifies for ARV treatment, however, is not straightforward. In fact, the criteria to qualify for HAART initiation, is currently in flux: whereas previous WHO guidelines recommended ARV treatment initiation as a CD4 immune cell count of 200 per milliliter (200/mL). As of November 2009, however, the WHO has revised these guidelines and currently recommends treatment initiation at a CD4 count of 350/mL. This has huge implications for access.

The "test and treat" model of ARV treatment, which is gaining ground in theory if not yet comprehensively in practice, recommends immediate treatment for all who test positive for HIV—and further stipulates annual testing to ascertain incidence and so to tackle treatment. If put into force across sub-Saharan Africa

---

52   There were long debates about Africans not using or able to use watches and time, which were seen as critical at the onset of antiretroviral therapy, which demanded strict schedules of pill-taking every day.

53   It should be noted that access to generics, as illustrated in the above analysis, has not always been straight forward. Even after some of the bitter battles fought, South Africa is currently paying more for some ARVs than do other African countries—due to an early tendering process that locked it into a payment scale well above those negotiated later and under more favorable conditions (notably the greater availability of generics on the international market)—though it is now negotiating new tenders and contracts, with the help of the Clinton Foundation which is advising Health Minister Aaron Motsoaledi.

in particular, adherence to these new guidelines will exponentially increase the number of people eligible for ARV treatment; a significant logistical challenge to access.

The consequences are already accumulating—illustrating again the external dependencies rife in the HIV/AIDS arena in sub-Saharan Africa, including South Africa. For instance, in Swaziland and Malawi, among other African countries, the application of these guidelines is completely contingent upon donor funding. The new guidelines significantly increase the number of those eligible for treatment—by 50 percent in Malawi alone.[54] Even South Africa relies on external funding for its HIV/AIDS program. The country has promulgated a new HIV/AIDS policy to ensure access to ARVs under the new WHO recommendations, but it only pertains to pregnant women, infants and those co-infected with TB. The South African Finance Ministry expected even that broadened access criterion to increase enrolment in its ARV program by roughly a million people—effectively doubling the country's case load. In order to pay for the expansion, South African President Jacob Zuma reopened the budget to acquire more funds for AIDS when it became clear that costs would be higher.[55] Despite this, South Africa continues to rely on the United States, the country's principle donor, to fund its fight against the pandemic.

The US gave South Africa an additional US$620 million for 2009[56] alone, to scale-up its health infrastructure and to help finance this extensive ARV roll-out. This skirts the fact that nearly US$ 1 billion of the HIV/AIDS budget are directly from PEPFAR. The Clinton Foundation might well advise the health minister, since South Africa currently still purchases more expensive medicines than most countries, a fall-out from some of the fights about generic access in 1998–2001.

Yet overall, funding is being flat-lined. PEPFAR in particular, the world's largest funder of HIV/AIDS programs, has capped its budget at 2009 funding levels. As a result, "US officials have asked some AIDS clinics overseas to stop enrolling new patients in a US-sponsored program that provides lifesaving antiretroviral drugs, in a bid to stem the rising costs of one of the most ambitious US assistance programs."[57] Though official policy does not limit the number of new patients being enrolled for treatment—a number that is rapidly increasing under the new WHO guidelines outlined above—in practice, this is exactly what is occurring. PEPFAR director Eric Goosby "signaled strongly that the United States will not push to implement the new [WHO HIV treatment] guidelines," which

---

54   International Treatment Preparedness Coalition 2010. "Rationing Funds, Risking Lives: World Backtracks on HIV Treatment." Quoted in "Same problems, less funding." 2010. *PlusNews* (4 May).

55   Dugger, C.W. 2010. "South Africa Redoubles Efforts Against AIDS." *The New York Times* (25 April).

56   Ibid.

57   "Boston Globe Examines How PEPFAR Budget Pressure Are Affecting AIDS Clinics in Africa." 2010. Henry J. Kaiser Foundation (13 April).

would start treatments earlier, "because that would triple the number of people eligible to receive the drugs and greatly increase costs."[58]

PEPFAR is not alone. A report by the International Treatment Preparedness Coalition (ITPC) noted that "a global pullback on commitments to fund and fight AIDS is resulting in restrictions on the number of people being enrolled into treatment programmes, more frequent drug shortages, and reduced national AIDS budgets." Consequently, "patients are being turned away from treatment programmes and AIDS drug stocks are running out because of government budget cuts and flat-lined funding from major donors."[59] The potential consequences for stemming the spread of the epidemic, with continues to induce roughly 1,500 infections a day in South Africa,[60] are dire.

Especially relevant to this analysis, though HIV/AIDS programs should arguably have *always* been the prerogative and responsibility of national governments for their citizens, this funding flat-lining is driving the argument for 'country ownership,' though not without the perverse consequences Mbeki tried to avoid: namely of national responsibility without the means of guarantee. PEPFAR's Goosby outlined a plan that included the "eventual transfer of responsibility for AIDS treatment to the patients' own governments; consolidating clinics, rather than opening more; and treating the sickest patients first." This resurgent emphasis on independence from external sources, especially of funding, might yet serve to shore up the domestic sovereignty and the sovereign statehood of a state such as South Africa, and enable it to (better) enact its responsibilities to respond, including to HIV/AIDS.

6.9 Responsibility and Sovereignty: Is There (Still) a GAP?

Thus South Africa has chalked up some successes, as iterated above, yet also faces lingering problems in its responsibility to respond to its HIV/AIDS epidemic. These challenges are part and parcel of its overarching attempts to fulfill its constitutional obligations and to deliver upon the tenets of sovereignty.

Moeletsi Mbeki, President Mbeki's brother and an eminent and respected political analyst, delivered a dour diagnosis to South Africa's economy, predicting already in November 2007 "a long, slow decline." He says, "if South Africa is to develop in the 21st century, and get rid of endemic poverty and high unemployment, the elite of this country cannot continue to enjoy the standards of living of the middle classes of the West without the equivalent productivity, which is the case

---

58   Ibid.

59   "Report looks at HIV/AIDS Funding in Developing Countries." Kaiser Family Foundation (27 April 2010).

60   Dugger, C.W. 2010. "South Africa Redoubles Efforts Against AIDS." *The New York Times* (25 April).

at present,"[61] or it will inevitably become more circumscribed in its sovereign statehood and more dependent upon external influence and funds—a scenario looking increasingly unlikely given the current state of global finance.

Regarding the HIV/AIDS epidemic in South Africa, on the one hand, some nominal progress has been and is being made. "Anti-AIDS measures are in all the business plans of all government departments. Just before me on SABC Africa this morning there was an interview with a researcher from the Wits medical faculty on their finding that boys and girls who are in secondary schools are less likely to get AIDS. Not unlikely but less likely."[62] Indeed, is this progress?

A precarious situation in the best of times, the burden of HIV/AIDS, illustrating as it does the GAP, notably as evidenced in the wake of the 2008 global recession, is particularly onerous now. Indeed, the sustainability of South Africa's HIV/AIDS response, notably its public roll-out, is constrained by the flat-lining of funding in the aftermath of the global financial crisis. Yet its responsibility to respond stands. So what is the final verdict?

6.10 Status 2013

As argued, the twin challenges of continuous funding and guaranteed access to ARVs threaten the South African response and the country's responsibility to respond to its HIV/AIDS epidemic.

First, though skeptical through the early 2000s when it might have benefited from external state and non-state interventions against HIV/AIDS, South Africa resisted and reacted almost only *involuntarily*. Only just before the financial crisis of 2008, did it finally throw in its lot and bow to the associated pressures aligned around it. These came notably from UNAIDS and the Global Fund, backed by the US Government, and supported by local activists such as the Treatment Action Campaign, to roll-out. Then, heeding this apparent wisdom, and under the guidance of the revised WHO guidelines released in 2009, South Africa acquiesced *voluntarily* to expand the roll-out of ARVs to its populace, assuming continued external support. Just then financial crisis caved, and with it a slowdown in external funding: illustrating in practice precisely the kind of unpredictability that the South African Government, by initially balking at such a comprehensive roll-out, had attempted to avoid. Having then, however, agreed, as South Africa Minister of Health, Dr Aaron Motsoaledi, acknowledged, the South African Government has "no choice but to keep spending."[63] "If we stop anything, we will just reverse all our gains."[64] Such a scenario might, ironically, look like a

---

61 "Gap Between Haves and Have-nots Yawns Wider." 2007. *PlusNews* (8 November).

62 Personal correspondence with Ambassador Thomas Wheeler, 21 January 2008.

63 Bryson, D. 2010. "AP Interview: S. Africa concerned at costs of AIDS." *Associated Press* (1 December).

64 Ibid.

counter-revolution: the very thing that returning exiles and the new generation of democrats in South Africa tried so hard to stave off at the beginning of this, what should have been, a new era of life as opposed to an epic battle against an epidemic of death.

Currently, South Africa is home to around 5.7 HIV-infected people, in a country of roughly 50 million. A new study by an international team of experts estimates that another five million South Africans will become infected over the next 20 years: regardless of prevention measures, or the preventative benefits of antiretroviral treatment. Yet paying for that treatment under South Africa's current National HIV/AIDS and STI Strategic Plan (set to run through 2015) is projected to cost the country US$88 billion over the coming two decades, with the number of new infections falling only from 500,000 to 350,000 annually. Even a more ambitious plan whose cost is estimated at US$102 billion over the same time period would only reduce the number of annual infections to 200,000.[65] In addition to the challenges presented by funding cuts, the sheer scale of the rate of infections means that neither plan represents a sustainable solution to South Africa's HIV/AIDS epidemic.

The reality of this situation is slowly dawning. Though it provides 80 percent of the funding that flows into its HIV/AIDS response—notwithstanding donor commitments—South Africa is only able to provide antiretroviral treatment for half of the population that requires it, or roughly 1.2 of the 2.2 million people who currently need it—a number that is set to increase with increased incidence and prevalence. The only effective way to curtail both the cost and the spread of the epidemic then is to stop its transmission in its tracks.

Failing that, South Africa is facing its second challenge: how to guarantee access to ARVs as long as they are necessary, which promises to be for at least another generation in this long-wave event. According to its provisions, the South African Government "has halved the price the government will pay for the life-saving drugs"; however, fixed dose combinations, which would decrease the pill burden, and also drive costs down further (especially in terms of the logistics of packaging, storage and distribution) "are still largely absent from the deal."[66] The tender itself is made possible by the fact that the government's ARV suppliers, 10

---

65   Ibid.

66   The delay in allowing fix-dose combinations under the deals is apparently due to "continued registration delays with the Medicines Control Council (MCC)," though in some instances these have been approve by the US Food and Drug Administration. This duplication is addressed in the chapter eight's recommendations. Furthermore, "according to Andy Gray, a senior lecturer at the department of therapeutics and medicines management at South Africa's University of KwaZulu-Natal, the tender has only included dual fixed-dose combinations, such as a tenofovir and emtricitabine, in limited amounts. The tender makes no provision for triple combination pills, including those that would add nevirapine [sometimes a problematic ARV due to its side-effects and propensity to foster resistance] to this combination to form South Africa's first-line regimen." See "New ARV tender halves drug prices." 2010. *PlusNews* (20 December).

pharmaceutical companies in long-standing relationships with the Government, will continue "to supply the national programme with ARVs although in different proportions."[67] The estimated savings come to roughly US$685 million from the end of January 2011, reversing a trend in which South Africa pays substantially more for its ARVs than do other countries—a situation stemming from and perpetuated by the pharmaceutical court case that ran from 1998–2001. These savings could mean that the Government could theoretically afford to treat twice as many HIV-positive South Africans: or according to the numbers above, then all of those who qualify for treatment. However, the tender makes no "provision for a reduction in drug prices should the prices of the active ingredients decline," which as in the past, would lock South Africa into paying more for drugs which it could—and arguably should—be able to access for less. This is a lingering legacy of South Africa's struggle to be seen and accepted as an established and legitimate player in international capital markets—a place of positive investment—and in the realms of protection of intellectual property rights: both spheres in which its focus on independence and sovereign statehood collided with the need to respond to its HIV/AIDS epidemic.

Once again, this very confrontation is brewing. In November 2010, European and Indian officials met in Brussels to "to thrash out the details of a Free Trade Agreement (FTA)," focusing on preserving "data exclusivity," which civil society activists contend "could mean tighter intellectual property protections that could reduce access to cheap Indian generic drugs"; the source of 80 percent of donor-funded ARVs found in Africa.[68] Though still shrouded in secrecy, the deal *could* mean that Indian generics' manufacturers would have to conduct their own clinical trials to prove the efficacy of their drugs; a redundancy that could delay poor countries' access by anywhere between five and 10 years," according to Michelle Childs, director of policy and advocacy for MSF's campaign for access to essential medicines.[69] This would significantly slow Africa and South Africa's—despite its new tender—ability to respond to its HIV/AIDS epidemic. While the EU contends that the new provisions will not endanger access to essential medicines, Childs argues that they are an example of TRIPS-Plus, tougher or more restrictive conditions than those required by TRIPS.[70] Given South Africa's contentious TRIPS-related past, this does not seem to bode well for the successful application of TRIPS or to the sustainable access to ARVs in South Africa. At the time of this writing, mid-2012, no final deal has been reached.

More than the funding crisis occupying South African Minister of Health Motsoaledi's thoughts, a dearth of ARVs—first-line, second-line, not to mention third-line drugs, single doses, and combinations—would severely hamper the

---

67 "New ARV tender halves drug prices." 2010. *PlusNews* (20 December).

68 "EU-India deal could threaten access to essential HIV drugs." 2010. *PlusNews* (9 November).

69 Ibid.

70 Ibid.

response to the country's HIV/AIDS epidemic. This is principally because, as the above analysis has shown, that response is predicated on treatment access. Despite the central role that prevention needs to play and continue to play, especially as it is increasingly admitted that treatment without prevention is no solution to the ever-expanding epidemic, and the South African Government's long-time reluctance to become dependent upon the treatment option, both in terms of rights in practice (funding and access to ARVs) and in terms of responsibility (with regard to its sovereign responsibilities), the key component in the fight against HIV/AIDS has become ARV treatment.

Interrupted or delayed, much less permanently denied, loss of access to ARVs would bring Mbeki's worst fears to bear, and would present a different kind of death-knell in the fight against HIV/AIDS: condemning millions to death, with governments restricted in their actions, held responsible and accountable by the logic and legality of sovereignty. The result could be an existential threat not only for infected individuals, but for the government rendered ineffectual and illegitimate as a consequence, at a loss to deliver upon its responsibilities though still saddled with their associated accountability.

So now, South Africa, like other national and international actors in an increasingly global arena, needs to bridge the GAP, clearly delineating lines of responsibility and accountability.

6.11 Conclusion

As the above analysis indicates, a GAP exists between tactical and ultimate responsibility and accountability between states and external state and non-state actors intervening in the realm of domestic sovereignty. South Africa's policy process to implement its responsibility to respond to its HIV/AIDS epidemic illustrates this. The country's policy process took a circular route to a response to the epidemic, influenced by internal and external factors, as well as local-global alliances. Though at times different actors assumed tactical responsibility in responding to HIV/AIDS, ultimate responsibility and accountability remain with the state. The result is the GAP.

This led to a process that has been meandering and muddled. The most critical consequence is the unabated spread of HIV/AIDS. Beyond that, however, is the crisis in sovereign responsibility it did not unleash, but revealed: a problem not unique to either South Africa or HIV/AIDS, but applicable to other countries grappling with the constraints of limited sovereign statehood and particularly the GAP, especially when confronting an incisive problem spanning local, national and global policy rubrics. As such, any solution to the HIV/AIDS crisis, and more significantly to the GAP in responsibility and accountability that it highlights, will have to take these into account.

These final assessments indicate that South Africa lies in the eye of the epidemic. The initial fury of the storm might be mitigated, but the impact has yet to hit in all of its prolonged, essential force. South Africa remains before its central challenge: to acknowledge and to act upon its constitutional and sovereign responsibilities to its populace regarding HIV/AIDS, and to do so in such a manner as to safeguard its sovereign statehood—in conjunction, not contention, with local-global alliances and external state and non-state actors.

Chapter 7
Comparative Applications of the GAP Hypothesis

As argued throughout this analysis, South Africa faces constraints from both its national and international policy environs particularly regarding its domestic sovereignty and its HIV/AIDS policy response. Looking once again through the lens proffered by the GAP, this chapter offers a comparative analysis of the room to maneuver and the policy results in Brazil and Uganda, which also faced significant HIV/AIDS epidemics, respectively. In testing the applicability of the GAP hypothesis, both comparisons focus on the similarities and differences in those countries' focus on the responsibility to respond to HIV/AIDS at the nexus of external actors' ad hoc engagement and intervention and the state's ultimate sovereign accountability.

Setting the stage for the comparison, it is necessary to reiterate that in South Africa's case, after it assumed the rights and responsibilities associated with sovereign statehood upon its democratic transition in 1994, the country faced—and still faces—a long struggle to fulfill these. Meeting the demands for the rights and responsibilities related to responding to the HIV/AIDS is no exception. In the striving, South Africa, and Brazil and Uganda as will be discussed below, embody and attempt to put into practice the theory that

> States, on their part, are obliged under international law to respect, protect, and fulfill the right to health, including the obligation to ensure accessibility, availability, and quality of health facilities, infrastructures, and delivery services. They are also obliged to give sufficient recognition to the right to health in national political and legal systems and to adopt appropriate national health policies. Every country in the world is now party to at least one human rights instrument that addresses health-related rights, including the right to health and a number of rights related to conditions necessary for health.[1]

A state is endowed with the responsibility to provide for the security and protection of its citizens, who accept and thereby legitimize state power—territorially and with regard to welfare—resulting largely in internal peace and at least the potential for prosperity.

---

1   Lisk, F. 2009. *Global Institutions and the HIV/AIDS Epidemic*. New York: Routledge Global Institutions: 79.

In order to protect life and to pursue prosperity, a state sets policy priorities. In South Africa, political-economic independence, provision of public housing and water, employment policies and crime-fighting have all be prioritized above HIV/AIDS. The accompanying implications went a long way in practically constraining the South African state's ability to enact fully its responsibility to respond in the realm of HIV/AIDS of its own accord. In other words, despite its focus on independence, South Africa wound up dependent upon assistance to address HIV/AIDS. This, in turn, spurred the circumscription, by local-global alliances and external actors, of its domestic sovereignty.

What does this mean?

As argued, responsibility to respond falls under the rubric of governance and governability, which are the prerogative and mandate of a sovereign state. The fact that evolving local and global actors and alliances assume the responsibility to respond to varying degrees has a number of implications, most notably on the ability of the state to enact its responsibility to respond—and to account for that.

First, this evolution has a precondition and consequence: where the state is unable or unwilling to render its responsibility to respond, local-global alliances can step into the void. In that case, the assumption of responsibility by exogenous internal and/or external actors serves a purpose. Second, these alliances exacerbate the loss of the state's control over its responsibility to respond and can become a precondition in themselves—a catch-22 cycle more or less vicious. Third, with and despite the assumption of aspects of the tactical, day-to-day responsibility to respond by various local-global actors and alliances, the legal, constitutional and governance responsibility continues to reside with the state. Fourth, this legal, constitutional governance responsibility is also the harbinger of ultimate accountability for and to the responsibility to respond.

This leads to the identification of a GAP between the function and ultimate assumption of the tenets of sovereignty as related to statehood. The resulting tension is rising as weak states proliferate and the lines of accountability blur. As illustrated and analyzed above, this is precisely what occurred in the case of HIV/AIDS in South Africa.

In the case of the HIV/AIDS epidemic in South Africa, this GAP is clear. As enshrined in the Constitution of democratic South Africa, "everybody according to the human rights of the United Nations is entitled to free or good health ... those are some of the fundamental human rights." Yet as the HIV/AIDS epidemic progressed, "they [the right to free or good health, in this instance to treatment and care for HIV/AIDS] weren't being given"[2] by the government.

Beset by competing priorities, budget constraints chosen or imposed, prescriptions to shore up independence and to avoid especially financial dependence, denial, dearth of commitment amidst an attempt to harness sustainable development into the future, the South African Government dallied—repeatedly.

---

2   Interview with Professor Ruben Sher, 8 March 2005.

On the one hand, "the people, the doctors would say why give people AZT [the first antiretroviral available to treat HIV] when they are going to die in any case? What about people with other disease? What about them?"[3] On the other hand, activists formed local and global alliances to ensure that those rights would be honored in the case of the epidemic, as immediately as possible. These "people were shouting 'drop the prices' [of antiretroviral medicines] and they were boycotting international companies … It was only through tremendous pressure through various activist groups that government came forward with ARVs. And I guarantee you if it was not for that pressure they [the government] would not have done it."[4]

Indeed, the National Health Council rejected a comprehensive application of the WHO's revised treatment initial guidelines on grounds of affordability.[5] Though stark, the Council's reservations were reasonable given South Africa's internal funding limits and the precariousness of dependence upon external funding. In order to address the latter, then Minister of Health, Barbara Hogan, called for international donors to "start making longer-term commitments, and to coordinate their assistance with other donors."[6] In making her call, the Minister acknowledged South Africa's inability to meet the funding requirements for its pledged HIV/AIDS program, regardless of which WHO treatment guidelines it applies. The country's shortfall has both domestic and external roots: domestically,

> Falling demand for and prices of commodity and mineral exports on which many African countries depend for revenue and spending, including public sector investment in health and other basic human needs; reduction in official development assistance, including to the Global Fund to Fight AIDS, Tuberculosis and Malaria, which has reported an estimated funding gap of $4 billion for 2010; decline in capital inflows including emigrant remittances on which extended families and relatives … depend for food and healthcare including AIDS' medicines.[7]

Similarly, internationally, Dr Fareed Abdulah, Africa director for the Global Fund to Fight AIDS, Tuberculosis and Malaria, "said that the Global Fund was 'extremely concerned' about its ability to continue raising sufficient funds to meet the constantly growing demand for its grants."[8] As a result, South Africa's

---

3   Ibid.

4   Ibid.

5   "Funding shortfall threatens treatment programmes." 2009. *PlusNews* (2 April).

6   "Hogan Closes Clear-the-Air Conference." 2009. *PlusNews* (3 April).

7   Personal correspondence with Professor Franklyn Lisk regarding impact of the global financial crisis on AIDS governance, and as communicated in draft statement prepared for clearance and issue under the signature of the UNAIDS Executive Director, May/June 2009.

8   "Funding shortfall threatens treatment programmes." 2009. *PlusNews* (2 April).

dependence upon external actors to fulfill its responsibility in the HIV/AIDS arena grows, alongside willful and imposed limits on its domestic sovereignty. In the end, however, regardless whether these constraints render the state capable or not, healthcare provision, including for HIV/AIDS, ultimately remains the responsibility of the state.[9] Echoing this, President Mbeki noted that "dealing with the epidemic essentially undermines Africa's long-sought and elusive autonomy, as the epidemic impedes development, particularly in the political and psychological senses."[10] Perhaps by not heeding it, by not dealing with it, he thought he—and Africa—could wrest development and autonomy from the clutches of the beast. Nearly three decades later, South Africa is still struggling to assert its domestic sovereignty in order to address the epidemic amidst a host of competing priorities and constrained by local-global alliances and external influences and dependencies.

This trajectory and its still-unfolding outcomes indicate that "states are inevitably weaker now than they were decades ago, and people have the right to bypass the state if only this can save them—both by appealing to international organizations and by building local institutions."[11] The consequence, however, particularly when the delegation of responsibility and accountability does not occur, is a further weakening of states.

"States are legally sovereign, as long as they do not limit their sovereignty by treaties with other states or supranational organizations,"[12] but even in the absence of such formal limiting, states cannot implement their responsibility to respond independently. Furthermore, states are required, by virtue of the tenets of their sovereignty, to act upon their associated legal obligations. "If they fail, they should be blamed, and individuals, NGOs, [and] states may help to obviate their shortcomings."[13] However, no mechanism holds these external state and non-state actors to account as they try to bridge the GAP between themselves and the state in which, on which, and around which they impart and impose their advocacy and intervention. As a result, although exogenous actors and alliances might render tactical responsibility to respond in certain crises and conditions, the accountability continues to rest with a state whose sovereignty is consequently compromised, limited.

While the actors and ensuing alliances in the AIDS arena in South Africa have saved and prolonged the lives of millions, delivering some immediate protection, the sustainability of such protection as prescribed by the tenets of sovereignty, is in jeopardy, not least because the local-global alliances and their funding in particular

---

9   It remains to be resolved, however, in the context of global health sovereignty, how and which states are responsible for the health of their citizens, at home or abroad, or those living within their borders generally.

10   Fredland, R.A. 2001. "A Sea Change in Responding to the AIDS Epidemic: Leadership is Awakened." *International Relations*, 15(6): 89–101.

11   Personal correspondence with Professor Vittorio Hösle, 22 January 2008.

12   Ibid.

13   Ibid.

are in peril in the wake of the recent global financial crisis. Nonetheless, the state remains accountable—whether it can deliver or not—for that same responsibility to respond. Its eventual, or continued, failure to enact that responsibility further circumscribes its sovereignty, and weakens it more. It is this GAP that appears as the eye of a whirlpool, a storm that increasingly characterizes the state of the relationship between states and non-state actors in an interconnected global order.

Though often presented as a unique case, in terms of its history, the severity of its epidemic, the country's unsuccessful battles for access to ARVs, the prominence of its former president's denial, and its relative wealth, is this exceptionality merited? What do the examples of Brazil and Uganda in their responses to HIV/AIDS illustrate? Do they evidence the GAP in responsibility and accountability exhibited in South Africa?

7.1 Brief Insights into HIV/AIDS and State Sovereignty: Brazil

Brazil's HIV/AIDS prevalence, at approximately 0.6 percent[14] of its population, remains below the threshold of 1 percent that defines the outbreak of an epidemic. Nonetheless, it correlates to about 730,000 infected Brazilians, who in turn constitute some 43 percent of Latin America's HIV/AIDS burden.[15] Affecting mainly intravenous drug users, men who have sex with men—and women, whether or not they acknowledge this—and sex workers, the spread of HIV/AIDS is not predominately fueled by heterosexual sexual networks as it is in South Africa. Still it poses a significant social and political problem.

Facing in some ways challenges similar to those confronted by South Africa, in terms of the impending threat and possible pervasiveness of the disease, Brazil has reacted slightly differently. It did so from both a different premise, but also under different national and international policy conditions that those which characterized South Africa's policy-making.

Brazil did not question the course of globalization. Nor, acknowledging and accepting the presence of the epidemic through a different historical prism, did Brazil attempt to ply national and international priorities into new shape before acquiescing to their demands and dictates. Instead, Brazil largely accepted the rules-of-the-game of global interdependencies and attempted to leverage these to its benefit.[16] "Given the increasingly global frames of disease control, the way

---

14   See www.avert.org [accessed: 10 July 2012].

15   In the 1990s, before the advent of anti-retroviral drugs to fight HIV/AIDS, Brazil's HIV/AIDS epidemic threatened to become the second-worse in the world after South Africa's. However, perhaps in part because of its political engagement and the roll-out of its universal anti-retroviral program, it was overtaken by India's epidemic which has the dubious honor of "second-place," while South Africa's remains the severest to this day.

16   In this context, and in the particular context of anti-retroviral access and price negotiation, it must be noted that Brazil's economy and market are far larger than those of

a state deals with AIDS reveals its statecraft: in the Brazilian case, engagement with—and submission to—the forces of globalization."[17] Brazil's case is that of a country which bowed to those forces of globalization, but which also bent them to its own will.

This strategic approach served Brazil well, if not perfectly. In 1996, just prior to South Africa's ill-fated pharmaceutical fight over patent rights and access to ARVs, Brazil passed a strong patent protection law, changing its domestic policy arena and challenging that dominant in international intellectual property rights. The passage of the patent legislation was in line with Brazil's adoption of TRIPS under the auspices of the WTO in 1995. In its aftermath, in November 1996, the country promulgated its first AIDS treatment law. Brazil's roll-out program in turn adhered to but also pushed the limits of the dictates of globalization, and reaped some benefits.

Contrary to the situation in South Africa, Brazilian AIDS activists[18] did not invoke TRIPS and its supposedly protective provisions as a means to accessing ARVs. Instead, they convinced the state to "draft two additional legal articles that would allow compulsory licensing of patented drugs in a public health crisis," legislation which created "a venue for state activism vis-à-vis the pharmaceutical industry."[19] Thus where in South Africa conflict over the state's response to the HIV/AIDS epidemic became an issue of sovereign concern, torn between internal and external influence and interventions, leading to constraints in the country's

---

South Africa, bringing with them considerably more clout in international trade and even intellectual property right negotiations than does the exceptional but nonetheless relatively small country at the tip of the African continent.

17   Biehl, J. 2007. *Will to Live: AIDS Therapies and the Politics of Survival*. Princeton and Oxford: Princeton University Press: 11.

18   Without going into the definition of "activist" in great detail, it is useful to note that activists, here in the HIV/AIDS arena, are in this instance a creature of globalization themselves. They are often locally rooted with global ties and able to exploit these to the benefit or detriment of the state within which they find themselves, and which remains responsible and accountable for the contents of its sovereign responsibility to respond —and to protect not only special interests, here those infected and affected by HIV/AIDS, but also broader society. See also Cox, R.W. 1992. "Towards a Post-Hegemonic Conceptualization of World Order: Reflections on the Relevancy of Ibn Khaldun." In *Governance without Government: Order and Change in World Politics* (ed.) Rosenau, J. and Czempiel, E.-O. Cambridge: Cambridge University Press: 145. As Biehl writes, "Neoliberal governmentality has taken a new shape. Rather than actively seeking areas of need to address, the new market-oriented state selectively recognizes the claims of organized interest groups that 'represent' civil society, leaving out broader public needs for life-sustaining assistance—in the domains of housing, economic activity, and so forth. To be 'seen' by the state, people have to join these groups and engage in lobbying and lawmaking." Biehl, J. 2007. *Will to Live: AIDS Therapies and the Politics of Survival.* Princeton and Oxford: Princeton University Press: 11. This applies, as has been shown, to South Africa as well.

19   Biehl, J. 2007. *Will to Live: AIDS Therapies and the Politics of Survival.* Princeton and Oxford: Princeton University Press: 57.

domestic sovereignty, the polemics surrounding the response to the epidemic in Brazil remained an internal policy prerogative.

Brazil was aided by its large market size, something that South Africa both in terms of its population and in terms of its purchasing power could not proffer. Brazil constitutes the eleventh largest pharmaceutical market in the world, no small prize, even if the prices of pharmaceuticals such as ARVs are slashed. Playing by select rules of the game of globalization alongside its market size, Brazil "won" a similar pharmaceutical fight that the small, arguably stubborn, less flexible and less savvy South Africa, lost.

Brazil, under then President Cardoso, a sociologist renowned for his development of dependency theory, understood the country's market power as a tool to enhance its domestic sovereignty, as opposed to an asset that could also be twisted against it.

> The AIDS policy evolved in a paradoxical space, caught between a downsizing of central government and the desire of politicians to create, in Cardoso's own words, 'new rules for the political game.' ... [Cardoso] spoke of the state as contingent in nature and of his own political efforts to find new ways, beyond protectionism, to frame the rules of accountability and to find a state voice vis-à-vis the market. 'One cannot judge a priori or simplistically whether globalization is good or bad. One must see and decide in practice what is good and what is bad about it. We had to open the economy, keep a strict budget, and stop using inflation as a tool for capitalization. The state guarantees competition and also pushes for changes in the global productive basis.' ... Speaking as someone who 'successfully' shepherded Brazil toward the global market, Cardoso insisted that the state retains sovereign power: 'It is a question of responsibility. Nobody orders you to do these reforms. To say that the World Bank or the International Monetary Fund [IMF] forces you to limit public spending, for example, is a phantasmagoria of those who don't know how things work. These institutions bring experiences to the negotiating table, and a country like Brazil has enough weight to accept them or not.'[20]

In Brazil's case, in return for its "successful" adoption of and acquiescence to the WTO TRIPS regulations, even alongside its passage of national emergency legislation, "pharmaceutical imports to Brazil have increased substantially."[21] Furthermore, "while Brazil experimented with new modes of regulating markets for lifesaving treatments, pharmaceutical companies took the conflicts over drug pricing and the relaxation of patent laws at the WTO as opportunities both to negotiate broader market access in Brazil and to open up unforeseen AIDS markets in other countries."[22] After its 1997–1998 pharmaceutical fight fiasco,

---

20   Ibid., 11.
21   Ibid.
22   Ibid.

pharmaceutical companies also targeted South Africa, its burgeoning HIV-infected population and ensuing state roll-out, in their push to expand access and acquire market share, a move which has—proven profitable.[23]

Yet all is not well with this result. Illustrating this point is the quagmire in which countries such as Brazil, South Africa, and Uganda (as will be discussed below), dependent upon external aid to fight disease, such as HIV/AIDS, find themselves, regardless of their strict adherence to the tenets of globalization. For instance, while the WTO and pharmaceutical companies have demanded that countries adopt TRIPS, "American pharmaceutical companies have at the same time successfully downplayed the WTO as they lobbied for strict bilateral and regional trade agreements that made local production of generic drugs unviable."[24] This alters the terms of trade, including of pharmaceutical products, enabling companies and countries to negotiate individualized agreements, imperiling the TRIPS provisions to enable access to drugs whether by patent, parallel import, voluntary or compulsory license, by citing of a national emergency.

As in South Africa, in order "to make the antiretroviral treatment rollout economically feasible, the [Brazilian] government had to invest in the production of generic drugs and engage in political battles over pricing with major pharmaceutical corporations."[25] At the same time, certainly due to its market size as well as its state-centric approach, Brazil successfully bargained down the price of drugs essential to the antiretroviral therapy, something South Africa's situation rendered impossible. In 2001, the same year that the South African court case ended with that state acquiescing not to invoke TRIPS provisions for compulsory licensing or parallel imports, Brazil won a "confrontation with the US Government over patent legislation."[26] Unlike South Africa, Brazil did not "completely compromise its regulatory functions as it negotiates loans, adjustment plans, and the transfer of technology with international agencies."[27] Though this approach would no longer benefit South Africa, it inspired other countries to invent and invoke trade and treatment models other than those imposed "from the North."[28] As such, Brazil's "AIDS policy ended up working as a kind of counterweight to the economic orthodoxy in place internationally,"[29] and "all these initiatives created an international dialogue on intellectual property and medicines, and in the process, Brazil helped to constitute a southern trade bloc at the WTO aimed at

---

23   Obviously the acquisition of market share has been aided by the pressure of antiretrovirals and their purchase by international organizations such as PEPFAR and the Global Fund, among others.

24   Ibid.
25   Ibid., 57.
26   Ibid.
27   Ibid.
28   Ibid., 72.
29   Ibid., 77.

creating a world-wide system of drug price differentiation."[30] Also, "as the AIDS policy unfolded, Brazil attracted new investments, leading to novel public-private cooperation over access to medical technologies,"[31] not always under the state's control: the same local-global alliances that beset South Africa, with the difference that these came *after* the state asserted and assumed control of most of its HIV/AIDS policy and program implementation.

Aided by slightly different circumstances, Brazil, amending some of the rules of the game of globalization, largely won in its response to the epidemic. In contrast, South Africa tried to apply the accepted economic orthodoxy in order to reap the benefits of playing by all of the rules of the game. Instead, it ended up outside of the local-global arch as opposed to inside it, with limited sovereign control over its response and ensuing consequences.

The Brazilian Government threw what authority and power it had behind a concerted effort to defend the lives of its citizens and to act out its responsibility to respond. But while advocating for a particular population, this was of a smaller order of magnitude vis-à-vis the general population, which much more economic might to support the effort. Though Brazil is also economically a very unequal society, it did not face the same social and democratic pressures with which South Africa, emerging as it was from the apartheid era, was confronted all at once. Thus while South Africa owed a 'debt' both monetary to the IMF and donors and psychological, thanks to the market boycotts that helped speed the end of the apartheid regime, amidst clamoring for all of the fruits of economic development and democracy simultaneously, haranguing its HIV/AIDS negotiations, Brazil faced none of those pressures. Thus while the South African Government found its efforts to determine the pace and breadth of its HIV/AIDS policy circumvented, the Brazilian Government remained in steadfast control.

After its initial efforts, starting in November 2006, Brazil began negotiating a price reduction with Merck for efavirenz, a new-generation ARV. In April 2007, it warned Merck that unless Brazil could buy efavirenz the same price offered to the Thai government, it would issue a compulsory license in seven days' time. On Thursday 3 May the Brazilian Government rejected Merck's offer of a 30 percent price reduction. It issued a compulsory license the following day, making good on its threat and employing all of the legal provisions in the TRIPS agreement.[32] "From an ethical point of view the price difference is grotesque,"[33] said current President Luiz Inacio Lula da Silva. "By reducing the price per day from US$1.56 to $0.45 by buying Indian generic products prequalified by the World Health Organization, the Brazilian government said it expects to save $30 million in 2007

---

30   Ibid.

31   Ibid., 11.

32   Alcorn, K. 2007. "Brazil issues compulsory license on efavirenz." *Kaiser Network* (7 May).

33   Ibid.

and \$237 million between now and 2012 (when the efavirenz patent expires)."[34] "And from a political point of view, it represents a lack of respect, as though a sick Brazilian is inferior," Lula da Silva added." Other actors defending competing interests did not see it that way.

> Daniel Christman of the US Chamber of Commerce said: "Brazil is working to attract investment in innovative industries that rely on IP [intellectual property], and this move will likely cause investments to go elsewhere. Ironically, the Brazilian decision comes on the heels of real progress. Last Monday, the Office of the US Trade Representative recognized Brazil's successful crackdown on counterfeiting and piracy, moving the country from the Priority Watch List to the Watch List in its annual 'Special 301' report.[35]

Yet despite this dire prediction of Brazil losing IP-related industry, the country appears to be thriving as an investment destination and successful South-South leader and member of the BRICS states.

Nonetheless, the battles are far from over. For instance it remains to been seen what the pending lawsuits before India's courts will mean for the manufacture and sale of generic medications, including ARVs. A decision in the Novartis case is expected on 22 August 2012. Thus, Brazil's erstwhile "success" in appropriating some of globalization's framework for its benefit is caught up in the same precarious struggle to rewrite the rules of the game and to address HIV/AIDS as is South Africa. At stake is not only the immediate response to the epidemic, but also the security and integrity of countries struggling to enact their domestic sovereignty and responsibility to respond. Indeed, as has been shown in the preceding analysis, the very nature of the pressures of the demands brought by local-global alliances can and does compromise the ability of the state to enact this domestic sovereignty and its associated responsibility to respond. The GAP lens offers a useful framework through which to evaluate the effect of national and international policy conditions on the creation of sustainable solutions to problems across different contexts, especially wherein the accountability for ultimate and tactical responsibility is a question.

7.2 Brief Insights into HIV/AIDS and State Sovereignty: Uganda

The relationship between HIV/AIDS, state sovereignty and the responsibility to respond differs between South Africa and Brazil, and again from Uganda. Whereas Brazil boasts a "success" in terms of its policy response to HIV/AIDS, and South Africa has struggled to (re)assert tactical alongside theoretical accountability, Uganda's case is again different. Here again, the GAP analysis can provide insight,

---

34   Ibid.
35   Ibid.

especially as Uganda is arguably wedged even more tightly between its domestic conditions and its (inter)national policy constraints than is South Africa.

According to sheer numbers and statistics, Uganda is proportionally more affected by the epidemic than is Brazil, but less so than is South Africa. It also has higher dependence upon external aid and is subject to a greater number of prescriptions from the global North than are either Brazil or South Africa. As a consequence, its domestic sovereignty is arguably much more compromised than that either of the other two countries mentioned here. Yet Uganda's trajectory in terms of HIV/AIDS is often lauded as a "success," even more so than that of Brazil, since its HIV prevalence rate appears to have fallen from roughly 15 percent in the mid-1990s to just over five percent (5.4 percent[36]) of the population as of 2007. However, the verdict is still out on both the cause and the durability of that reduction. Uganda still faces a serious concern in the form of its HIV/AIDS epidemic and associated strains upon its responsibility to respond.

As Uganda's HIV infection rate rapidly rose throughout the 1990s, the country's President, Yoweri Museveni, struck a comparatively progressive approach against the epidemic rarely seen in Africa. In particular, he publicized and promoted behavior change to stem the tide of the swelling epidemic, emphasizing the home-grown Ugandan initiative of "zero-grazing" to discourage multiple, concurrent sexual partners, whose networks are largely now viewed as the fuel of the epidemic. In light of the President's outspokenness and the initial fall in infections, it seems reasonable to assume that ordinary Ugandans heeded his advice. Indeed, the decline in HIV prevalence in Uganda coincided with "a plunge in the proportion of people with casual sexual partners—everything from informal girlfriends and boyfriends, to one-night stands, visits to sex workers, and short-term, impermanent affairs"[37] in apparent confirmation of the application of the policy of "zero-grazing."

> [I]t stood to reason that partner reduction would have had a more powerful effect [than condoms]. If the network of concurrent relationships serves as a superhighway for HIV, partner reduction would be like a sledgehammer, breaking up the highway into smaller networks, and destroying the 'on-ramps'—the casual relationships that let HIV onto the superhighway in the first place.[38]

However, while it does appear that the transmission rate of HIV in Uganda slowed from the late 1990s, there is no conclusive evidence that this is causally linked to behavior change with regard to sexual partnership networks. Though many analyses make this assertion, most of them ignore the role and impact of

---

36   See www.avert.org for more statistics, including the breakdown by urban and rural population.

37   Epstein, H. 2007. *The Invisible Cure: Africa, The West, and the Fight Against AIDS*. New York: Farrar, Straus and Giroux: 175.

38   Ibid., 176.

the deaths of thousands of Ugandans erstwhile involved in such sexual networks. Death, and thereby the removal of links in the chains of those sexual networks, is bound to have had a profound impact on the rate of HIV incidence.[39] In seeming confirmation of this correlation, as sexual networks become established in a new generation, one which does not bear the memory of the suffering and deaths of those that have gone before, Uganda's incidence rate is again on the rise.

In the interim, ARVs entered the scene. As they entered the collective consciousness especially of donors, these, notably on the international level, paid less heed to the merits of partner reduction and the policy of "zero-grazing."

> It is possible that the implications of the findings from Uganda—that Africans had fought this epidemic on their own through frankness and common sense, compassion for the afflicted, and a shift in sexual norms and attitudes surrounding sexual relationships and the rights of women—were the last thing UN bureaucrats would have wanted to hear. It meant that fighting AIDS would require an approach with which they were quite unfamiliar, and for which their existing expertise might not be paramount.[40]

In "every UNAIDS document I could find that had been produced in the decade since the agency was established in 1996, I found almost no mention of partner reduction and none whatsoever of Zero Grazing."[41] UNAIDS' "Best Practice" collection of briefing documents ignored such a possible response to the epidemic, mentioning "condom programs, voluntary testing and counseling, STD treatment services, and many other things."[42] In order words, the best practice model imposed notably external interventions based on a medical response to HIV/AIDS as opposed to one more holistic.

---

39   A new study conducted in Zimbabwe has just revealed this relationship, linking primarily AIDS-related deaths, with some assistance from hard-to-measure behavior change, with a decline in incidence. See Leach-Lemens, C. 2010. "HIV fall in Zimbabwe due to deaths and behaviour change, not migration." *Aidsmap* (4 June). See also Navario, P. 2010. "Zimbabwe's Second Wave?" *Huffington Post* (19 May).

40   Epstein, H. 2007. *The Invisible Cure: Africa, The West, and the Fight Against AIDS*. New York: Farrar, Straus and Giroux: 181.

41   Ibid., 177.

42   Ibid. Also, the issue of partner reduction is usually couched under the rubric of "be faithful" in the ABC mantra. However, "be faithful," or fidelity, has, perhaps astoundingly, more than one possible interpretation. Fidelity can mean, to some of those practicing it, that a person's main, long-term, partner does not find out about any others. This has important implications, since it is most often in such long-term, apparently faithful partnerships, that precautions against the transmission of HIV are not taken, and in such partnerships that HIV tends to be spread most reliably. See Timberg, C. 2007. "Speeding HIV's Deadly Spread: Multiple, Concurrent Partners Drive Disease in Southern Africa." *The Washington Post Foreign Service* (2 March).

PEPFAR reinforced this approach. Cited for its "success," but largely ignoring its terms, Uganda was chosen to receive assistance. It heeded local and global demands to accept hundreds of millions of dollars in PEPFAR funding to provide primarily for ARVs to shore up the response to the epidemic.

> President Bush, in his public speeches, identified Uganda as his model for the successful implementation of a newly minted US policy of ABC. [Mostly without the condoms] In fact, evaluations of US AIDS funding noted that Uganda had received an unusually high share of the resources. Thus, one might understand that President Museveni felt particularly obliged to the US government and to President Bush.[43]

As a condition of the aid, the country also agreed to advocate ABC—abstinence, be faithful and condomize—though with an emphasis on the first two points. This tuned down and drowned out completely any mention of "zero-grazing." Already at the International AIDS Conference of 2004 held in Bangkok, President Museveni went on record with a revised stance on AIDS prevention. Museveni refuted the effectiveness of condoms, calling them un-masculine, and thereby undermining 20 years of hard-won acceptance of condoms and a central means, within ABC, of HIV prevention.[44] He expressed his gratitude to US President George W. Bush, thanking him for the US$94 million in PEPFAR funds Uganda received for the fiscal year of 2004–2005. Indeed, US funding to Uganda increased "by 50 percent between 2004 and 2005 and Uganda was scheduled to receive [US]$58 million from PEPFAR in 2007."[45] While the funding provided bolsters Uganda's means to address and treat HIV/AIDS, it also posed a number of problems.

Most notably, its volume threatened to overwhelm the structures meant to absorb and administer it. For example, with regard to the US$258 million allotted to Uganda for 2007,

> [I]t seems Uganda was expecting only about [US] $235 million and when an extra $22.2 million was forthcoming they were not quite sure what to do. 'We had to go through the process of planning again ... It is becoming difficult to absorb more funds ... All partners are at the limit,' says a dismayed member of PEPFAR's field staff.[46]

Such incapacity would only increase Uganda's dependence upon external contributions, both in terms of finance but also in terms of skills, notably administration and implementation. As a result, it threatened to eclipse the state

43   Susser, I. 2009. *AIDS, Sex, and Culture: Global Politics and Survival in Southern Africa.* West Sussex, UK: Wiley-Blackwell: 50.

44   Ibid., 51.

45   Ibid.

46   Ibid.

and undermine its domestic sovereignty and ability to assume its responsibility to respond. Thus while the PEPFAR funds flowed to Uganda, "the contributions of the Ugandan government to AIDS treatment and prevention have remained stable—only around 5 percent of the total."[47] Therefore, "clearly, the sharp difference between what the Ugandan Government has contributed to AIDS funds and the millions contributed by PEPFAR suggests the importance of this funding to President Museveni and possibly even to the stability of his regime."[48] This means that Uganda's HIV/AIDS budget and capacity is essentially outsourced, rendering it dependent upon external funding, decision-making and intervention, severely compromising the country's sovereign responsibility to respond and to be feasibly accountable.

This trajectory reveals the extent of the external influence exerted upon national states to adopt a particular approach in responding to the HIV/AIDS epidemic and to the ensuing relationship of dependency; regardless of whether such interventions are appropriate or effective. This is evident even in the case of the promotion of ARVs, which have the obvious merit of prolonging the lives of those who are HIV infected and treated with them, but carry the attendant disadvantage of possibly prolonging the epidemic by enabling, through that longevity, lax prevention efforts and the continual transmission of HIV.[49] Therefore, though finally, in 2006, UNAIDS began to stress reduction of multiple sexual partnerships as a key goal for AIDS prevention, particularly in Africa. By then, however, the epidemic had spread exponentially across Africa especially, and even in Uganda transmission rates were once again on the rise.

These developments, especially of dependency and the GAP indicators, in Uganda, share some similarities with those in South Africa, but stand in notable contrast to those in Brazil. In Uganda, as in South Africa, while the state assumed responsibility to provide protection in the form of healthcare broadly and antiretroviral treatment specifically under the auspices of its domestic sovereignty, the enactment and fulfillment thereof became inextricably tied to external influence and interventions. In Brazil on the other hand, as described above, the state has remained the central decision-maker and actor in the country's HIV/AIDS program. Whereas Uganda's ability to deliver upon its sovereign responsibility to respond has been compromised amidst this dependency, Brazil has better been able to act out its sovereign provisions.[50] So in two out of three cases involving

---

47   Ibid.

48   Ibid.

49   As a societal and sexual disease, these are the inherent dangers of the continual spread of HIV/AIDS, short of quarantine, which, though applied in Cuba, is both against human rights' edicts, and inherently impractical.

50   The emergence of such parallel systems is beginning to receive attention. See, Piller, C. and Smith, D. 2007. "Gateses' charitable gifts have unintended consequences." *Tribune Newspapers: Los Angeles Times* (16 December); and McCoy, D., Kembhavi, G., Patel, J. and Luintel, A. 2009. "The Bill & Melinda Gates Foundation's grant-making

the responsibility to respond to HIV/AIDS, the domestic sovereignty of states is further compromised and limited by external involvement, thereby jeopardizing the implementation of that responsibility and associated accountability.

Drawing on these comparisons as seen through the lens of the GAP, it is possibly to conclude that each of these countries, South Africa, Brazil and Uganda, bore and continue to bear the ultimate responsibility to respond to their HIV/AIDS epidemics. Whether they can act on their own, in both theory and practice, has depended on the relative weight of the epidemic not only vis-à-vis other priorities but in relation to the social and economic costs to be carried ultimately by the state. Where the relation was low, as in Brazil, the state could assume near complete control. Where it was higher, as in South Africa, compromise led to circumvented decision-making and fragmented implementation: the very hallmarks of the GAP.

> Early on the South African government told aid agencies and donors that it would decide what aid is needed and how it would be administered. The result is that the UN and its agencies run what is at present a unique program, essentially an experiment, along those lines. They are not the lead agency, but respond to what SA needs/requests rather than forcing programs on the country.[51]

This stance stands in stark contrast to the take-it-or-leave-it and circumvention of the state approach implied by Ambassador Rasool and chronicled throughout this analysis. Yet it is gaining traction, and not only with the UN, but also with PEPFAR's country programs, for example. Though not—yet—implemented across the board, this shift towards 'country ownership' promisingly constitutes an initial rope across the GAP, forming as it does a line of clearer designation of responsibility and accountability leading back to the ultimately responsible and accountable state. Where it was outsourced, as in Uganda, the assumption of tactical responsibility outweighed both the relation and the theoretical ultimate responsibility—as PEPFAR and other donors wind down their programs, however, the GAP question of just that final accountability is reemerging.

Whether the GAP framework is applicable beyond the case of HIV/AIDS is the next question.

7.3 Additional Applications

Can the GAP analysis be applied to other crises that challenge state domestic sovereignty and responsibility to respond?

As the above analyses have illustrated, enacting domestic sovereignty is a complicated exercise. So, too, is marrying the theoretical and tactical responsibility

---

programme for global health." *The Lancet*, 373(9675) (9 May): 1645–1653. See also recommendations in Chapter 8.

51   Personal correspondence with Ambassador Thomas Wheeler, 18 January 2008.

to respond with the ultimate accountability to do so. While exercising sovereignty has always been an enterprise prone to various restrictions, those are ever-increasingly tied to external influences, aided and abetted by local-global alliances. Local as well as external actors and influences converge into alliances to address a priority, and failing to elicit a desired state response, might set up parallel structures of response bypassing it. The outcome can undermine domestic sovereignty, and limit its sovereignty, further undermining its ability to enact its responsibility to respond for which it retains ultimate accountability. This shift results in the GAP. The consequences are far-reaching, especially with regard to the allocation of responsibility and accountability.

As seen in the case of HIV/AIDS in South Africa, the epidemic has progressed and the state's domestic sovereignty is and has been increasingly circumscribed. The South African state has become beholden to the local-global alliances in its midst—demanding HIV treatment, sourcing funds, procuring it, pitting financing for HIV/AIDS at times against other pressing priorities and the pull of foreign direct investment—resulting in a downward spiral of dependence and diminished ability to act upon its responsibility to respond. With the trend toward "country ownership," an arguably weakened South Africa finds itself again facing an upward climb to reconnect its tactical with its ultimate responsibility and accountability to respond.

Is it the only state facing such a challenge? Can its lessons be applied elsewhere?

Here two possible examples of the application of the GAP framework are explored. The first looks at its applicable to the responsibility to respond to migrant access to healthcare; the second to that of universal access to water.

In the case of managing migrant health, where health is deemed a universal human right, and the responsibility for it lies with sovereign states, the GAP exists between the responsibility of the source and the recipient country for migrant access to healthcare. At present, this is unchartered territory. For example, Zimbabweans who cross the border into South Africa are stateless in terms of healthcare and cannot access public healthcare unless with forged identification documents. By contrast in Spain, migrants (had) automatically had six months of healthcare access before being required to document employment to maintain that access; a short-term bridge of the GAP. However, in the latter case, this access has been cut due to the current financial straits in which the country finds itself in 2012, illustrating the dire need for a more sustainable solution in allocating responsibility and accountability.

The health of incoming migrants has consequences for the sedentary populace, as well as vice versa. Therefore, the lack of clarity in terms of determining the responsibility for the healthcare of migrants exacerbates disease transmission—both into the recipient country and back into the source country—and takes an avoidable human toll, not only on health but also on economic productivity. Also given that, for instance, there are more Malawian doctors in London than in all of Malawi, it would seem only reasonable that the United Kingdom support the health of migrant Malawians. As an added bonus, such immigrant doctors might be better able to recognize and treat diseases stemming from their place of origin than domestic doctors: a real boon in a world increasingly facing the global transmission of disease. Therefore, regulating or transferring healthcare responsibility between states would serve to cover the GAP between responsibility jurisdictions. In order to bridge the GAP, responsibility and accountability could be shared between states and non-state actors to allow access for migrants in both source and recipient countries. Such an arrangement would go a long way toward resolving this particular healthcare dilemma, promoting productive migration while protecting both migratory and sedentary populations.

In the case of access to water, the crisis and the benefits of regulation are also comparable. The GAP, in fact, is more obvious. Water is also a universal human right, and one which people need to access everywhere, therefore making water availability and access everywhere a necessity. The guarantee that that necessity be met depends upon states as well as non-state actors who control the source, flow, cleanliness, points of access, and delivery of water. As a commodity that often crosses borders, and is variously owned by public and private providers, water is subject to numerous jurisdictions. Ultimately states are responsible for guaranteeing continuous, safe, and affordable access. This results in another instance of the GAP.

For example: to use South Africa again, the state state is responsible for guaranteeing its populace's right to water. However, Johannesburg's water comes from across the border in Lesotho where it flows from rivers dammed by the World Bank-funded Highlands Water Project, where it displaced thousands of people. Lesotho as a whole also has less water security, despite being the source of Johannesburg's supply, than does the city. However, in the city, water provision, and therefore access, is managed by a French company, Suez. If people in Soweto (a township on the southern outskirts of Johannesburg) do not pay for their water, Suez will terminate their access. This is illegal under the provisions of global water governance as promulgated by the UN. The state should have to intervene, because it is the state, not the company, and not the UN, which retains the duty to provide for its populace's water. The South African state, however, has little leverage to make the for-profit company comply.

At present no global enforcement mechanism exists to make a company meet a state responsibility. Short of nationalization, no mechanism exists under which South Africa could revoke Suez's license to provide water: and seeing what the threat of such a compulsory license under TRIPS led to the case of HIV/AIDS, such a move by the state would likely lead to a crippling global response and further stymie the country's ability to meet its responsibility to respond, in this case to its populace's right to water.

Thus the analysis shows that the GAP is applicable beyond the case of HIV/AIDS. It also highlights the need for a global system of regulation to bridge it and to provide for the responsible accounting of the responsibility to respond.

7.4 Conclusion

As observed at the outset of this analysis, an arch of *almost* single-minded focus on sovereign statehood links democratic South African presidents Mandela, Mbeki and Zuma. Former President Mbeki and Minister of Finance Manuel put a premium on the independence of South Africa's domestic sovereignty, arguably to the point of harming an effective response to the HIV/AIDS epidemic. Current President Jacob Zuma, has, against expectations, continued to carry the torch. He is being met with much more positive resonance.

> The Zuma government and his Minister of Health, Dr Aaron Motsoaledi, are now developing a national HIV strategy that aims at preventing further cases, treating those who are infected, and weaning the nation of foreign assistance for not only AIDS but all of the country's health needs. In short, South Africa aims to be the first African nation to build health for all, *independent of foreign donors.*[52]

Indeed, also as the trend towards "country ownership" picks up, South Africa has promulgated a policy document on a National Insurance Scheme, an effort being met at the global level by a series of initiatives aimed at designing and adopting universal health insurance. The critical challenge remains to bridge the GAP.

Zuma's goal, however, faces some of the same critical challenges that dogged the Mbeki administration: a promise to treat all of those who require ARVs, coupled with ongoing dependence upon foreign aid to finance drug purchases—whose price stands to rise even as the necessary amounts expand as more people require them and as increasing numbers need second- and third-line medications—amidst the continued volatility of the South African rand. Zuma's focus on independence has, however, much like Mbeki's, not been able to shield the country from internal and external interventions curtailing primarily its domestic sovereignty, especially the state's ability to enact its responsibility to respond, on its own terms.

In the case of South Africa, the trajectory of HIV/AIDS coincides with the transformation of a nation: a nation throwing off the shackles of apartheid, transiting through revolution, and striving to evolve into a responsible democracy. "Ironically, in terms of the AIDS epidemic, the 1994 victory over apartheid allowed the opening of borders to migrant labor from the rest of southern Africa, which may actually have accelerated the spread of the virus."[53] Shown to be applicable to South Africa, "the history of countries throwing off tyrannical regimes tends to

---

52   Author's emphasis. Council on Foreign Relations 2009, Global Health Update (23 December). As of 2010, South Africa is again receiving increased aid from PEPFAR. This puts it in the precarious position of being dependent, with particular risk due to the financial crisis and funding flat-lining.

53   Susser, I. 2009. *AIDS, Sex, and Culture: Global Politics and Survival in Southern Africa.* West Sussex, UK: Wiley-Blackwell: 81.

follow a pattern," of "euphoria, accompanied by utopian pledges for the future."[54] As former President Mbeki acknowledged, "the new rulers find the business of governing more difficult and messier than they could ever have imagined":[55] "the new administration had to learn the rules of the inherited bureaucracy and to negotiate with provincial hierarchies."[56] Indeed, amidst and despite the severity of the HIV/AIDS epidemic, "Hein Marais stresses the enormous energies required for the transition. Throughout the 1990s, as central ANC leaders focused on issues of housing, racial equality, and income, concern with AIDS became marginalized."[57] The struggles of governance, of agenda-setting, and of implementation of policy, of meeting responsibility to respond, are, furthermore, far from resolved.

It can thus be concluded that South Africa finds itself in the precarious, but not unique, position of being a sovereign state whose responsibilities are, at least at times, assumed by non-state actors. This assumption of tactical responsibility, which occurs both with and without the consent of the sovereign state, is not accompanied by a similar transfer of ultimate responsibility and accountability, which remains the remit of the state. This, as has been argued, is the GAP. "Since most sovereign states confer extensive powers, and a monopoly of military power ('the sword of war') and police power ('the sword of justice'), on their officials, that raises fundamental questions of accountability and answerability."[58] This means that no effectual linear relationship between rights and responsibilities, and accountability, exists at the national or global level, or between them: an increasingly widespread phenomenon which poses a considerable existential threat to the *legitimacy* of as well as the enactment of the tenets of sovereignty, most notably its attendant responsibility to respond.

Aspects of this situation also reflect the notion of dependency. The notion of dependency emphasizes the incongruence between what governments *should* do and what they actually can do, when their 'doing' is contingent upon outside support that they can do little to determine. For instance, states might try to de-

---

54   Russell, A. 2009. *The Battle for the Soul of South Africa*. Hutchinson: Introduction.

55   Ibid.

56   Susser, I. 2009. *AIDS, Sex, and Culture: Global Politics and Survival in Southern Africa*. West Sussex, UK: Wiley-Blackwell: 81.

57   Ibid.

58   Jackson, R. 2007. *Sovereignty*. Cambridge: Polity Press: 18. "What is required is not only the support of other individuals and private organizations but also and even more so the recognition of human rights by authoritative and credible public organizations with powers of enforcement and the will to act accordingly. Here is where the sovereign state enters the equation. State involvement is crucial because, as Thomas Hobbes pointed out long ago, 'the laws of nature, in the state of nature, are silent.' An organized state authority with sufficient will and power is required to give natural law an authoritative voice that will be heard and heeded by most people. Thomas Paine agrees with Thomas Hobbes and claims that the sovereign state exists primarily for that purpose. He speaks of 'the end of all political associations' as 'the preservation of the natural and imprescriptible rights of man'." 119.

link from the world economy "by expropriating foreign capital and/or controlling its entry" asserting control of domestic sovereignty, by "cutting down imports, etc., with associated redistributive measures."[59] South Africa attempted some of these measure through the proposed the RDP. Yet, as has been shown throughout this analysis, internal and external pressures counteracted these impulses, pushing for acquiescence to the global rules of the game. Mandela weathered the loss of 'confidence' inherent with any attempt at such de-linking. The South African Government then promulgated GEAR. Thus, South Africa accepted the necessity of the International Monetary Fund's endorsement as creditworthy to shore up that confidence, and submitted, for instance, to the IMF review in July 2007. Instead of de-linking, South Africa heeded calls for increased integration into global political-economic structural hierarchies and accepted circumscribed domestic sovereignty.[60] Though not completely dependent as a result, this trajectory illustrates South Africa's circumscribed independence nonetheless.

This contemporary curtailing and limiting of its domestic sovereignty posits two possible trajectories for the foreseeable future: a reassertion of state-centric sovereignty alongside the wresting of control over responsibilities to respond from local-global alliances and external actors with less dependence upon them; or, a restructuring of global allocation of sovereign responsibility and accountability, along the lines of those proposed by R2P. In the latter instance, voluntary measures would become compulsory, and the 'international community' would be endowed not only with responsibility in theory, but with responsibility and accountability in practice.[61] Both possibilities present challenges and opportunities.

> The gap between how power is exercised in Africa and international assumptions about how states operate is significant and, in some cases, growing. State consolidation in Africa is not merely an academic issue but is, instead,

---

59   Seers, D. 1981. *Dependency Theory: A Critical Reassessment.* London: Frances Pinter (Publishers) Ltd: 135.

60   Ibid., 140. "What ultimately sets the boundaries on the policies of delinking governments are the political interests of these countries," including the interests of domestic—international constituencies as seen in the HIV/AIDS arena. In addition, in accepting this circumscribed domestic sovereignty on the macroeconomic level, the country paid a double price: it gave up many of the egalitarian policies inherent in the RDP and even in the redistribution pillar of GEAR, and saw South African poverty actually increase in the first decade of democracy.

61   Ibid., 130. "The first approach notes that state sovereignty involves heavy responsibilities, and that the primary responsibility of sovereign states is to protect people within their own borders." ... "The legal foundations of the responsibility to protect are obligations inherent in state sovereignty, which is the source of international law."

> Enacting these obligations is critical to the future of tens of millions of people who are at risk from the insecurity that is the inevitable by-product of state decline and failure.[62]

Regarding the former, and poignantly in the case of the HIV/AIDS epidemic response, South Africa arguably attempted such an approach of reasserting its full domestic sovereignty. As such, the South African Government attempted to secure the opportunity of being "more in control of its own future" by establishing "priorities and programs of its own choosing."[63] At the same time, however, it recognized the challenge posed by HIV/AIDS, and the positive role played by local-global alliances "to combat the devastating aspects of the disease that can potentially harm any government's development."[64] Consequently, inversely to its attempts, South Africa found itself caught ever more tightly between its ability to exercise its circumscribed domestic sovereignty.

In the latter instance, the local-global alliances and the international community as such—represented by the Global Fund, UNAIDS and the UN, among others—did act upon responsibilities pertaining to HIV/AIDS, not least in providing testing and treatment access. However, by that very generosity they also foisted expectations upon South Africa which the state could not—alone—meet. Far from assuming responsibility to respond, these external actors and their actions emphasized South Africa's dependency upon them and actually reinforced the country's circumscribed domestic sovereignty. This furthered weakened the South African state, without contending with the emerging cleavage between tactical responsibility and ultimate responsibility and accountability to respond. In the current reckoning, this GAP remains. However, there are ways to bridge it. Proposals to that effect are the focus of the next and final chapter of this book.

---

62   Herbst, J. 2000. *States and Power in Africa.* Princeton, New Jersey: Princeton University Press: 4–5.

63   Fredland, R.A. 2001. "A Sea Change in Responding to the AIDS Epidemic: Leadership is Awakened." *International Relations,* 15(6): 89–101.

64   Ibid.

Chapter 8
Conclusion and Recommendations

In conclusion it should be possible to answer the questions asked at the outset: How did South Africa meet its responsibility to respond to its HIV/AIDS epidemic between 1981 and 2011? In particular, what can be concluded about South Africa's HIV/AIDS response in light of its responsibility to respond? Whereto the responsibility to respond? What lessons can be applied from the analysis of South Africa's response to its HIV/AIDS epidemic to bridging the GAP that ensues between tactical and ultimate responsibility to respond?

What can be done to bridge the GAP? Two scaffolds seem to appear. The one rests on the delegation by the state to external, non-state actors of responsibility and accountability for their response. The other builds upon a system of coordinated *shared* governance. This consists of legal delineation of responsibility and accountability among all participating actors at the local, national and global governance levels, as required to sustain sovereign statehood and the responsibility to respond. Can it be concluded that South Africa is following either of these approaches? What lessons can the South African experience impart for other states facing similar crises amidst increasing local-state-global fragmented responsibility to respond?

As premised above, South Africa's sovereign statehood endows upon it the responsibility to provide for the security and welfare and well-being of its populace. In order to strengthen this guarantee, it is answerable to itself, as well as to the international community of sovereign states. However, the reverse, that either the international community of sovereign states or any external actor is responsible to the state in which they act, is not the case.

This lopsided reality is clearly on display in the South African response to HIV/AIDS.

HIV/AIDS, and the evocative responses it engendered, has become not only a state crisis, but a global concern. Affected states, external state partners, and local-global advocacy and activists alliances all vie to respond to the pandemic. Yet the ultimate responsibility to respond remains within the rubric of sovereign statehood. While attempting to strengthen the response to the epidemic, the scores of external—and ultimately non-responsible and unaccountable—actors can actually weaken the state.

This has been particularly evident in the aftermath of the 2008 global financial crisis. When the external aid upon which HIV/AIDS interventions depend evaporates, the affected state is left not only with unmet expectations of medical care, but also with baton of responsibility and accountability it might be too weak to carry. Its domestic sovereignty and sovereign statehood is thereby compromised.[1] And yet strong, competent statehood is a prerequisite for effective implementation of the responsibility to respond. Indeed exquisitely ironically, given the circuitous route outlined in the preceding analysis, as PEPFAR's Goosby indicated, the sustainability of current and future HIV/AIDS responses is increasingly contingent upon effective national, notably domestic sovereignty and national assumption of the responsibility to respond.

It is relevant here to reiterate that the reference to the 'responsibility to respond' refers to the three central tenets of the expanded definition of sovereignty—territorial sovereignty, security of welfare, and accountability to the international community for fulfilling the first two prescriptions. It is based on the assumption of internal, or domestic, sovereignty as ascribed to the nation-state,[2] as per Krasner and Hösle.[3] This definition of the responsibility to respond is particularly applicable in the case of HIV/AIDS in South Africa. Notably, "external sovereignty seems to be a logical consequence of inner sovereignty":[4] so South Africa's external assertion of its sovereign statehood vis-à-vis the international community of sovereign states in effect depends upon its internal, its domestic sovereignty. Yet given the external interventions motivated by the necessity of a response to HIV/AIDS and imparted to and imposed upon the South African state, this domestic sovereignty is compromised. What then, given that "inner sovereignty without external sovereignty seems incomplete and inconsequential. On the other hand, external sovereignty endangers precisely what has been achieved by inner sovereignty:

---

1   See also Rosenau, J.N. 1992. "Governance, order, and change in world politics." In *Governance without Government: Order and Change in World Politics* (ed.) Rosenau, J. and Czempiel, E.-O. Cambridge: Cambridge University Press: 3: "During the present period of rapid and extensive global change, however, the constitutions of national governments and their treaties have been undermined by the demands and greater coherence of ethnic and other subgroups, the globalization of economies, the advent of broad social movements, the shrinking of political distances by microelectronic technologies, and the mushrooming of global interdependencies fostered by currency crises, environmental pollution, terrorism, the drug trade, AIDS, and a host of other transnational issues that are crowding the global agenda. These centralizing and decentralizing dynamics have undermined constitutions and treaties in the sense that they have contributed to the shifts in the loci of authority. Governments still operate and they are still sovereign in a number of ways; but, as noted above, some of their authority has been relocated toward subnational collectivities. Some of the functions of governance, in other words, are now being performed by activities that do not originate with governments."

2   As opposed to the "responsibility to protect" as enshrined by the ICISS, which refers to the responsibility to protect against war crimes, crimes against humanity, and genocide.

3   This is not to be confused with the ICISS definition of "the" responsibility to project in cases pertaining to crimes against humanity, war crimes and genocide.

4   Hösle, V. 2004. *Morals and Politics.* Notre Dame: University of Notre Dame Press: 493.

namely, peace through the hierarchizing of decision-making structures"?[5] Were South Africa not bowed by and bound to external actors, it could not deliver upon its HIV-related responsibilities, endangering its domestic sovereignty. Nonetheless, in the final instance, the South African state remains accountable for its responsibility to respond—whether it can meet this or not. Consequently, South Africa sought a way out, a means of assuming only the responsibility it could account for: alone.

> In a dangerous world marked by overwhelming inequalities of power and resources, sovereignty is for many states their best—and sometimes seemingly their only—line of defence ... For many states and peoples, it is also a recognition of their equal worth and dignity, a protection of their unique identities and their national freedom, and an affirmation of their right to shape and determine their own destiny.[6]

However, this 'solution' did not last. In a world of limited statehood beholden to local-global alliances, it could not last.

So South Africa finds itself in the situation outlined above of uninvited interventions against HIV/AIDS which contributed to the curtailing of its domestic sovereignty. Despite its resistance, its reservations that were proven correct by the by consequences of the global financial crisis, South Africa is circumscribed in its domestic sovereignty. This has come to be primarily as a result of the state's reluctance to act and to the responding rally by local-global alliances of advocates and activists seeking the rights as guaranteed in the Constitution. Yet this outcome was not completely inevitable.

The state could have acted out another part. South Africa might have capitalized on external interventions through 2007, including favorable returns on capital market investments (as opposed to waiting for greater foreign direct investment in its own economy) reaping the benefits of a wave of essentially free HIV/AIDS funding, and then launching its own, independently financed HIV/AIDS response. But to act such would have been to read the future. Instead, South Africa attempted to go-it-alone through 2007, only to find itself dependent just as the promise of continuously financed dependency which the previous interventions seemed to promise evaporated.

Now, some of that dependency forcibly severed, South Africa still holds the reigns of domestic sovereign responsibility to respond. It is suddenly overreached.

Who will hold the external actors to account for the responsibility to respond of the state in which and on which and around which they act?

---

5 Ibid.

6 See International Commission on Intervention and State Sovereignty (ICISS) 2001. "The Responsibility to Protect." Ottawa: International Development Research Centre.

8.1 Whereto the Ultimate Responsibility to Respond?
Tactical Recommendations

The local-global alliances described above form an arch which contributes to and exacerbates the GAP between a sovereign state and external state and non-state actors' ability to enact and account for the responsibility to respond. In the case of HIV/AIDS in South Africa such an arch resulted in internal activism tied to external intervention jeopardizing South Africa's domestic sovereignty. One outcome has been hundreds of thousands of lives saved.[7] Another outcome, however, has been the creation of a system of governing alliances, networks, parallel to that of the sovereign state but without sovereign safeguards of responsibility and accountability. In this instance "the government ... has simply disqualified itself from a meaningful role in the fight against AIDS. The void has been filled to a small extent with NGOs running limited programs in parallel to the government's half-hearted attempts."[8] That void invited the emergence of local-global alliances which continue to constrict not only a state's sovereign statehood, but also the state's sovereign ability to respond. This leads to the GAP.

Challenging South Africa's non-linear and particularly chaotic response to HIV/AIDS, especially surrounding the controversy of Mbeki's "denialist" stance toward the epidemic, South African activists, led by the TAC reacted. They staged demonstrations, filed legal briefs accusing the then health minister Manto Tshabalala-Msimang and then President Mbeki of genocide,[9] and illegally imported antiretroviral drugs. Through its activism, TAC formed local-global alliances with international AIDS organizations, such as MSF which put pressure on the South

---

7   See Chigwedere, P., Seage, G.R., Gruskin, S., et al. 2008. "Estimating the Lost Benefits for Antiretroviral Drugs Use in South Africa." *Perspectives: Epidemiology and Social Science, Journal of Acquired Immune Deficiency Syndrome*, 49(4) (1 December) for estimates on the cost of delayed anti-retroviral therapy in terms of human lives in South Africa.

8   Personal correspondence with Mariette van Beek, formerly of the World Bank, 24 January 2008.

9   A charge of genocide falls directly under the rubric of the ICISS's responsibility to protect. In the case of a state's failure to so protect its people, the ICISS guidelines recommend that the "international community" intervene to guarantee this protection itself. Though the charges against Mbeki and Tshabalala-Msimang were dropped, and not pursued in theoretical or practical debate vis-à-vis the rights and responsibilities stipulated by the notion of sovereignty itself, the accusations themselves bring to the fore the entire argument put forward in this book: that a sovereign state, setting its priorities and seeking to enact these within national and international contexts, challenged by local-global alliances which can constrain domestic sovereignty, finds its ability to act upon its responsibility to respond in the first instance undermined, with longer-term consequences for its sovereignty statehood as well. This last point is illustrated in the withdrawal of external actors and assistance and the retention of responsibility and accountability by a partially neutered state without adequate capacity to act.

African Government to respond to HIV/AIDS—in a certain manner. Involvement in the South African AIDS arena by the Global Fund, PEPFAR, UNAIDS, and the private sector, including the GBC, increased the pressure. When the South African Government caved to their demands to deliver a particular response to the HIV/AIDS epidemic, though it had attempted alternative responses both before and in the meantime, it did so along some of the main lines demanded by these alliances and actors. The fact that such external interventions infringing upon and limiting a state's independence can include "programs by major international financial institutions [and arguably other such influence-wielding organizations] whose recipients often feel they have no choice but to accept,"[10] certainly applies to South Africa's case in perception and practice. Consequently, South Africa ceded, both willingly and unwillingly, some of its domestic sovereignty to the agenda of one important cause, the fight against HIV/AIDS. In doing so, it further curtailed its own ability to assume actively the associated responsibilities and accountability to respond. However, its sovereign statehood retained the ultimate responsibility and accountability.

Despite this evidence, some argue that compromised or limited sovereignty is a fiction. They contend that state sovereignty is reinforced as opposed to undermined, by local-global alliances. By implication they would not see a GAP between the tactical assumption of some tasks belonging to the rubric of sovereignty,[11] and ultimate responsibility and accountability. But how then would ultimate responsibility and accountability flow between external actors and the sovereign state?

By the logic of those who see local-global alliances strengthening the state that flow materializes in the act of the state's "participation" in negotiations regarding the external assumption of responsibility to respond they argue that its sovereignty is enhanced.[12] This is not entirely different from the notion of delegation of responsibility and accountability, discussed in more detail below. However, the very act of negotiation implies that the state does not have control, nor authority over the external taking-over of elements of state responsibility to respond. As such, as opposed to the state being the arbiter of its responsibility to respond, where such participation is "allowed" by external actors, the latter might take on tactical, generally short-term assignments to intervene, but not assume ultimate, legitimate

10   International Commission on Intervention and State Sovereignty (ICISS) 2001. "The Responsibility to Protect." Ottawa: International Development Research Centre.

11   It should be noted that this relationship exists whether the efficacy in terms of external interventions are effective or not; but the pressure brought to bear on the sovereign state is greater when the domestic claim to effective capacity is weak—as in the case of South Africa's non-linear, delayed and often ineffective response to HIV/AIDS—and that of external interventions is stronger—as in the apparent cases of interventions by PEPFAR and the Global Fund, for instance.

12   Personal correspondence with Dr Viviane Brunne, at the Population Activities Unit (PAU), of the United Nations Economic Commission for Europe (UNECE), January 2009.

responsibility and accountability. The state then that realizes it must answer for its responsibility to respond, finds itself right in the chasm created by the GAP. It does best then to reject such negotiation, in order to be able to account for what responsibility to respond it can effect. Mbeki's rejection of external financial aid quoted above clearly illustrates this.[13] Such processes illustrate and substantiate the claim that sovereignty is circumscribed by the emerging GAP between state and external state and non-state actors in the assumption of responsibility and accountability. Indeed, they show that local-global alliances that are not subject to the delineation of responsibility and accountability as borne by the sovereign state weak its sovereign statehood. In other words, despite external interventions, including those imposed by the arch alliances described above, which in some cases (where they are effective) fulfill the tasks of a non-acting government, the responsibility and accountability for those, as well as their sustainability and associated moral culpability, remains with the sovereign state. This means that the state's ability to enact its responsibilities is at once co-opted and undermined and yet that the state remains held to account in both the present and the future. In the case of HIV/AIDS then, while external actors imposed policies and programs on South Africa, both willingly accepted, and willfully opposed compromising the state's domestic sovereignty, South Africa retains the constitutional and sovereign responsibility for carrying out those policies and programs on which people's lives depend, regardless of whether it still harbors the tools to effectively do so.

A solution that bridges the GAP would be welcome, and is vital. Is the illustration of possible negotiation, which hinges on the state's capacity to engage in such and to gain an advantage for itself, the only possible option? What light can comparisons shed on other possibilities?

Options and opportunities abound in the ongoing responses against HIV/AIDS and in the continuing challenges of and to state sovereignty to vouchsafe the responsibility to respond. With this in mind, the following concluding insights and recommendations are offered pertaining to the HIV/AIDS epidemic directly; to health systems; and to governance structures, notably for sharing, not shedding sovereignty, more broadly.

Thus, for "those concerned with the world's health will be glad that development assistance for health has risen from US$5.6 billion in 1990 to US$21.8 billion in 2007," on the and also "concerned that the influence of intergovernmental agencies is being crowded out by donor-driven funding patterns that may not be fully responding to country needs,"[14] can hope that a solution is in sight which takes both into account, accountably. So where

---

13   Despite his similar prioritization of domestic sovereignty, President Zuma has accepted unprecedented levels of PEPFAR funding, with no sure sustainable South African financial commitment once PEPFAR departs as it has announced, and also South Africa's first World Bank loan to fund a coal-fired energy plant since 1994.

14   "Who runs global health?" 2009. *The Lancet*, 373(9681) (20 June): 2083.

Inequalities in health services, reduced quality of services because of pressures to meet targets, decreases in domestic spending on health, misalignment between GHIs [Global Health Institutions] and country health needs, distraction of government officials from their overall responsibilities for health, the creation of expensive parallel bureaucracies to manage GHIs in countries, the weak accountability of a rapidly expanding GHI-funded non-governmental sector, and increased burdens on already fragile health workforces.[15]

exist, bridges can be built to span the GAP. These need to rest on three pillars: sustainable HIV/AIDS interventions, which do not neglect other health needs and rights' demands; health systems' reform that manages both shedding and sharing of responsibilities; and global governance reordering, which likewise acknowledges, allocates and assumes tactical and ultimate responsibility to respond.

First, the primary focus of anti-HIV/AIDS initiatives should be their sustainability. This is premised on the clear delineation of ultimate responsibility and accountability of those actors and entities responding to the epidemic with medical prevention, treatment, and care. It also takes into account the capacity and capability medical personnel, infrastructure and budgetary support. Attention should also be paid to tuberculosis and topical diseases, as in the GSK patent pool, and as advocated by the Obama Administration's Global Health initiative as well.

Building on the strong efforts of President Bush, we will carry forward the fight against HIV/AIDS. We will pursue the goal of ending deaths from malaria and tuberculosis, and we will work to eradicate polio. We will fight—we will fight neglected tropical disease. And we won't confront illnesses in isolation—we will invest in public health systems that promote wellness and focus on the health of mothers and children.[16]

Despite external pledges, internal financial commitment is crucial, particularly in light of the state's sovereign responsibility and accountability, for health.

Furthermore, priority-setting and policy-making should remain within the real domestic sovereignty of the state. For instance, the Partnership Frameworks introduced in the 2008 PEPFAR reauthorization act redefine the role between the US Government and PEPFAR's partners. Emphasis is placed on increased "host country" autonomy in decision making, to promote "harmonization" with national AIDS plans, and to strengthen country "capacity, ownership, and leadership."[17] Signing these agreements is critical, as guidelines stipulate that no new funding above 2008 levels will be allocated until they are in place. Malawi became the first country to establish a Partnership Framework on 18 May 2009.

---

15   Ibid.

16   "Text of Obama's Speech in Ghana." *The Associated Press*, 11 July 2009.

17   See http://www.avert.org/pepfar.htm [accessed: 5 July 2009].

Yet the Partnership Frameworks allude to a lingering problem: first, while the frameworks might boost country involvement and ownership vis-à-vis PEPFAR, similar agreements are required of countries by the foreign ministries, or ministries administering foreign aid, of the UK, Netherlands, and other countries: the bureaucratic capacity and expertise associated with such processes is enormous,[18] taxing already stretched capabilities that would be better served by a mechanism of coordinated and pooled local, national, and global requests for and receipt of funding. Second, despite such agreements, "giving" recipient countries greater ownership, it is important to avoid the primacy of the constituency of the giving country in the allocation of responsibility and accountability for the use and effectiveness of the funding.[19]

Likewise, the plethora of participants in HIV/AIDS efforts needs to be pared down. This pruning and streamlining should emphasize clear coordination and delineation of tasks, of funding, and of responsibility and accountability. Specifically, superfluous duplication and bureaucracy should be culled between the US Centers for Disease Control, the USFDA, the Global Fund, World Bank, WHO, and UNAIDS. As opposed to proffering separate drug approval processes, for instance, they should be streamlined into one: to certify and facilitate access to medicines, patented and generic, to reduce duplicity of programs and projects, to increase local involvement and reduce bureaucracy, and therein to increase effectiveness, responsibility, and accountability across entities and throughout governance levels. In this context, it is important to speed up and avoid duplication of pharmaceutical approval processes between the WHO and the FDA, replacing the "fast-tracking" initiative with a permanent process.

Similarly, neither the disease nor the fight against it should be owned or steered by a unilateral approach, but should be addressed in a consciously, multi-lateral, multi-pronged division of labor and resources in public, NGO and private sectors. As James Chin, formerly an epidemiologist at the WHO/GPA and currently a clinical professor of epidemiology at the University of California– Berkeley, argues, UNAIDS, for example, has ignored evidence of the ineffectiveness or failure especially of its prevention policies, thus focusing on and persuading donors to put billions of dollars into the wrong interventions. In doing so, it—willingly—promoted "a range of myths that have more to do with

---

18   Overall the paperwork requirements and the number of site visits, which detract from real service delivery, especially medical counseling and treatment: An average of four-monthly reports and additional visits, by direct donors and associated interested parties, per organization funded [by PEPFAR] currently detracts from actual work. Even more astounding at the country-level, a study in the 1990s found that a typical African country prepared 2,400 donor reports every quarter and hosted 1,000 meetings a year. See Brainard, L. (ed.) 2007. "Security by Other Means." CSIS and the Brookings Institution: 40.

19   For additional inspiration see Kidder, T. 2009. "A Death in Burundi." *The New York Times* (22 July).

political correctness than science."[20] It is also vital to avoid creating parallel health systems, since these serve to undermine both functional state capacity, including that of its health care cadre, as well as its the effective responsibility to respond of its sovereign statehood. Overall responses should be designed and implemented with as well as for specific states and affected (sub-) epidemics.

These can and should be based on collaborations—between private and public healthcare facilities, between national and international donors and experts—including across borders. Where this is not the case, "you have donors funding programmes on either side of a border, but not figuring out ways to facilitate cross-border treatment ... National governments need to realize that denying treatment to migrants is counterproductive to their own HIV and AIDS efforts."[21] Illustrating the need for this is that

> A further important finding by the WHO team is that GHIs have not taken the independent evaluation of their programmes sufficiently seriously. For initiatives that have many well-known researchers on their boards and advisory committees, this is an extraordinary failure. GHIs have been flying blind, apparently indifferent to knowledge about the effects of their investments in countries.[22]

A prime example of this is the Gates Foundation.

> The Gates Foundation funds a wide range of contributors to global health, extending from UN agencies to global health partnerships, the World Bank, universities, and non-profit and non-governmental organisations. All the key contributors to global health have an association with the Gates Foundation through some sort of funding arrangement. Coupled with the large amount of money involved, these relations give the foundation a great degree of influence over both the architecture and policy agenda of global health.[23]

As evidence published in *The Lancet*[24] points out, the beneficiaries of Gates' funding are first and foremost global health partnerships, research institutions and universities, none of which are responsible and accountable to the people and

---

20   Lisk, F. 2009. *Global Institutions and the HIV/AIDS Epidemic*. New York: Routledge Global Institutions: 135.

21   "Entry, treatment, rights denied." 2009. *PlusNews* (23 June). This is particularly pertinent to inter-African migrants, such as Zimbabweans in South Africa, as well as migrants into the UK, for example.

22   "Who runs global health?" 2009. *The Lancet*, 373(9681) (20 June).

23   McCoy, D., Kembhavi, G., Patel, J. and Luintel, A. 2009. "The Bill & Melinda Gates Foundation's grant-making programme for global health." *The Lancet*, 373(9675) (9 May): 1645–1653.

24   Ibid.

states which they aim to serve: the recipients of the 20 largest individual grants awarded by the foundation between 1998 and 2007, or 65 percent of total funding, was shared by 20 organizations, including five global health partnerships—such as the Global Fund to Fight AIDS, Tuberculosis and Malaria and GAVI Alliance, which together received a quarter of all funding through ten grants. The next largest funding allocations went to public awareness and advocacy organizations, followed by universities, all of which were in the developed world—of the eight total universities, moreover, five were in the USA, and three were in the UK. The lowest levels of funding went to government agencies—of which the US National Institutes of Health received the most—and for-profit companies.[25] These examples highlight clearly the reality of emerging and "recent changes to collaboration in global health [which] have been characterized by the emergence of loose horizontal networks, where it is unclear who is making decisions and who is accountable to whom."[26] Furthermore,

> The support of vertical, disease-based programmes can undermine coherent and long-term development of health systems, and its sponsorship of global health policy networks and think tanks can diminish the capabilities of Ministries of Health in low-income and middle-income countries. Additionally, the foundation's generous funding of organizations in the UK and USA accentuates existing disparities between developed and developing countries while neglecting support for the civic and public institutional capacities of low-income and middle-income countries.[27]

Thus, while widely lauded for its initiatives in HIV/AIDS, tuberculosis, and malaria, the Gates Foundation is itself a part of, and contributes to the creation of the alliances and parallel structures analyzed here, which bypass the states in which it works, undermining domestic sovereignty, and imperiling the ability of the state to assume responsibility to respond. Finally,

---

25   In addition, "Governments of developing countries with ongoing IMF programs find that they are unable to utilize available funds from donors, such as Global Fund grants, to recruit additional health professionals or to increase salaries and provide other incentives for experienced doctors and nurses who would otherwise go abroad or move to the private sector. This could happen where an IMF country program, in the interest of financial stability, imposes a ceiling on government wage bills or a freeze on public sector recruitment, which in effect conflicts with the need to strengthen the public health workforce as required for responding effectively to HIV/AIDS and other health problems." See Lisk, F. 2009. *Global Institutions and the HIV/AIDS Epidemic*. New York: Routledge Global Institutions: 147.

26   McCoy, D., Kembhavi, G., Patel, J. and Luintel, A. 2009. "The Bill & Melinda Gates Foundation's grant-making programme for global health." *The Lancet*, 373(9675) (9 May): 1645–1653.

27   Ibid.

> The current pattern of global economic governance is thus affecting global health governance in two ways: first, through its direct impact on national capacity to respond to health and other development problems, and second, through the creation of conditions that encourage interventions by international financial institutions in the economies of marginalized countries on the basis of global governance structures and rules that were established for a different purpose, time, and context.[28]

This is not a sustainable solution.

Such lies in an integrated approach with complementary national and global responsibilities and accountability—allocated and assumed where it is actually possible to be enacted.

This means culling unnecessary and duplicative bureaucracy at the national level, such as between South Africa's entities 'responsible' for HIV/AIDS response from the Cabinet on down, as well as, as outlined above, at the international level, such as the UN; the Donor Forum; the World Bank's Africa HIV/AIDS Incentive Fund.[29] After such a streamlining process, the above-mentioned responsibility and accountability should be meted out according to: focused, evidence-based, prioritized, and costed strategies to combat HIV/AIDS; a multi-sectoral approach in key sectors, including inter-regional health systems, education and prevention programs; better monitoring and evaluation of the AIDS response, in particular of implementation and impact of feedback loops; coordination of donor funds to increase effectiveness of the global response within countries; and the rhetorical and real assumption of national authority, alongside clear mandates of the transfer thereof, and of the associated responsibility and accountability, to the auspices of the 'international community' and its responsibility to respond. In order for this last provision to function, a number of changes are necessary to existent governance structures—not to mention to their underlying conceptualization.

The restructuring critical to health systems' functioning and to the HIV/AIDS epidemic response is equally pertinent and applicable to global governance systems more broadly: to the crisis of the GAP between state and external state and non-state responsibility and accountability.

> One of the parameters operates at the macro level as the boundary for the overall structures of the global system, which is considered to be undergoing a transformation from the long-standing state-centric, anarchical system to a new set of bifurcated arrangements wherein a multi-centric world composed

---

28   Lisk, F. 2009. *Global Institutions and the HIV/AIDS Epidemic*. New York: Routledge Global Institutions: 149.

29   Through which the Bank offers knowledge and technical assistance to non-borrowing countries.

of diverse 'sovereignty-free' collectivities has evolved apart from and in competition with the state-centric world of 'sovereignty-bound' actors.[30]

Indeed, as this analysis has indicated, guaranteeing the health, health sovereignty and domestic sovereignty of citizens and states are no longer—and can no longer be—the sole responsibility of the states which remain ultimately accountable for them. Yet the regulation of this responsibility and concomitant accountability has not become part of global governance in a systemic way. This book has argued that this disconnect constitutes the GAP. It has made the case that the identification of this problem heralds a widening chafe in governance that needs to be addressed.

Bridging it can be done in two ways that mirror the dimensions of the problem itself: tactical and theoretical. Since this book has focused on the case study of HIV/AIDS response in South Africa, its tactical recommendations likewise pertain to practical solutions to the problem of the responsibility to respond to that particular problem.

8.1.1 Recommendation: Prevention and Treatment

It is a naïve surprise that, despite considerable global attention to HIV/AIDS, so little has been achieved in slowing the pace of the pandemic in sub-Saharan Africa, [which] reflects denial and neglect of the effects of profound social forces and human behavior on the environment and how these have contributed to the emergence and spread of new plagues. Failure to recognize the pervasive social, economic, behavioral and political aspects of HIV/AIDS, both in terms of its origins and its control, is self-defeating. The complexity of the scientific endeavor required to understand the pathobiology of the disease, and to develop appropriate treatment and vaccines, is more than matched by the complexity of understanding and dealing with the social underpinnings of HIV/AIDS and other plagues locally and globally.[31]

---

30   Rosenau, J. and Czempiel, E.-O. (eds) 1992. *Governance without Government: Order and Change in World Politics*. Cambridge: Cambridge University Press: 281–282. See also Spät, K. "Inside Global Governance: New Borders of a Concept." *Critical Perspectives on Global Governance* (CPGG), available at http://www.cpogg.org/paper%20 amerang/Konrad%20Spaeth.pdf [accessed: 28 July 2009]: 9: "perceived problems are designated to the global and then characterized as unsusceptible to an effective solution at the state level. By this double move, the order and authority inside of the state is taken outside into the 'global' and substituted by a governance beyond the state."

31   Benetar, S. 2005. "The HIV/AIDS pandemic: A sign of instability in a complex global system." In *Ethics and AIDS in Africa: The Challenge to our Thinking* (ed.) van Niekerk, A.A. and Kopelman, L.M. South Africa: David Philips Publishers; and personal correspondence with Solomon Benetar, 2007 and 2008. See also, Grill, B. and Hippler, S. 2009. *Gott, AIDS, Afrika: Das tödliche Schweigen der katholischen Kirche*. Bastei Lübbe: 26.

Despite decades of attempts accompanied by setbacks, it is possible to slow the HIV/AIDS epidemic, and eventually to defeat it altogether.

8.1.2 Primacy of Prevention

The pivotal recommendation is prevention first, second and last. After all of the discussion devoted to ARVs—why? The foremost reason lies in simple statistics: for every two people who access ARVs, another five become infected with the HI-virus. This is a patently unsustainable solution, rendered all the more so due to the long-term funding cuts as a result of the 2008 financial crisis. Additional reasons include the rising tide of drug-resistance strains of HIV which require second- and third-line ARVs. These are on the one hand more expensive than first-line drugs and so less available; and on the other hand, due to a number of pharmaceutical companies paring back or eliminating their HIV/AIDS research units all together, not even developed or likely to be developed. Finally, even if all people, all over the world who require or will require ARVs would have access to them, the logistical and practical prospects of millions more people dependent upon daily drug regimens for the rest of their lives renders such a response implausible and impractical. Furthermore, the implications of such an approach for the health and lives of millions of men, women and children living with a still-deadly disease for the foreseeable future, for communities and societies, and for governments are almost beyond the realm of comprehension.

Effective prevention itself rests on three pillars: increased knowledge of HIV and its routes of infection, treatment and care to mitigate transmission and to serve as an incentive to seek help—but also as a reminder of the interminable nature of the disease—and care: care to search for knowledge of infection, care to not acquire or to pass on the virus, and care to assume responsibility and accountability to follow through at the individual, community, institutional and governmental levels, all day and all night, every day and every night.

In order to translate these pillars into practice, the following is proposed:

First, the focus should be on life beyond merely living. A life lived free of HIV is a life lived more freely. The "Scrutinize" campaign launched by Matchboxology in South Africa takes this approach, urging (condom-users) to "flip HIV to HIV victory!" offers a valuable lesson in stark contrast to the ways the disease and its prevention are usually approached. As a case in point: in 2004, the convener of the American Chamber of Commerce in Johannesburg's HIV/AIDS Committee suggested that youths be enticed to remain HIV negative with the coming attraction of the World Cup tournament 2010 to be held in South Africa. A participant[32] responded incredulously that many of these young people, especially those at risk for HIV due precisely to a lack of education and employment and consequently exhibiting a corresponding sense of despondence over their life prospects, lacked

---

32   Disclaimer: the author is the unnamed participant.

food security over the course of the next week. Far from their minds would be whether they died of a virus in roughly 10 years, with or without the World Cup, which such impoverished youths would not be able to afford to watch in any case. Instead, Matchboxology's strategy acknowledges and accepts the reality of HIV/ AIDS, pays primarily attention to prevention, the ultimate weapons against further spread of HIV, and promotes survival and life, as opposed to dwelling on fear and death.

Second, prevention, especially educational campaigns, should take into account sociological contexts and structural factors, and also pay heed to the appropriateness of communications. As early as 1987, Professor Sher noted that US-designed anti-AIDS campaigns, focusing primarily on homosexual transmission, were ill-suited to South Africa, where a burgeoning heterosexual epidemic rendered them all but obsolete. This initial error, perpetuated by US-conceived and South Africa-funded campaigns Lovelife, Soul City and Khomanani, which conduct most of their advertising and educational outreach in English, in a country with 11 official and innumerable other spoken languages, quite possibly proved fatal, as it served to thwart attempts to address and deal with HIV/AIDS, which upon its initial high-profile discovery was deemed a white, heterosexual, US/European disease.

Third, as in treatment and a searched-for vaccine, prevention has no 'silver-bullet.' Solutions that are presented as such, male circumcision, for instance, should be taken with a grain of salt. Though some studies have shown that it can reduce the infection rate in men by as much as 50 to 60 percent, the verdict is out on how much it protects men's partners. In fact, a study reviewed in *The Lancet* on 18 July 2009 reported that HIV incidence in women whose HIV-infected partners were circumcised was not statistically different from that of women whose partners were not: in other words, male circumcision might protect the male partner from acquiring infection, but provide no such protection, or even increase risk of infection, for the female partner.[33] Yet, in an ongoing nod to the internal-external alliances described in detail above and promoting particular responses to the HIV/ AIDS epidemic, on 20 July 2009, the *New York Times* chastised South Africa for failing to roll-out circumcision, noting that "circumcision has been proven to reduce a man's risk of contracting HIV," and that though South Africa appears to be—again—dragging its feet on implementing the circumcision guidelines recommended by the WHO, "some other African nations are championing the procedure and bringing it to thousands."[34] As the *Lancet* study indicates, however, caution is warranted, especially as more than half of those infected in South and

---

33   Wawer, M.J. et al. 2009. "Circumcision in HIV-infected men and its effect on HIV transmission to female partners in Rakai, Uganda: a randomised controlled trial." *The Lancet*, 374(9685) (18 July): 229–237. See also Baeten, J.M., Celum, C. and Coates, T.J. 2009. "Male Circumcision and HIV Risks and Benefits for Women." *The Lancet*, 374(9685) (18 July): 183–184.

34   Dugger, C.W. 2009. "South Africa is Seen to Lag in HIV Fight." *The New York Times* (20 July).

southern Africa now are women: their protection and the responsibility of national governments and global governance for both women and men should be equally paramount. Circumcision alone does not seem to be the be-all, end-all embodiment of that protection.

8.1.3 The Promises of Treatment

Another element of prevention involves treatment, which is also no cure-all, but which offers a chance to ameliorate the symptoms of HIV/AIDS and to curb the spread of the epidemic. Treatment, particularly ARV treatment, promises to extend lives and improve its quality, if not to turn HIV/AIDS into a chronic manageable disease. It does so by suppressing viral loads, allowing the human immune system to rebuild and remain robust after initial infection, and thereby to postpone the onset of AIDS. Low viral loads also generally translate into lower rates of transmission, potentially thwarting the spread of the epidemic—in the case of adequate ARV coverage. Here the first stumbling blocks amass: lack of adequate personnel to administer ARVs, lack of ARVs themselves and their generic versions; lack of access to and uptake of testing, which is the entry point for treatment initiation. "It's absolutely phenomenal how testing has been escalated over the last five years, but the argument that more testing will lead to more people on treatment earlier is not coming to fruition":[35]

> Donor projects want to know how many people tested and know their status, ... [but] who cares if they tested and know their status if they don't do anything with the information. The people who run those testing programmes must be able to demonstrate that those people entered into a system of care or it's pointless.[36]

Though not pointless, the problem is persistent, and increasingly complex. For example, in addition to the indicated lack of influence of an HIV test, recent studies have revealed that in some instances, testing positive tends to lead to behavior change,[37] whereas testing negative has the opposite effect, and even spurs riskier behaviors, leading to increased incidence. Finally, those who access treatment owe their lives to the assumed responsibility and accountability of states and the international community—which, as has been shown, do not always rise

---

35   "Time to Rethink Testing." 2009. *PlusNews* (26 June).

36   Ibid.

37   Reliable and conclusive data on these trends are hard to find, and the advent of anti-retrovirals tends to change the equation, in sometimes unpredictable ways. While on the one hand, ARVs can themselves be a prevention tool, they can also lead to the perception that AIDS is a chronic, manageable disease, which in turn can help incite risky behaviors, among HIV-negative and HIV-positive people, leading to infection, and between multiple HIV-positive people, leading to supra-infection, drug resistance, and lack of ARV efficacy.

to the occasion, at the cost of many of those lives.[38] Starkly illustrating this is the 2010 PEPFAR decision to flat-line it's funding at 2009 levels and decrease annual budget allocations in the coming years, which has

> Already led PEPFAR-supported clinics in South Africa to begin turning away patients. In addition, UNITAID, the international drug purchasing facility, is to phase out drug funding, leaving Zimbabwe, Mozambique, the Democratic Republic of Congo (DRC) and Malawi without funding for costly second-line ARV drugs by 2012 ...

> Dr Eric Goemaere, MSF Medical Coordinator in South Africa, called donor backtracking a 'moral betrayal.' 'Years ago, countries in this region [southern Africa] were unsure that they could afford treatment, but they were told [by the international community], 'Set ambitious targets, we will follow with the money.'[39]

Now that is patently not the case.

Additional caveats abound; among them the real risk of drug resistance. Drug resistance occurs naturally in all HIV patients accessing ARVs. This poses problems to long-term treatment, especially as this involves second- and third line drugs, which are more expensive than the more readily available first-line drugs. In addition, drug resistance can be accelerated in a number a ways; for instance when people share drugs and when an infected person on ARVs develops drug resistance and then transmits drug-resistance strains of the virus to another person. Further complicating efforts at treatment amidst rising resistance is the use of ARVs to prevent the transmission of HIV. While this might work in instances where uninfected people taking ARVs as prevention are exposed to non-drug-resistant strains of HIV against which those drugs can work preemptively. In other cases, such as people already unknowingly infected with HIV using ARVs as a 'prevention' method or becoming exposed to already drug-resistant strains of the virus, such use of ARVs could fuel the rapid development and lethal spread of further drug resistance strains.[40]

---

38 "PEPFAR's biggest success—support for more than 2 million people on HIV treatment—is also its largest liability ... with more than 2 million people on HIV treatment in PEPFAR's partner countries, 3 it is counterintuitive and dangerous to devote resources to starting people on treatment without commensurate effort to support them." See Navario, P. 2009. "PEPFAR's biggest success is also its largest liability." *The Lancet*, 374(9685) (18 July): 184–185. Preparing to support indefinitely, an ever-rising number of HIV/AIDS infected persons, threatens to turn PEPFAR, or similar programs, into a whole-scale developmental project, supplanting health systems, and states' and their responsibilities, which is neither desirable, practical, nor sustainable.

39 "Dependency: Lost funding means lost lives." 2010. *PlusNews* (27 May).

40 "ARVs for prevention? Proceed with caution, say researchers." 2010. *PlusNews* (25 May).

In an optimistic scenario PrEP [pre-exposure prophylaxis] reduced HIV infection risk by 75 percent when used by 60 percent of the target population, 5 percent of which were unknowingly already infected. Under such conditions, 2.5 percent of the population would have drug-resistant HIV strains after 10 years. A pessimistic scenario assumed that PrEP reduced HIV risk by only 25 percent and reached just 15 percent of the population, 25 percent of which were already infected. In this case, 40 percent of the population would experience drug-resistance after 10 years.[41]

The scenarios emphasizes the importance of regular HIV testing, which in turn leads to a conundrum—of needing to test in order to assess status in order to access ARVs which promise life, with contingencies. Even if all of the available resources went to treatment, arguably also a means of indirect prevention,[42] this would do nothing to stem the tide of rising incidence.

Addressing each of these prevention recommendations requires a clear understanding of the evolving epidemic at hand, as well as medical and political clout and commitment. Finally, it also requires money: money to spend on education, on training, on testing and on treatment; money to spend on the right—appropriate, effective—education, training, testing and treatment; money to sustain the right education, training, testing and treatment. South Africa has just increased its HIV/AIDS budget by 33 percent, and PEPFAR is contributing another 900 million rand [US$120 million] through 2012.[43] The status of funding after that point remains an open question.

Thus the questions remain: this funding, its inherent dependency at the state and individual level, sustainable? Who is responsible? Who is accountable? The answers lie in the analysis of sovereign statehood and in its conclusion of circumscription bodes ill for the guarantee of ultimately responsive responsibility.

There can also be positive prognosess on the trajectory of response to the HIV/AIDS epidemic. The emphasis on life and behavior change as noted in the first prevention recommendation can resurrect the hope of successfully addressing HIV/AIDS. This should also be facilitated in practice by measures and means that promote life and lives beyond HIV/AIDS: investment in vocational training and tertiary education to support the knowledge economy, and particularly education,

---

41   From a study by Ume Abbas, of the Cleveland Clinic Foundation in Ohio, US, working with colleagues from the University of Pittsburgh, cited in "ARVs for prevention? Proceed with caution, say researchers." 2010. *PlusNews* (25 May).

42   See also De Cock, K., Gilks, C.F., Lo, Y.-R. and Guerma, T. 2009. "Can antiretroviral therapy eliminate HIV transmission?" *The Lancet*, 373(9657) (3 January): 7–9; Garnett, G.P. and Baggaley, R.F. 2009. "Treating our way out of the HIV pandemic: could we, would we, should we?" *The Lancet*, 373(9657) (3 January); and Fauci, A.S. 2009. "A Policy Cocktail for Fighting HIV." *The New York Times* (16 April).

43   "Straight talk with South Africa's Health Minister." *PlusNews* (14 May).

training and retention of medical personnel;[44] in food security, especially for land and agricultural reform, including knowledge transfer and training, subsidized fertilizer and seeds,[45] and transfer of land rights.[46] Coupled with this should be investment in infrastructure to link farms to markets, not only within South Africa, but regionally as well, initiatives which can and should be replicated across sectors, including, for instance, in the innovation, production and distribution of medical drugs. Such reforms put into practice would go a long way toward improving the lives of rural populations, to reducing the economic pressures on migration, and the associated risks of HIV/AIDS.

8.1.4 Health Systems' Strengthening

Beyond HIV/AIDS, the health structures critical to the response to the epidemic as well as to broader health-related concerns, need to be evaluated and revamped notably in light of the GAP between the responsibility and accountability inherent in the responsibility to respond.

> Since both the international community and the recipient countries are locked into a system that is unable to produce development consistently or predictably, the solutions need to recognize that the current system of institutions and incentives must be changed on both sides ... 1) official aid needs to become much more selective and competitive, delivered with few if any strings to prove, developmental governments in recognition of the fact that funding is fungible and that an overabundance of uncoordinated donors can crush local ownership and boost transactions costs ... .Second, we suggest that large-scaled aid programs be explicitly seen as a temporary (albeit medium-term) development tool.[47]

This shift should include provisions through which the funder can be held accountable to those receiving the funding at least as much as to those doing the funding. Recipients need a means to police the efficacy of the funding they receive; in essence, buy (with, in the case of ARVs, their lives: both in living

---

44   Due to fiscal constraints, both internally and externally imposed, South Africa reduced its tertiary academic medical facilities, including research and teaching hospitals, in favor of primary care clinics, many of which exist on paper but not in practice. In addition, like many southern African countries, South Africa struggles to provide healthcare services to its rural populations, and to retain doctors and nurses across the country. This increases South Africa's dependency upon international research and medical technology, including HIV/AIDS testing kits and anti-retroviral medications, as well as on medical professions in the private and NGO sectors.

45   This has been done in Malawi, with success.

46   This has been the case too often in South Africa, and as disastrously seen in Zimbabwe.

47   Bräutigam, D.A. and Knack, S. 2004. "Foreign AIDS, Institutions, and Governance in Sub-Saharan Africa." *Economic Development and Cultural Change*, 52(2): 277–278.

thanks to the funding, but also in dying, if the funding is withdrawn without a suitable replacement).

As indicated at the end of the above prevention recommendation, possible responses to HIV/AIDS should include a wide swath of reforms not limited to directly addressing the medical aspects and impacts of the epidemic. One of the critical, overlapping, areas ripe for intervention is in health systems' reform, especially around treatment.[48] This concerns the production and procurement of generic drugs especially. Possible response options include local innovation, production and distribution, patent pools, and regional bulk purchasing.

8.1.4.1 Local innovation, production and distribution
A critical reason for the difficulties in access and the dearth of appropriate drugs to treat HIV/AIDS in (South) Africa is related to drug development and distribution. In the past, and for the most part in the present, Africa has not had the capacity to innovate in drug development or production, or to distribute and deliver it to the populations that need it most, particularly in rural areas. Coupled with this is the need for investment in infrastructure and capacity, particularly in terms of the training and retention of medical personnel.

The current lacks are significant. They pertain not only to access to existing imported branded or generic drugs, but also to the innovation of drugs tailored for the predominant strains of HIV in Africa: these are different from those prevalent in Europe and the US, those against which most available drugs have been developed. Recently, however, the tide seems to have started to turn, with Africa preparing to take a direct role in its drug development chain.[49]

For example, South Africa has Aspen Pharmacare, which produces and markets generic ARVs based on acquired recipes,[50] and likewise, the Quality Chemicals plant in Uganda has also received WHO pre-qualification.[51] The Ugandan plant will eventually produce both HIV as well as malaria drugs, which, with the WHO approval of the drug standards, it will be able to sell for profit to international agencies such as the United Nations. In fact, the EU, UNAIDS and the African Union (AU) are currently supporting this and similar developments in the Democratic Republic of Congo and Ethiopia.[52] The AU, furthermore "wants to promote regional rather than local production," arguing that "if the countries

---

48   Similar variants of some of these recommendations were offered at the 18th International AIDS Society Conference held in Vienna, Austria, 18–22 July 2010.

49   Some support for health systems is coming from Chinese loans, though Western and international donors and investors are also taking a greater interest, as evidenced in the stated priorities of the Obama Administration's Global Health Initiative.

50   As opposed to its own innovation.

51   The pre-qualification is for its manufacturing technology, not yet for its drug products, which will require separate approval to be able to be sold.

52   Anderson, T. 2010. "Tide turns for drug manufacturing in Africa." *The Lancet*, 375(9726) (8 May): 1597–1598.

that are producing can work together we could, as a continent, have more access to the medicines."[53]

> African countries are likely to start producing generic medicines, such as for the main three infectious diseases (HIV/AIDS, tuberculosis, and malaria). The [Chinese] loans will also be spent on particular projects that would use Chinese goods, technologies, and services. It can be used to boost manufacturing, invest in infrastructure and other productive investments, or to set up science and technology parks.[54]

Analysts anticipate that US$73 million in new Chinese loans will be earmarked for pharmaceutical development and healthcare, including treatment of HIV/AIDS, as well as malaria. Part of the money is also expected to benefit the training of 3,000 doctors.[55] These investments promise not only a boost for HIV patients and governments who will be able to access ARVs at a substantial savings, but also for local and regional industry and economic development. A related source of savings and a spur to local innovation lie in patent pools.

8.1.4.2 Patent pools

A number of deals are in the making with regard to both relaxing patent restrictions and to creating patent pools to aid access to HIV/AIDS medications and other drugs. On 14 July 2009, GlaxoSmithKline announced its intent to waive patent restrictions to allow generic drugs firms to copy its HIV drugs, including Abacavir, a second-line drug. Glaxo also said it "would share its research and patent portfolios for HIV drugs with Pfizer, an American rival, in the hope of accelerating drug development."[56] Similarly, Novartis, in partnership with the Institute for OneWorld Health, intends to operate with flexibility to benefit the poor, focusing on developing drugs against secretory diarrhea. The Institute for OneWorld Health also has a deal with Roche involving lifting patent restrictions. In addition, another related collaboration exists between Cambia, an Australian non-profit, and Queensland University of Technology, together with the Global Initiative for Open Innovation, which, with money from the Gates Foundation, "will combine open-access software and sophisticated search features to make

---

53　Byaruhanga, J., health officer at the AU Commission in Addis Ababa, quoted in Anderson, T. 2010. "Tide turns for drug manufacturing in Africa." *The Lancet*, 375(9726) (8 May): 1597–1598.

54　Brautigam, D. (American University, Washington, DC, USA), quoted in Kenyon, G. 2010. "Hopes for African generics from Chinese credit." *The Lancet Infectious Diseases*, 10(5) (May): 300.

55　Kenyon, G. 2010. "Hopes for African generics from Chinese credit." *The Lancet Infectious Diseases*, 10(5) (May): 300.

56　"All Together Now." 2009. *The Economist* (16 July).

the confusing thicket of drugs patents accessible to researchers the world over."[57] Finally, in a culmination of these efforts, GlaxoSmithKline (GSK) launched a patent pool, which South Africa's Technology Innovation Agency (TIA) became the first to join on 12 May 2010.[58]

The GSK patent pool, which aligns with the US Food and Drug Administration's definitions of neglected diseases, includes more than 2,300 existing patents as well as related knowledge on 16 tropical diseases, including tuberculosis and malaria. It does not include ARVs, whose patent-sharing would go a long way towards increasing access to them. However, even there some progress is underway: Katy Athersuch, a medical innovation and access advisor to MSF, said that South Africa's involvement in the GSK patent pool could boost other patent pools, "such as those proposed by UNITAID, [which first proposed a patent pool in July 2008, to increase availability of and access to ARVs] the UN drug procurement facility, and UNAIDS."[59] Such patent pools promise almost immediate generic production, thanks to existing drug recipes. It also brings with it the brain-power behind possible future drug development. Both boons would go a long way not only to addressing the current need for treatment in the fight against HIV/AIDS, but also for that in the long-term, especially in terms of addressing increasing drug resistance: "in 20 percent of ARV patients at MSF's clinic in Khayelitsha, a township outside of Cape Town, first-line treatment failed after five years, and second-line regimens would fail in 25 percent of patients within two years."[60] Though patent pools face challenges; for instance that participation in them remains voluntary, and that bilateral and multilateral trade rules and intellectual property rights legislation, including TRIPS, are not always amenable to them.[61]

Indeed, the spectre of patents and patent-rights is again raising its head. "The United States is using trade threats to coerce countries into adopting intellectual property laws that will increase the cost of medicines," particularly India with regard to its manufacture of generic medications, placing it on a 'priority watch list' reminiscent to the measures taken against South Africa in 1998. Furthermore, the US and EU may circumvent the TRIPS agreement by making provisions that, for instance, limit the circumstances under which compulsory licenses may be issued, or extend the life of patents beyond 20 years. Of particular concern are negotiations around a "Broad-based Trade and Investment Agreement" between India and the EU, negotiations for which are still under way in 2012. Activists fear such an agreement may impose TRIPS-plus-type conditions on India's manufacture and export of generic medicines.

---

57   Ibid.
58   "Government is first to join major patent pool." 2010. *PlusNews* (12 May).
59   Ibid.
60   Ibid.
61   See "HIV generics under threat from tighter patenting rules." 2010. *PlusNews* (2 August).

Nonetheless, the parallel suggestion of and even progress towards patent pools bodes well for the increased sharing of the secrets of drug recipes and of new innovation. Finally, they also raise the stakes—and potential rewards—for African companies entering the fraught fray of drug development.

8.1.4.3 Regional bulk purchasing

In order to make the most of patent pools and local innovation, production and distribution of drugs, including ARVs, a regional system of bulk purchasing would serve South and southern Africa well. This would prove especially true if more drugs are developed in the region, at affordable prices, and if governments invest in both the necessarily linked infrastructure and coordinated regulation of trade.[62] Bulk purchasing would maximize the benefits of local production and take advantage of related price reductions. It would also add an incentive to pharmaceutical companies, investors and purchasing entities to tailor drugs to a wider market, and to ensure that those drugs can be distributed and dispersed within it.

In order for bulk purchasing to pack the greatest punch it is vital that it be based upon a procurement strategy, including FDA/WHO approval and provision mechanisms for second-line drugs, at the global, regional, and national levels. This should be the case not only for HIV drugs, but also for tuberculosis drugs, whose efficacy is being compromised by drug resistance and multi- and extra-drug resistance, and which are the leading killers of HIV-infected persons. Furthermore, in addition to drugs, bulk purchasing should include diagnostics, and also prevention aids, notably condoms, and the female condom.[63]

Yet the best bulk purchasing, the most comprehensive patent pools and the highest caliber of innovation will do little to stem the tide of the HIV/AIDS epidemic without the healthcare personnel to use and apply them.

8.1.4.4 Health care personnel recruitment

Illustrating the challenges inherent with health care personnel recruitment, PEPFAR's original act included a provision that the "President should establish a program to demonstrate the feasibility of facilitating the service of United States health care professionals in those areas of sub-Saharan Africa and other parts of the world severely affected by HIV [and] AIDS, tuberculosis, and malaria."[64] While the assistance and support of US health care professionals in underserved regions is a possible and even useful short-term solution to shortages, it is not a mainstay in the long-term. Far more important is the training and retaining of local health care professionals, which should occur in cooperation with national governments and ministries of health, with the private sector and also with

---

62   The Southern African Development Community (SADC) is working on this.

63   There are generally never enough male condoms in sub-Saharan Africa, and the availability of the female condom is very circumspect.

64   Available at www.pepfar.gov.

international programs and recruiters which siphon off such health care workers to wealthier regions. Taking doctors and nurses from HIV/AIDS-stricken regions to work in elder care and hospitals in the richer world is certain not to aid the fight against HIV/AIDS. Individuals should have a choice, but in particular HIV/AIDS programs should emphasize and make available incentives, means and support for local professionals to contribute locally. As US President Obama said in his speech in Ghana on 11 July 2009,

> In recent years, enormous progress has been made in parts of Africa. Far more people are living productively with HIV/AIDS, and getting the drugs they need ... Yet because of incentives—often provided by donor nations—many African doctors and nurses go overseas, or work for programs that focus on a single disease. And this creates gaps in primary care and basic prevention. Meanwhile, individual Africans also have to make responsible choices that prevent the spread of disease, while promoting public health in their communities and countries.[65]

In a sign of progress, PEPFAR's new Partnership Agreements, mentioned above and discussed below, present possibilities for host countries, together with donor, also recruiter, countries, to combat these initiatives.

Also, in at least a partial response, on 17 May 2010, representatives of the 193 Member States of the World Health Organization met to deliberate on a draft global code of practice on the international recruitment of health personnel. Though also voluntary, the code would "promote coordination of national policies for ethical recruitment, while balancing the rights and obligations of source countries, destination countries, and migrant health personnel."[66] These should be supplemented by agreements between host and recruiter states to channel funding to train and *retain* especially doctors, nurses and pharmacists, shortages of which chronically undermines the capacity of healthcare infrastructures and hampers initiatives to adequately respond to and provide HIV/AIDS treatment and care across southern Africa.[67]

Particularly interesting to this analysis are the codes' proposed key principles. These are that states have the sovereign right: to strengthen their health systems to progressively realize the right to health, with particular attention to the needs

---

65 "Text of Obama's Speech in Ghana." 2009. *The Associated Press* (11 July). The new WHO program also notes that for every 100 doctors Ethiopia trains annually, 50 go abroad.

66 Taylor, A.L. and Gostin, L.O. 2010. "International Recruitment of Health Personnel." *The Lancet*, 375(9727) (15 May): 1673–1675.

67 The Gates Foundation came under fire in East Africa for offering incentives to medical personnel, drawn from the public sector, to treat HIV and AIDS through its Foundation's grantees. Such practices not only undermine the public health response to HIV/AIDS, but also health care delivery more broadly.

of developing and transitional countries; to protect the rights of migrant workers; to promote mutual benefits of recruitment; to encourage workforce planning to reduce the need for recruitment; to develop national and international data gathering systems and support research; and to prohibit discrimination.[68] These recommendations fall directly within the remit of bridging the GAP in governance responsibility and accountability identified in this analysis.

8.2 Theoretical Recommendation: Share, not Shed

All of the tactical recommendations above illuminate the bastion of the ultimate responsibility to respond at the sovereign state. Here I suggest that a possible theoretical solution to safeguard that ultimate responsibility while recognizing that tactical support outside of the state will likely remain necessary. The solution might take one of three forms.

First, a stably governed state (this would not apply to fragile or failed states, but could be applied to areas of limited statehood, where the state, even nominally, possess the recognition of legitimate authority and ultimate responsibility), cognizant of and committed to its sovereign responsibilities, but constrained in its ability to implement them—all, and all at once—such as South Africa, might contract with external state and non-state actors to facilitate their delivery. These contracts would necessarily be time-limited, and necessarily subject to independent monitoring and review. They would also have to be terminable at any time, and the state would have to have resource to charge and seek redress (also in order for the state to be able to meet its obligations even if lacking its own capacity for the during of the time necessary to find another solution) in the case of a breach of contract, as the state would bear the ultimate responsibility for their satisfactory implementation. In order for this to work, such an independent monitoring and review mechanism would have to be developed within existing global institutions, such as the WHO, who would be signatories to the contract. (There is little value in creating new, global oversight institutions in each of the probable policy sectors, to say nothing of those not yet anticipated.)

Second, the state could share responsibility, such as is the case in private-public-partnerships (PPPs), but with the added amenity that recipients of the policy implementation would have direct recourse to the responsible party. In other words, if PEPFAR were not a contracted deliverer of a service (assuming), where South African citizens would address their state in the event of its failure to deliver, but an equal partner, South African recipients of its intervention would be able to pursue claims against it with its decision to flat-line funding.

Third, regional governance bodies, such as the African Union and ASEAN, would be equipped with embellished authority, initially in terms of oversight

---

68   Taylor, A.L. and Gostin, L.O. 2010. "International Recruitment of Health Personnel." *The Lancet*, 375(9727) (15 May): 1673–1675.

and eventually in terms of intervention (though even the EU is far from this in practice). Finally, a trigger system, whereby a state fails to or is unable to meet its sovereign responsibilities could activate a globally-based suzerain to regulate the delivery of that responsibility while supporting the state's evolution towards effectively accepting and being able to implement its ultimate responsibility and accountability. This suzerain would have to be subject to the same monitoring and review mentioned in the first proposal. In other words, global governance needs to evolve from ad hoc governance to a system that shares, does not shed, sovereignty; organized and run coherently.

8.2.1 Evolutions in Sovereignty

As the example of the South African response to HIV/AIDS shows, sovereign responsibilities and accountabilities once ascribed to states are not completely (if they ever were) under their control. Indeed, increasingly, external state and non-state actors are taking on some of the tasks formerly reserved for the realm of sovereignty. Insofar as this increases access to and provision of healthcare, boosts economic development and improves social welfare and mitigates political strife, this shift should be welcomed—there is little good, in a globally interconnected world, in condemning millions to ill-health amidst poverty, whose consequences reverberate in diseases spread across porous borders, spurring (economic) migration, and strife in an intensifying vicious cycle. As such, external state and non-state actors persuading states, even poorer ones, to act to improve healthcare, or even bullying them, can act as a good. But where they assuming some erstwhile state functions and also poaching some state capacity to act, and do so without accountability and even impunity—what happens when they change their priorities and depart—their actions portend a danger. That danger is that sovereign responsibility and accountability are not provisioned especially over the longer-term, despite having raised expectations that they and the goods they promise, will be delivered.

As such, the GAP exists been state responsibility and global responsibility. This is once again evidenced in the case of South Africa. Domestically, South Africa's Constitution protects the right to health, and holds the state responsible for its implementation.

> Everyone has the right to have access to health care services, including reproductive health care; sufficient food and water; and social security, including, if they are unable to support themselves and their dependants, appropriate social assistance. The state must take reasonable legislative and other measures, within its available resources, to achieve the progressive realisation of each of these rights. No one may be refused emergency medical treatment.[69]

---

69 Constitution of the Republic of South Africa. 1996. Chapter Two, Bill of Rights, paragraph 27.

A similar provision actually exists on the level of global governance, where

> Governments have a responsibility for the health of their people which can be
> fulfilled only by the provision of adequate health and social measures. A main
> social target of governments, international organizations and the whole world
> community in the coming decades should be the attainment by all peoples of
> the world by the year 2000 of a level of health that will permit them to lead a
> socially and economically productive life.[70]

Furthermore, as Richard Horton, argues that "The purpose of government is to
uphold the dignity of its people,"[71] which, he maintains

> Shows why health ought to be a core political concern. It allows us to incorporate
> disability, not only preventable mortality, as a central priority of the health
> system. It invites us to consider the political structures needed to deliver health
> as a capability, not merely as health, and how we might hold those political
> structures accountable for their promise to deliver capability as an outcome.

But which 'political structures' can be held both responsible and accountable for
guaranteeing access to and provision of health and healthcare? Those based on
state sovereignty? Or another sovereign arrangement?

With regard to state sovereignty, it must be asked whether it is even possible for
a state to fulfill its theoretical obligations. What does it mean that, for instance in
the case of human health, threats to and which cross increasingly porous borders,
as well as those posed by external actors, be they state or non-state, interfere with
the rules and rights of persons to access healthcare inside an ostensibly sovereign
state? Is the ostensibly sovereign state capable of guaranteeing the security and
welfare of its citizens under such complex conditions?

This last question begs an answer to the final of the trio of sovereign state
obligations, that of its accountability to the "international community." This
means that states must answer for their responsibility in providing and protecting
the rights of their citizens, including the right to health and healthcare, and to
answer not only to those citizens, but also to an "international community" of
equally sovereign states, an amalgam which could, in theory, intervene where and
when a state failed to meet such responsibilities (with both positive and negative
consequences, as alluded to above). Were this to work in practice, it could serve
as a kind of "Article V" protection for the rights of all citizens; but it could
also undermine the sovereignty of the ostensibly protecting state, which, if that
international community were to renege on its intervention, would have disastrous

---

70   From the Declaration of Alma-Ata, paragraph V.
71   Horton, R. 2013. "Why governments should take health more seriously." *The
Lancet*, 381(9871) (23 March).

consequences for that same security and health protection the intervention was meant to provide in the initial instance. So what do to?

Two key elements emerge here that pertain to the resolution of the crisis inherent in the bifurcation of responsibility and accountability in (global) healthcare. First, despite myriad global governance "regimes," consortia of sovereign states at the level of international governance, no formal provisions are made for, on the one hand, a smooth assumption of sovereign responsibilities and accountability if a state fails to meet its obligations and these are in some capacity assumed by external actors and agents. This leads to the second problem, namely, that there are no operable plans for reestablishing and reasserting sovereignty when the amalgam of the international community fails to meet obligations it assumed. The result is an ad hoc governance system, but one that fails spectacularly in delineating responsibility and accountability, and thereby fails to guarantee human security at both a local and a global level. It is an ad hoc system which remains the ultimate guarantor of responsibility, held to account locally and globally, largely irrespective of its capabilities, and equally without regard for the shifting sands of governance alliances all around it.

8.2.2 Share, not Shed

The question then, is how to resolve these tensions? How can the South African Government, or any government and state, facing a profound and possibly prolonged crisis, govern its citizens' rights in a guaranteed manner, the working assumption being that the state is ultimately responsible for and accountable to its citizens for that rights' delivery? Is it necessary that the state also be in charge and in control of all aspects of that rights' delivery, as in this South African instance, of access to and provision of ARVs to an HIV-infected populace? In other words, does guarantee of (sovereign) responsibility and associated accountability need to be conjoined to the ultimate sovereignty of the state? Or can the two be untangled? Can the lines of responsibility and accountability be redrawn to implicate external state and non-state actors? What would such an arrangement look entail?

These insights lead to two potential solutions to the presented problem. First, given the current plethora of global regimes and state reliance on them and assorted external and state and non-state actors to meet their sovereign responsibilities, one possibility would be to integrate these once and for all into a global government. This would have to rest not only on a universal declaration, but also on a binding constitution with competing centers of power, but be ultimately uncontested. It would have the benefit of unequivocally assuming the role of being the bastion of both responsibility and accountability for all of the world's citizens. It has the drawback of being (in the current state of world affairs) thoroughly idealistic and impossible to implement. For better or worse, and despite its limitations, this possible solution shows perhaps most apparently, the endurance of the fundamental order of sovereign statehood in the currently operational international system.

The second possible solution derived from these insights is to both consolidate state sovereignty and to render it more flexible. This means both strengthening states, but also enabling them to meet their obligations on a guaranteed basis—and where necessary, still with external support. This would entail reasserting, on the one hand, and re-affirming, on the other hand, state sovereignty, while explicitly delineating lines of responsibility and accountability for the provision of sovereign 'goods' as opposed to leaving these to be delivered on an ad hoc basis. In other words, this solution advocates equipping states and the international community of states with both the language and the tools to govern by globally accountably not merely inter*nation*al governance. This would have the benefit of leaving the current international order intact, while nonetheless tacking the current gap between responsibility and accountability at the global governance level. There would be a "change from an international system which was multinational, needing coordination for certain things, to a global health system in which national states had to cede some autonomy and take on transnational responsibility" to resolve "the tension between the national state and the globalizing world [that] needed to be dealt with."[72] This reorganization would, subtly, but significantly, bridge the gap between ultimate *state* responsibility and accountability to an ordered sharing thereof with the international community of states, where

> International is the coordination of nations to do health. Global was saying that there was a certain transcendence of nations that was needed in governing health. If we can understand the subtle difference between the two, we're beginning to understand the transition that I think we all find ourselves in managing health.

This rendering might result in a form of shared governance where the sovereignty of individual states is shored up as the ultimate guarantor of its provisions of physical security, welfare and health, and international accountability, while not leaving compromised [6], failing or even failed states in the lurch when they cannot deliver: consequently, it seems plausible to contend that while the state can retain ultimate authority over its sovereign responsibility and accountability, it is not imperative that it also be in charge and in control of all aspects of the provision of its citizens' rights—with one important caveat: it must preside over the power to revoke any discharge[73] of responsibility to external actors, and be able to hold these to account. In the current global governance arrangement, this is not an institutionalized possibility. There is no way for the South African Government to hold PEPFAR to account for its decision to flat-line its funding, and the ensuring consequences of that decision on South African ARV recipients, dependent on a (nonexistent) guarantee of PEPFAR funding. Instead, these citizens turn to the state for the ultimate guarantee of their right to health, but the state is unable either

---

72   Rasool, E. 2012. South African Ambassador to the US Remarks to Council on Foreign Relations (CFR) (9 January), emphasis added.

73   Personal communication with Tanja Börzel, Freie Universität Berlin, January 2013.

to deliver or to ensure that the actor that assumed some ad hoc responsibility for ARV provision be held to account. The ad hoc nature of such an arrangement then, needs to be revamped in order to link not only immediate culpabilities, but more importantly, to govern the sustainable link between guaranteed and ultimate sovereign responsibility and accountability.

Neither one of these solutions is likely to be adopted without a debate. However, a *voluntary* code of practice, while a good start, will not address the GAP between dislocated functional responsibility and state's ultimate responsibility and accountability to respond. There needs to be a link between the two. In addition, this link needs to take into account accountability by external actors to the state in, on and around which they operate. Any, however necessary, shift in the global statist order, is going to presage a contest, "largely a battle about the redistribution of power within a new governance arrangement, a new distribution of votes within a new governance arrangement."[74] Such shared sovereign responsibility and accountability in turn is only able to function if two criteria are met: first, if states still bearing ultimate sovereign responsibility for the security and economic conditions conducive to the welfare of their populaces are liable to the international community of sovereign states echoing R2P, and second, if that international community, not only of sovereign states but also of non-state actors, is equally liable to the states and populaces on which their interventions act. Without such a clear delineation of responsibility and accountability, state sovereignty is likely to continue to be circumvented and circumscribed—an unaffordable outcome in a system which continues to rely on states' ultimate responsibility and accountability in order to function (legitimately). A re-assertion of sovereignty will thus at the end of the day, rest upon the recognition, allocation, and assumption of responsibilities and accountability associated with it nationally and globally—central to the definition of state sovereignty.

8.3 Conclusion: Bridging the GAP

A critical choice abounds: between renewed national responsibility and accountability married to the ability of their enactment, and rejuvenated global responsibility and accountability vested with both the authority and accountability. On the national level furthermore, state structures should be able to feasibly claim and reclaim the supremacy of their policy-making and implementation: to avoid the parallel structures which sap their authority, capacity and accountability. On the global level, states operating as part of the 'international community' as well as institutions should be held mutually accountable to both themselves and to the collective.

---

74   Rasool, E. 2012. South African Ambassador to the US Remarks to Council on Foreign Relations (CFR) (9 January).

In conclusion, in a still-state centric international political system, the assumption of a state's ultimate responsibility and accountability stands. There is scant evidence upon which to argue that this system will undergo any significant shift toward dissolving such vital statehood and state-centered sovereignty. Therefore, the ultimate sovereign responsibility and accountability of each state to its citizens is likely to remain intact.

However, whether each state can guarantee this ultimate responsibility and accountability, as the case study of a well-developed and well-functioning country illustrates, is up for much more debate. The difference lies in the guaranteed ability (in terms of financing and capacity, as well as political will) and the ultimate recourse of citizens to access their rights. Thus while leaving the latter principle intact, the former needs revision.

Therefore it is time to rethink governance—national, international, global —as shared governance, and in particular as the shared governance of sovereign responsibility and accountability. This is going to presage a battle, "largely a battle about the redistribution of power within a new governance arrangement, a new distribution of votes within a new governance arrangement."[75] Such shared sovereign responsibility and accountability in turn is only able to function if two criteria are met: first, if states still bearing ultimate sovereign responsibility for the security and economic conditions conducive to the welfare of their populaces are liable to the international community of sovereign states a la R2P, and second, if that international community, not only of sovereign states but also of non-state actors, is equally liable to the states and populaces on which their interventions act. Without such a clear delineation of responsibility and accountability, state sovereignty is likely to continue to be circumvented and circumscribed—an unaffordable outcome in a system which continues to rely on states' ultimate responsibility and accountability in order to function (legitimately). A re-assertion of sovereignty will thus at the end of the day rest upon the recognition, acknowledgement, allocation, and assumption of responsibilities and accountability associated with it bi-directionally: in other words, from states unto their citizens as well as to the international community, but also the international community unto the states and citizens upon with they act.

Two approaches, based on the varying flexibilities of order described above, to bridging the GAP emerge as potentially feasible. These are to shed or to share governance. The first is for the state, as the ultimate harbinger of sovereign responsibility and accountability, to *shed* its authority to external actors to address a particular problem. This would work under two conditions: a) that those external actors, state and non-state, assume that authority in function, and accept their accountability to the delegating state; and b) that the delegating state possess the power as well as the authority to enforce its delegation. The second, *shared* governance, involves the coordination of state and non-state actors at the

---

75   Ibid.

global level to likewise address a particular problem. This would require a global mechanism for allocating responsibility as well as a global system of accounting.

Each approach has pros and cons. Delegation is clearer on the lines of responsibility and accountability, whereas shared governance is just that, shared. It is predicated on the coordination of responsibility and accountability but without an obvious final arbiter. Shared governance, however, could draw on the resources of numerous state and non-state entities, not only for problem intervention but also as an enforcement mechanism, whereas delegation must rely on an essence of goodwill in the absence of weak state's power to coerce compliance.

Delegation might also employ elements of suzerainty: in shedding some of its sovereignty to an external sovereign, replete with the accompanying responsibility and accountability. The key here would be to delegate to one suzerain, as opposed to a conglomeration. In this instance, the state would forfeit neither its Westphalian sovereignty, i.e. the international recognition of its sovereignty and participation in the international community of sovereign states, nor its entire domestic sovereignty, but merely those elements of it that it is not able to render alone.[76] However, the suzerain would assume ultimate responsibility and accountability for those elements of sovereignty under its control. This system might work to solve the immediate problem in the interest of accounting, but it would have to clarify how a state would rescind the delegation and reclaim its full sovereignty. The alternative would be further weakening of the state, which, as seen in the preceding analysis, remains the final repository of sovereign responsibility and accountability.

Shared governance, by its very definition, could not employ elements of suzerainty, as it would have to negotiate, to *share* authority, including responsibility and accountability with both the state as well as with the advocating and acting external state and non-state actors involved in solving a particular problem to forge a system of *shared governance.* This would also have to be an enforceable system which allocates sovereign responsibility and accountability among all governing actors. This arrangement would feature devolved lines of authoritative responsibility and accountability. It could still impose incentives for cooperation, as well as impart sanctions in its absence: offering a compliance mechanism that delegation cannot. However, given its limited authority over the allocation of responsibility and accountability, this otherwise promising mechanism could be compromised. The R2P doctrine is a case in point. Meant to invoke an international—arguably shared governmental—response to the understated 'problem' of genocide, crimes against humanity, and war crimes through an escalating scale of responses from sanctions to interventions, it has shown few teeth, failing as it does to designate definite responsibility and accountability on the part of an order of shared governance compelled to comply.

---

76 As opposed to the case of Bosnia which after the Balkan wars of 1992–1995 was forced to cede its sovereignty to EU suzerainty.

Thus both shedding and sharing governance need a mechanism to hold the limited suzerain in the first instance, and the conglomeration of shared governance in the second, to account effectively. That mechanism could take the form of overlapping governance circles of alliances of state and non-state actors converging on and over the state. In this arrangement, the state bears—and is borne by—its ultimate responsibility and accountability. In other words, the state would be the delegator (one overlapping circle; of which there might be many) and sharer (another overlapping circle) and final arbiter (the state at the center of this system) of sovereign responsibility and accountability. By eliminating some of the reigning hierarchy inherent in the current system of global (regime) governance, this system based on overlapping circles of governance with a particular focus on allocating and ensuring the assumption of responsibility and accountability would not weaken but strengthen sovereign statehood and the delivery of the tenets of sovereignty. As such, this system would differ from that current in action, wherein state and global governance first because it would level that existing hierarchy, and second because it would be based not only on mutual benefit but on mutual responsibility and accountability. Whereas the present system consists of concentric circles in which the state, as the final harbinger of responsibility and accountability sits as an island amidst a sea of actors circling all around it, this proposed arrangement would separate the state out, and vest it with the authority to manage its responsibility and accountability, if necessary, in conjunction with other actors. It would be an arrangement in trade but a trade arrangement in sovereignty.

Merging *delegation* and *shared governance* would result in an overlapping system of still state-centric governance that nonetheless is flexible enough to assign tasks outside of its direct control. It might look like this:

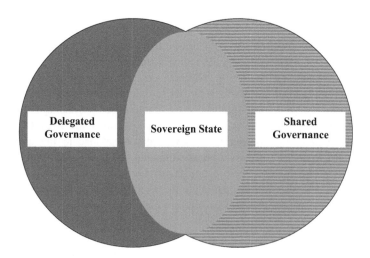

Figure 8.1   Bridging the GAP

Thus in the proposed order, the shedding side of the overlapping model would have to feature compulsory country ownership of the policy process, and donor/partner alignment with country priorities. In addition, it would require corresponding funding management, with provisions of country buy-in to incentivize independence and to keep the lines of responsibility and accountability clear. For instance, health funding could be supplemented and matched between national and external sources. Even with shedding of tactical responsibility, e.g. for the provision of ARVs, the state would retain knowledge of and control over funding allocation, notably for the event of flat-lining of external funding, the state would also have the opportunity to seek other external sources and/or to sanction the states or non-state actors reneging on their responsibility.

In other words, the state, bearing ultimate responsibility and accountability, could re-assume these, and even enact a corresponding punishment, e.g. in shifting terms of trade, on the external entity failing to meet its delegated responsibility. Such state action, however, requires support, too.

On the shared governance side, it would have to specify oversight of the lines of responsibility and accountability. This would have to take the form of accountability to the states in which, on which, and around which such shared—whether delegated or negotiated—governance operates. It must enable the recourse by the state (as above) to ensure that those lines remain operational. The implementation of such negotiated governance presupposes reform in the global institutions with the clout to act as enforcement mechanisms, namely, the UN, specifically the Security Council and/or a beefed up General Assembly; the World Trade Organization, whose TRIPS-Plus provisions must be made accountable not only to the shared conglomerate, but to the states; the World Bank; the International Monetary Fund; and also within the emerging centers power, whose rise will likely change the playing field of governance responsibility to respond notably but not exclusively in the global South. These would have to field the allocation and assumption of the responsibility to respond.

As showcased in theory above, reforms should harmonize the two alternative approaches outlined to designate both temporary and final harbingers of responsibility, and not only to empower but also to compel compliance mechanisms into action. One such attempt taking place in the health sector under the auspices of the Joint Action and Learning Initiative on National and Global Responsibilities for Health (JALI), a manifesto on global health governance was presented to the World Health Organization the week of 14 May 2012 and aims to inspire a grassroots-to-global movement. Included among pledges meant to be binding over the long-term are to clearly delineate responsibility and accountability in global health and governance, are prescriptions to explicitly

> Define state responsibilities for the health of all its inhabitants, regardless of nationality, gender, race, sexual orientation, immigration, or other status; to promote equity; to ensure equal access to quality health services, especially for

the most marginalized in society; and to extend social health protection and ensure that no one is impoverished by health spending.[77]

Define the responsibilities of states to the health of people beyond their borders, including through pooling and allocating sustainable resources to health; ensuring adequate investment in research and development; and not harming the health of people in other countries (for example, as a result of pollution and climate change).[78]

If adopted, the manifesto, a first step toward a Framework Convention on Global Health (FCGH) might prove to be a ways and means towards shared global governance.

Lacking reforms towards overlapping circles of governance, the GAP between state sovereignty and external state and non-state responsibility and accountability will grow. The structures and systems that can bridge the GAP rest on two pillars: a presumption still of sovereign statehood along with its necessity in meeting the responsibility to respond, and its increasing interdependence with external state and non-state actors to deliver. Building upon the pillars of shed and shared governance would clarify lines of responsibility and authority in order to provide for and sustain the guarantees to bridge the GAP.

---

77   "Health for All: Justice for All: A Global Campaign for a Framework Convention on Global Health," paragraph 10c. Joint Action and Learning Initiative on National and Global Responsibilities for Health (JALI). Private communications with Larry Gostin and Eric Friedman at JALI at the O'Neill Institute for National and Global Health Law at Georgetown University. Annamarie Bindenagel Šehović contributed to the drafting of the JALI Manifesto. See http://www.law.georgetown.edu/oneillinstitute/global-health-law/jali.cfm.

78   Ibid.

Bibliography

Books, Documents, Newspapers, Reports and Working Papers

"A glimmer of hope for microbicide research." *PlusNews*, 10 February 2009.

"A little money gets big results." *PlusNews*, 25 August 2008.

"A long paper trail to accessing ARVs." *PlusNews*, 7 November 2007.

"A new and improved PEPFAR under Obama?" *PlusNews*, 21 January 2009.

"Abbott Reduces Price of Kaletra/Aluvia in Low and Low-Middle Income Countries to $1,000." [Press Release] 10 April 2007. Available at http://www.abbott.com/global/url/pressRelease/en_US/60.5:5/Press_Release_0442.htm.

"Africa to feel pain of crisis for years." *The Mail and Guardian*, 16 January 2009.

"AIDS and Public Opinion in South Africa." *Afrobarometer*, Briefing Paper No. 14 (August 2005).

"AIDS Groups File Complaint over Merck AIDS Drug Access in South Africa." Available at www.wcl.american.edu/pijip/documents/complaint.pdf?rd=1.

"AIDS in Africa: The spread and effect of HIV-1 infection in sub-Saharan Africa." *The Lancet*, 359 (2002): 2011–2017.

"AIDS taboo broken in Uganda—now for the drugs." *The Mail and Guardian*, 24 November 2007.

"AIDS: How the virus passed to humans." *The Economist*, 24 June 2007.

"AIDS: Questions for Development." *IDS Policy Briefing*, 32 (July 2006).

"AIDS: The not-so-fair sex. Women may be more responsible for spreading HIV than has been suspected." *The Economist*, 30 June–6 July 2007: 79.

"AIDS: Time to grow up." *The Economist*, 22–28 September 2007.

"AIDS-related deaths in South Africa: 2 180 024 at noon on July 4th." AIDS Barometer in *The Mail and Guardian*, 4 July 2007.

"Alarm over drug recall." *PlusNews*, 12 August 2008.

"All Together Now." *The Economist*, 16 July 2009.

"Annual Report 2006/2007." Development Bank of Southern Africa. Available at www.dbsa.org [accessed 22 September 2010].

"ARV and TB drugs taken together halve deaths." *PlusNews*, 19 September 2008.

"ARVs as prevention tool sparks debate." *PlusNews*, 7 August 2008.

"ARVs for prevention? Proceed with caution, say researchers." *PlusNews*, 25 May 2010.

"At last, policy on AIDS may change." *The Economist*, 9 December 2006.

"Bishop Kevin Dowling: 'The best available means we have to protect life is the condom'." *PlusNews*, 21 August 2008.

"Bleak outlook for future AIDS funding." *PlusNews*, 20 February 2009.

"Board Concludes Article IV Consultation with South Africa." Public Information Notice (PIN) No. 07/94 (The International Monetary Fund, 6 August 2007).

"Boost for local AIDS research." *PlusNews*, 29 July 2009.

"Braced for two presidents." *The Economist*, 13 December 2007.

"Brazil rejects patent on an essential AIDS medicine." [Press Release] Doctors without Borders, 19 September 2008. Available at http://www.msf.org.au/media-room/press-releases/press-release/article/brazil-rejects-patent-on-an-essential-aids-medicine.html [accessed 22 September 2010].

"Brazil's AIDS programme—A conflict of goals: helping patients, or science." *The Economist*, 12–18 May 2007.

"Brazilian President Silva Issues Compulsory License for Merck's Antiretroviral Efavirenz." *AIDSMap*, 9 May 2007.

"Broken promises." AIDS Barometer in *The Mail and Guardian*, 26 September 2007.

"Changing the Guard in HIV Treatment." *Pharmaceutical Business Review Online*, 12 April 2007.

"Civil society demands more partnership with governments." *PlusNews*, 13 June 2008.

"Clinton Foundation closes deal to slash cost of second-line ARVs." *PlusNews*, 7 August 2009.

"Condom Stockouts Threaten Prevention Efforts." *PlusNews*, 6 July 2009.

"Countries pay widely varying prices for ARVs." *PlusNews*, 9 September 2009.

"Cross-border healthcare response needed." *PlusNews*, 3 April 2009.

"Current Impressive World Economic Growth Must be Sustained, and Benefits Extended to All." UNCTAD (4 July 2007). Available at www.unctad.org.

"Dependency: Lost funding means lost lives." *PlusNews*, 27 May 2010.

"Does HIV/AIDS still require an exceptional response?" *The Lancet Infectious Diseases*, 8 (2008): 457.

"Donor AIDS money weakening health systems." *PlusNews*, 15 August 2008.

"Drugs battle at WTO." 2001. Available at http://archives.cnn.com/2001/WORLD/meast/11/12/wto.drugs/index.html?related.

"Drugs not widely available." AIDS Barometer in *The Mail and Guardian*, 15 March 2007.

"Economic downturn puts treatment of millions at risk." *PlusNews*, 29 April 2009.

"Economic Transformation for a National Democratic Society." South African Policy Document, 30 March 2007. Available at www.anc.org.za/show.php?/include=docs/discus/2007/econ_transformation.html [accessed 22 September 2010].

"Entry, treatment, rights denied." *PlusNews*, 23 June 2009.

"Epidemic outpacing response says UNAIDS." *PlusNews*, 24 April 2008.

"EU-India deal could threaten access to essential HIV drugs." *PlusNews*, 9 November 2010.

"Europe's Aid to Sub-Saharan Africa: Better Results Needed." *The Lancet*, 373(9662) (31 January 2009): 434.

"Foreign Direct Investment Inflows to Africa Hit Historic High, but flows are geographically and sectorally concentrated." In UNCTAD World Investment Report 2006. Available at www.unctad.org.

"Foreign Direct Investment Rose by 34% in 2006." UNCTAD (9 January 2007). Available at www.unctad.org.

"Funding shortfall threatens treatment programme." *PlusNews*, 2 April 2009.

"Gap Between Haves and Have-nots Yawns Wider." *PlusNews*, 8 November 2007.

"Gevisser on AIDS: A complicity of opposites." *The Mail and Guardian*, November 2007.

"Global FDI Inflows Rise for Second Consecutive Year." UNCTAD, 16 October 2006.

"Global Fund facing shortfall." *PlusNews*, 6 February 2009.

"Global Fund money gets stuck with health department." *PlusNews*, 3 December 2008.

"Government is first to join major patent pool." *PlusNews,* 12 May 2010.

"Government under pressure to introduce new PMTCT regimen." *PlusNews,* 24 January 2008.

"Govt looks at dual HIV-prevention strategy." *The Mail and Guardian*, 31 July 2007.

"Grim Outlook for an AIDS Vaccine." Editorial in *The New York Times*, 30 March 2008.

"Health Dept awards R3.6 tender for ARVs." *BuaNews/SAGN*, 1 July 2008.

"High inflation in South Africa." *The Economist*, 1 April 2008.

"HIV and AIDS and STI Strategic Plan for South Africa, 2007–2011." Draft 9, The South African Department of Health, 14 March 2007.

"HIV biggest threat to pregnant women." *PlusNews*, 11 August 2009.

"HIV has been in humans for 100 years, study says." *The Associated Press*, 1October 2008.

"HIV incidence rising in 50+ age group." *PlusNews*, 3 March 2009.

"HIV Prevalence in Private Security Industry at 16%." *The Mail and Guardian*, 24 January 2008.

"HIV Prevention series." *The Lancet*, 372 (2008): 831–844.

"HIV/AIDS and the Public Agenda." *Afrobarometer*, nos 12, 14 and 45. Available at http://www.afrobarometer.org [accessed 17 July 2012].

"HIV/AIDS, Security and Democracy." Seminar Report. The Hague: Clingendael Institute, 4 March 2005.

"HIV/AIDS/STD Strategic Plan for South Africa, 2000–2005." The South African Department of Health, February 2000.

"HIV/AIDS: A Global Disaster." *The Lancet*, 372 (2008): 2.

"HIV/AIDS: Not One Epidemic but Many." *The Lancet*, 354 (2004): 1–2.

"Hogan Closes Clear-the-Air Conference." *PlusNews*, 3 April 2009

"Hope in a shipping container clinic." *PlusNews*, 25 August 2008.

"How drug patenting fails the world's poor." *The International Herald Tribune*, 21 May 2006. Available at http://www.iht.com/articles/2006/05/21/business/who.php.

"How much bang for the PEPFAR buck?" *PlusNews*, 7 April 2009.

"ICBC to buy $5.6 billion stake in South African Bank." *Reuters*, 25 October 2007.

"Implementation of the Comprehensive Plan on Prevention Treatment and Care of HIV and AIDS." Fact Sheet, South African Department of Health (23 November 2005).

"Improving the quality of HIV services globally." *The Lancet Infectious Diseases*, 735(8), Issue 12 (2008).

"Is There a Better Way to Say 'Opportunistic Infection'?" *Plusnews*, 2 July 2008.

"Knowing is not enough." *PlusNews*, 9 December 2008.

"Krankheit und Armut im suedlichen Afrka. Die Versorgung von AIDS-Kranken mit Medikamenten als effizientes Mittel der Armutsbekaempfung." BMZ Spezial 140, Bundesministerium fuer wirtschaftliche Zusammenarbeit und Entwicklung, June 2006.

"Leadership determines AIDS performance." *PlusNews*, 25 September 2008.

"Leading Edge: AIDS 2005—light at the end of the tunnel?" *The Lancet Infectious Diseases*, 4 (2004): 385.

"Local ARV manufacturers want state support." *PlusNews*, 12 October 2007.

"Lost funding means lost lives." *PlusNews*, 27 May 2010.

"Mainstreaming Local Government Responses to HIV and AIDS: A Case Study of the City of Cape Town's HIV/AIDS/TB Multi-Sectoral Strategy." Islanda Institute, 2007.

"Major improvements needed to retain patients on ARVs." *PlusNews*, 16 October 2007.

"Make circumcision safer, say researchers." *PlusNews*, 2 September 2008.

"Male circumcision—a gamble for women?" *PlusNews*, 8 August 2008.

"Manto concerned over cost of new-generation ARVs." *The Mail and Guardian*, 7 August 2007.

"Mark R. Dybul on HIV/AIDS Generic Antiretrovirals." Press release of special briefing, issued by the Office of the Spokesman, US State Department, 3 November 2007.

"Mbeki Praises Manto" *The Mail and Guardian*, 31 August 2007.

"Mbeki: EU trade deals harm Africa unity." *The Mail and Guardian*, 6 March 2008.

"Medicines and Related Substances Control Act 101 of 1965 after amendment by the Medicines and Related Substances Control Amendment Act (Act 90 of 1997)."

"Money delayed is ARVs denied." *PlusNews*, 19 November 2008.

"Multi-Country AIDS Program seeks epidemic's drivers." The World Bank: 14 June 2007. Available at www.worldbank.org.

"New ARV tender halves drug prices." *PlusNews*, 20 December 2010.

"New health minister has work cut out for her." *PlusNews*, 26 September 2008.

"New health minister to champion AIDS treatment." *PlusNews*, 2 October 2008.

"New hope for health in South Africa." *The Lancet*, 372 (2008): 1207–1208.

"New Ideas at 4th National AIDS Conference." *PlusNews*, 1 April 2009.

"No simple formula for universal access." *PlusNews*, 3 August 2009.

"Nozizwe says Manto sabotaged her work." *The Mail and Guardian*, 14 September 2007.

"Obama expands health agenda, but not funding." *PlusNews*, 8 May 2009.

"Offene 'Baustellen' von Global Governance in Theorie und Praxis." In Senghaas, D. and Roth, M. (eds) *Global Governance für Entwicklung und Frieden: Perspektiven nach einem Jahrzehnt.* Bonn: Stiftung Entwicklung und Frieden, 2006: 240–247.

"Optimistic UNAIDS sets ambitious goals." *PlusNews*, 10 February 2009.

"Our Commitment: The World Bank's Africa Region HIV/AIDS Agenda for Action 2007–2011." International Bank for Reconstruction and Development and the International Development Association, 24 June 2007.

"Overworked and under-protected." *PlusNews*, 4 December 2008.

"Pharmaceutical companies accused of collusion." *The Mail and Guardian*, 11 February 2008.

"Pharmaceuticals, Patents, Publicity ... and Philanthropy?" *The Lancet*, 373(9665) (28 February 2009): 693.

"Press Briefing on Access of Poor Countries to HIV/AIDS Treatments." UNAIDS, 25 June 2001.

"Press Conference by Secretary-General's Special Envoy on AIDS in Africa." UNAIDS, 22 June 2001.

"Public Opinion and HIV/AIDS: Facing Up to the Future?" *Afrobarometer*, Briefing Paper No. 12, April 2004.

"Public Sector Anti-Retroviral Treatment (ART) South Africa (Phase I)." IDRC, March 2004–September 2005.

"Quality of Health Care Depends on Geography." *PlusNews*, 7 July 2009.

"Question & Answer: Cabinet's decision on the Operational plan." 19 November 2003.

"Question marks over ARV tender." *PlusNews*, 29 February 2008.

"Questions about new prevalence survey." *PlusNews*, 9 September 2008.

"Rapid HIV tests not infallible." *PlusNews*, 16 October 2008.

"Responsibility to Protect: An Idea Whose Time has Come—and Gone? An Idealistic Effort to Establish a New Humanitarian Principle is Coming Under Attack at the United Nations." *The Economist*, 25 July 2009.

"Risky sex on drugs a challenge for HIV prevention." *PlusNews*, 3 December 2007.

"Routine HIV testing a long way off." *PlusNews*, 14 January 2009.

"SA government ends Aids denial." *The Mail and Guardian*, 28 October 2006.

"SA Lives lost as state coffers run dry." *PlusNews*, 25 February 2009.

"SA slowly shakes image as Aids pariah." *AFP/Sapa/SAGN*, 13 August 2008.

"SA worried about affordability of AIDS fight." *The Mail and Guardian*, 7 March 2008.

"Scrutinize: An in-your-face HIV prevention campaign." *PlusNews*, 4 March 2009.

"Securing our Future." Report of the Commission HIV/AIDS and Governance in Africa: An Initiative of the Secretary-General of the United Nations. Geneva: United Nations Economic Commission for Africa, 2008.

"Seizure of drug shipment threatens ARV access." *PlusNews*, 13 March, 2009.

"Sex by the side of the road." *PlusNews*, 4 August 2008.

"Skipping class, skipping treatment." *PlusNews*, 30 September 2008.

"Socio-economic determinants of HIV/AIDS pandemic and nations efficiencies." *European Journal of Operational Research* 176(3) (1 February 2007): 1811–1838.

"South Africa and AIDS: Sacking the wrong health minister. Doubts resurface about Thabo Mbeki's commitment to combating AIDS." *The Economist*, 18–24 August 2007.

"South Africa heads into elections in a sorry state of health." *The Lancet*, 373(9660) (24 January 2009): 285–286.

"South Africa: In the (beetroot) soup again. More allegations against the hapless health minister." *The Economist*, 25–31 August 2007.

"South Africa: Mbeki's big mistake." *International Herald Tribune*, 26 October 2005.

"South Africa: The economic and political consequences of the black middle class." *The Economist*, 1 November 2007.

"South Africa's Exodus." *The Economist*, 13 June 2007.

"South Africa—End of Mbeki." *The Economist*, 25 September 2008.

"South African AIDS Activists Dismayed over President's Praise of Health Minister." *The Mail and Guardian*, 1 September 2007.

"South African Generic Drug Maker to Produce Country's First Generic Antiretroviral Drug." *Henry J. Kaiser Family Foundation International News*, 7 August 2003. South African National Department of Health website, available at www.doh.gov.za [accessed 28 July 2009].

"South Africa—violence." *The Economist*, 25 September 2008.

"Straight talk with South Africa's Health Minister." *PlusNews*, 14 May 2010.

"Street-smart." AIDS Barometer in *The Mail and Guardian*, 8 March 2007.

"Sweet or sour." AIDS Barometer in *The Mail and Guardian*, 19 April 2007.

"Tailor prevention programmes, says UNAIDS." *PlusNews*, 3 December 2008.

"TB failures threaten HIV treatment gains." *PlusNews*, 8 August 2008.

"Text of Obama's Speech in Ghana." *The Associated Press*, 11 July 2009.

"Thabo Mbeki." *The Economist*, 20 January 2005.

"Thailand ignonriert Patentschutz bei Aidsmedikament." *Financial Times Deutschland*, 30 November 2006.

"The changing political economy of sex in South Africa: The significance of unemployment and inequalities to the scale of the AIDS pandemic." *Social Science and Medicine*, 64(3) (February 2007): 689–7000. Available at http://dx.doi.org/10.1016/j.socscimed.2006.09.015 [accessed 4 January 2007].

"The effect of migration on HIV rates." *PlusNews*, 13 September 2007.

"The long road to male circumcision" *PlusNews*, 8 December 2008.

"The person may change, but the policy lingers on." *The Mail and Guardian*, 11 December 2007.

"The Public Agenda: Change and Stability in South African's Ratings of National Priorities." *Afrobarometer*, Briefing Paper No. 45, June 2006.

"Theories and Models for Analyzing Public Policy." In *Improving Public Policy* (eds) Cloete, F. and Wissink, H. Pretoria: Van Schaik, 2000.

"There is Hope. Together in Partnership we can overcome HIV and AIDS." Statement of Cabinet on a Plan for Comprehensive Treatment and Care for HIV and AIDS in South Africa." 8 August 2003, released by Government Communications (GCIS), 19 November 2003.

"Time running out for treatment targets." *PlusNews*, 2 April 2009.

"Time to Rethink Testing." *PlusNews*, 26 June 2009.

"Transitions and trends in policymaking in democratic South Africa." *Journal of Public Administration*, 36(2) (2001): 125–144.

"Treatment as prevention: The next frontier." *PlusNews*, 6 August 2008.

"Two Cheers on Global AIDS." Editorial in *The New York Times*, 18 June 2007.

"UN calls for SA to do more in AIDS fight." *The Mail and Guardian*, 17 October 2007.

"United States Leadership against HIV/AIDS, Tuberculosis and Malaria Act of 2003." [act establishing the President's Emergency Plan for AIDS Relief, PEPFAR].

"Universal access—the race is on!" *PlusNews*, 3 April 2009.

"Universal HIV testing could eliminate HIV within a decade—WHO." *PlusNews*, 27 November 2008.

"Unplugging bottlenecks in ARV distribution." *PlusNews*, 10 December 2008.

"Waiting for grants." AIDS Barometer in *The Mail and Guardian*, 12 April 2007.

"Waiting to hear if treatment will start earlier." *PlusNews*, 5 August 2009.

"We can save more babies, say researchers." *PlusNews*, 20 November 2008.

"We shall overcome, says Mbeki." *The Mail and Guardian*, 8 February 2008.

"WHO narrows down second-line ARV options." *PlusNews*, 7 February 2008.

"Who runs global health?" *The Lancet*, 373(9681) (20 June 2009): 2083.

"Win some, lose some: The battle against AIDS is becoming a war of attrition. Which side is on top is not yet clear." *The Economist*, 9 August 2008.

"World Bank Emphasizes Tailored, Multi-Layered Approach in Africa AIDS Fight." 27 November 2007. Available at www.worldbank.org.

"World Investment Report 2006—FDI from Developing and Transition Economies: Implications for Development." UNCTAD, 2006. Available at www.unctag.org.

"Wrestling for Influence." *The Economist*, 3 July 2008.

Achmat, Z. "Crimes of the great denialist." *The Mail and Guardian*, 27 September 2008.

Alcorn, K. "Brazil Issues Compulsory License on Efavirenz." *The Kaiser Family Foundation*, 7 May 2007.

Alexander, N. *An Ordinary Country: Issues in the Transition from Apartheid to Democracy in South Africa.* Piertermaritzburg: University of Natal Press, 2002.

Altman, D. "AIDS and Security." *International Relations*, 17(4) (2003): 417–427.

Altman, D. "Government responses." *International Affairs HIV/AIDS Special Issue*, 82(2) (March 2006).

Altman, L.K. "A Doctor's World: At Meeting on AIDS, Focus Shifts to Long Haul." *The New York Times*, 19 August 2008.

Altman, L.K. "Behavioral Approaches Overlooked in AIDS Fight." *The New York Times*, 6 August 2008.

Altman, L.K. "Leaving Platform That Elevated AIDS Fight." *The New York Times*, 30 December, 2008.

Altman, L.K. "Researchers look to pill, taken daily, to avert HIV." *The New York Times*, 4 August 2008.

Altman, L.K. "Rethinking is Urged on a Vaccine for AIDS." *The New York Times*, 26 March 2008.

ANC 52nd National Conference Revolutionary Morality policy discussion document, "The ANC and Business." Sec. 6.

ANC 52nd National Conference Revolutionary Morality policy discussion document, "Challenges and Opportunities Facing Workers and Unions: The Role of the ANC." Sec. 9. Available at www.anc.org.za [accessed 22 September 2010].

ANC 52nd National Conference Revolutionary Morality policy discussion document, "The RDP [Reconstruction and Development Plan] of the Soul." Sec. 7. Available at www.anc.org.za [accessed 22 September 2010].

ANC 52nd National Conference Revolutionary Morality policy discussion document, "Role of the Working Class and Organized Labor in Advancing the National Democratic Revolution." Sec. 10. Available at www.anc.org.za [accessed 22 September 2010].

ANC 52nd National Conference Revolutionary Morality policy discussion document "Social Transformation." Sec. 11. Available at www.anc.org.za [accessed 22 September 2010].

ANC 52nd National Conference Revolutionary Morality resolution 58. Available at www.anc.org.za [accessed 22 September 2010].

ANC 52nd National Conference Revolutionary Morality resolution 60. Available at www.anc.org.za [accessed 22 September 2010].

ANC 52nd National Conference Revolutionary Morality resolution 63. Available at www.anc.org.za [accessed 22 September 2010].

ANC 52nd National Conference Revolutionary Morality resolution 64. Available at www.anc.org.za [accessed 22 September 2010].

Appel, M. "Robust Growth in Economy—IMF." *BuaNews (Tshwane)*, 6 August 2007.

Asamoah-Odei, E., Garcia, J.M. and Ties Boerma, J. "HIV prevalence and trends in sub-Saharan Africa: No decline and large subregional differences." *The Lancet*, 364 (2004): 35–40.

Ashoff, G. *Entwicklungspolitischer Kohärenspruch an andere Politiken.* Aus Politik und Zeitgeschichte, 48/2007, 26 November 2007.

ASSA2003. "New South Africa AIDS Model." 28 November 2005. Available at www.assa.org.

Avert. Available at www.avert.org [accessed 9 June 2009].

Ayodele, T. "Drug patents are beside the point." *The Mail and Guardian*, 6 May 2008.

Baeten, J.M., Celum, C. and Coates, T.J. "Male Circumcision and HIV Risks and Benefits for Women." *The Lancet*, 374(9685) (18 July 2009): 183–184.

Barber, L. and Russell, A. "Interview with Thabo Mbeki." *The Financial Times*, 3 April 2003.

Barber, S. "The U.S. Does Need to 'Butt Out' of Regional Crisis." *Johannesburg: Business Day*, 6 June 2008.

Barnett, T. "A Long-Wave Event. HIV/AIDS, Politics, Governance and 'Security'." *International Affairs HIV/AIDS Special Issue*, 83(2) (2006): 297–313.

Barnett, T. and Prins, G. "A report to UNAIDS." *International Affairs HIV/AIDS Special Issue*, 82(2) (March 2006).

Bartsch, S. and Kohlmorgen, L. "The Role of Southern Actors in Global Governance: The Fights against HIV/AIDS." *GIGA Working Papers*, 46 (2007).

Bearak, B. "Post-Apartheid South Africa Enters Anxious Era." *The New York Times*, 6 October 2008.

Bell, C., Devarajan, S. and Gersbach, H. "Thinking about the Long-Run Economist Costs of AIDS." *The Macroeconomics of HIV/AIDS* (ed.) Haacker, M. (Washington, DC: International Monetary Fund, 2004).

Benatar, S.R. "Global Health: Where to Now?" *Global Health Governance*, II(2) (Fall 2008/Spring 2009). Available at www.ghgj.org [accessed 9 July 2009].

Benatar, S.R. "Moral Imagination: The Mission Component in Global Health." *PLoS Medicine*, (December 2005). Available at www.plosmedicine.org.

Benatar, S.R. "South Africa's transition in a globalizing world: HIV/AIDS as a window and a mirror." *International Affairs*, 77(2) (2001): 347–375.

Benatar, S.R. "The HIV/AIDS Pandemic: A Sign of Instability in a Complex Global System." *Journal of Medicine and Philosophy*, 27(2) (2002): 163–177.

Benatar, S.R. "The HIV/AIDS Pandemic: A Sign of Instability in a Complex Global System." In *Ethics and AIDS in Africa: The Challenge to our Thinking* (ed.) van Niekerk, A.A. and Kopelman, L.M. South Africa: David Philips Publishers, 2005.

Benatar, S.R. and Fox, R.C. "Meeting Threats to Global Health: A call for American leadership." *Perspectives in Biology and Medicine*, 48(3) (Summer 2005): 344–361.

Bendavid, E. and Bhattacharya, J. "The President's Emergency Plan for AIDS Relief in Africa: An Evaluation of Outcomes." *The Lancet*, 150(10) (19 May 2009).

Beresford, B. and Davis, L. "ARVs Hogan acts." *The Mail and Guardian*, 17 November 2008.

Bernstein, M. and Sessions, M. "A Trickle or a Flood: Commitments and Disbursements for HIV/AIDS from the Global Fund, PEPFAR, and the World Bank's Multi-Country AIDS Program (MAP)." Washington, DC: Center for Global Development HIV/AIDS Monitor, 5 March 2007.

Bertozzi, S.M., Laga, M., Bautista-Arredondo, S. and Coutinho, A. "Making HIV prevention programmes work." *The Lancet*, 372 (2008): 831–844.

Biehl, J. *Will to Live: AIDS Therapies and the Politics of Survival*. Princeton and Oxford: Princeton University Press, 2007.

Biersteker, T.J. "The 'Triumph' of Neoclassical Economics in the Developing World: Policy Convergence and Bases of Governance in the International Economic Order." In *Governance without Government: Order and Change in World Politics* (ed.) Rosenau, J. and Czempiel, E.-O. Cambridge: Cambridge University Press, 1992.

Bindenagel, A. "Not Living, Not Dying Alone." *The Globalist*, 27 May 2005.

Birdsall, N. and Hamoudi, A. "AIDS and the Accumulation and Utilization of Human Capital in Africa." In Haacker, M. (ed.) *The Macroeconomics of HIV/ AIDS*. Washington DC: International Monetary Fund, 2004.

Bond, P. "From Racial to Class Apartheid: South Africa's Frustrating Decade of Freedom." *Monthly Review*, March 2004.

Bond, P. "Johannesburg's Water Wars: Soweto versus Suez." *le passant ordinaire*, 48. Available at http://www.passant-ordinaire.com/revue/48–611-en.asp [accessed 13 July 2009].

Bond, P. "US Policy toward South Africa and Access to Pharmaceutical Drugs." Available at http://www.cptech.org/ip/health/sa/.

Booysen, S. "Transitions and trends in policymaking in democratic South Africa" *Journal of Public Administration*, 36(2) (2001): 125–144.

Börzel, T. "Was ist Governance?" 19 December 2006. Available at http://www.polsoz.fu-berlin.de/polwiss/forschung/international/europa/team/boerzel/Was_ist_Governance.pdf [accessed 11 November 2010].

Boyd, M., Emery, S. and Cooper, D.A. "Antiretroviral roll-out: the Problem of Second-Line Therapy." *The Lancet*, 374(9685) (18 July 2009): 185–186.

Brainard, L. (ed.) *Security By Other Means*. CSIS and The Brookings Institution (2007).

Braml, J., Risse, T. and Sandschneider, E. (eds) "Einleitung: Staatliche und supranationale Akteure in Räumen begrenzter Staatlichkeit." In "Einsatz für den Frieden. Stabilität und Entwicklung in Räumen prekärer Staatlichkeit." *Internationale Politik*, Band 28 (2010).

Bräutigam, D.A. and Knack, S. "Foreign AIDS, Institutions, and Governance in Sub-Saharan Africa." *Economic Development and Cultural Change*, 52(2) (2004): 255–285.

Breitmeier, H. "Weltordnung im Umbruch: Verrechtlichung und Privatisierung in der Weltgesellschaft." In Senghaas, D. and Roth, M. (eds) *Global Governance für Entwicklung und Frieden: Perspektiven nach einem Jahrzehnt*. Bonn: Stiftung Entwicklung und Frieden, 2006: 104–130.

Brown, D. "Setback in AIDS fight: Test subjects may have been put at extra risk of contracting HIV." *The Washington Post*, 21 March 2008.

Brühl, T. and Rittberger, V. "From International to Global Governance: Actors, Collective Decision-making, and the United Nations in the Twenty-First Century." In *Global Governance and the United Nations System* (ed.) Rittberger, V. Tokyo: United Nations University Press, 2001.

Bruni, F. "Why Obama Isn't Saying 'I Do' to Same-Sex Marriage." *The New York Times*, 8 May 2012.

Bryson, D. "AP Interview: S. Africa concerned at costs of AIDS." *Associated Press*, 1 December 2010.

Calland, R. *Anatomy of South Africa: Who Holds the Power?* Cape Town: Zebra Press, 2006.

Cameron, A., Ewen, M., Ross-Degnan, D., et al. "Medicine prices availability and affordability in 36 developing and middle-income countries: a secondary analysis." *The Lancet*, 373(9659) (17 January 2009): 240–249.

Cameron, E., Clayton, M. and Burris, S. "A tragedy, not a crime." *The International Herald Tribune*, 7 August 2008.

Carreyrou, J. "Inside Abbott's Tactics to Protect AIDS Drug." *The Wall Street Journal*, 3 January 2007.

Cawthorne, P., Ford, N., Limananont, J., et al. "Comment: WHO must defend patients' interests, not industry." *The Lancet*, 369 (2007): 974–975.

Cawthorne, P., Ford, N., Wilson, D. et al. "Reflection and Reaction. Access to drugs: The case of Abott in Thailand." *The Lancet Infectious Diseases*, 7 (2007): 373–374.

Chaisson, R E. and Martinson, N.A. "*Tuberculosis in Africa—Combating an HIV-Driven Crisis,'* New England Journal of Medicine, 358(11) (13 March 2008): 1089–1092.

Chigwedere, P., Seage, G.R., Gruskin, S. et al. "Estimating the Lost Benefits for Antiretroviral Drugs Use in South Africa." *Perspectives: Epidemiology and Social Science, Journal of Acquired Immune Deficiency Syndrome*, 49(4) (1 December 2008).

Chin, J. "The Myth of a General AIDS Pandemic: How billions are wasted on unnecessary AIDS prevention programs." *Campaign for Fighting Diseases*, Discussion Paper No. 2 (January 2008).

Chin, J. "UNAIDS myths on AIDS pandemic costing billions—new report." UNAIDS, 20 May 2008.

Cohen, M.S., Mastro, T.D. and Cates, W. "Universal Voluntary HIV Testing and Immediate Antiretroviral Therapy." *The Lancet*, 373(9669) (28 March 2009): 1077.

Cohen, R. "Mbeki's Shame." *The International Herald Tribune*, 3 July 2008.

Corbett, E.L., Steketee, R.W. ter Kuile, F.O. et al. "AIDS in Africa: HIV-1/AIDS and the control of other infectious diseases in Africa." *The Lancet*, 359(2002): 2177–2187.

Cox, R.W. "Towards a Post-Hegemonic Conceptualization of World Order: Reflections on the Relevancy of Ibn Khaldun." In *Governance without Government: Order and Change in World Politics* (ed.) Rosenau, J. and Czempiel, E.-O. Cambridge: Cambridge University Press, 1992.

Creese, A., Floyd, K., Alban, A. and Guinness, L. "Cost-effectiveness of HIV/AIDS interventions in Africa: A systematic review of the evidence." *The Lancet*, 359(2004): 1635–1642.

Csete, J. "AIDS and Public Security: The Other Side of the Coin." *The Lancet*, 369 (2007): 720–721.

Czempiel, E.-O. "Governance and Democratization." In *Governance without Government: Order and Change in World Politics*, eds. Rosenau, J. and Czempiel, E.-O. Cambridge: Cambridge University Press, 1992.

DaimlerChrysler HIV and AIDS policy, accessed in South Africa, 2003.

Dawes, N. "Manuel lines in the sand." *The Mail and Guardian*, 9 February 2009.

De Cock, K., Gilks, C.F., Lo, Y.-R. and Guerma, T. "Can antiretroviral therapy eliminate HIV transmission?" *The Lancet*, 373(9657) (3 January 2009): 7–9.

De Cock, K.M., Mbori-Ngacha, D. and Marum, E. "AIDS in Africa: Shadow on the continent: Public health and HIV/AIDS in Africa in the 21st century." *The Lancet*, 360 (2002): 67–72.

De Waal, A. *AIDS and Power: Why There is No Political Crisis—Yet.* London and New York: Zed Books, 2006.

Debiel, T., Lambach, D. and Pech, B. "Geberpolitiken ohne verlässlichen Kompass?" *Aus Politik und Zeitgeschichte*, 48 (26 November 2007).

Dingwerth, K. and Pattberg, P. "Global Governance as a Perspective on World Politics." *Global Governance*, 12 (2006): 190–197.

Dowsett, G.W. "Cultural, Social, Ethical and Legal Issues of Male Circumcision Scale-up for Prevention." Australian Research Centre in Sex, Health & Society, La Trobe University (unpublished, 2007).

Dugger, C.W. "Clash over HIV treatment rekindled in South Africa." *The New York Times*, 9 March 2008.

Dugger, C.W. "Clinton foundation announces a bargain on generic AIDS drugs." *The International Herald Tribune*, 9 May 2007.

Dugger, C.W. "Clinton makes up for lost time in battling AIDS." *The New York Times*, 29 August 2006.

Dugger, C.W. "Condoms made in U.S. shape foreign aid policy." *The New York Times*, 29 October 2006.

Dugger, C.W. "South Africa is Seen to Lag in HIV Fight." *The New York Times*, 20 July 2009.

Dugger, C.W. "U.S. agency's slow place endangers foreign aid." *The International Herald Tribune*, 7 December 2007.

Dugger, C.W. "U.S. Plan to Lure Nurses May Hurt Poor Nations." *The New York Times*, 24 May 2006.

Epstein, H. *The Invisible Cure: Africa, The West, and the Fight Against AIDS.* New York: Farrar, Straus and Giroux, 2007.

Erdmann, G. "Südafrika—afrikanischer Hegemon oder Zivilmacht?" German Institute of Global Area Studies (GIGA) Institut für Afrika-Kunde No. 2 (2007).

Evans, G. "Facing Up to Our Responsibilities." *The Guardian*, 12 May 2008.

Farmer, P. *Pathologies of Power: Health, Human Rights, and the New War on the Poor.* Berkeley, California: University of California Press, 2005.

Fauci, A.S. "A Policy Cocktail for Fighting HIV." *The New York Times*, 16 April 2009.

Felix, B. "AIDS seen as a new threat to African democracy." *The Mail and Guardian*, 4 June 2007.

Fleischer, T., Kevany, S. and Benatar, S.R. "Will the National Health Insurance ensure the national health?" *South African Medical Journal*, 100(1) (January 2010).

Fourie, P. "AIDS Policy-making in Contemporary South Africa." In Zondi, S. and Le Pere, G. (eds) *Strategic Responses to HIV/AIDS in Southern Africa.* Johannesburg: IGD [forthcoming].

Fourie, P. "The Relationship between the AIDS Pandemic and State Fragility." *Global Change, Peace & Security (Australia)*, 19(3) (2007).

Fourie, P. *The Political Management of HIV and AIDS in South Africa: One Burden Too Many?* London: Palgrave Macmillan, 2006.

Fredland, R.A. "A Sea Change in Responding to the AIDS Epidemic: Leadership is Awakened." *International Relations*, 15(6) (2001): 89–101.

French, H.W. "African nations excluded from global discourse." *The International Herald Tribune*, 21 June 2007.

Frenk, J. "Strengthening Health Systems to Promote Security." *The Lancet*, 373(9682) (27 June 2009): 2181–2182.

Gallo, R.C. "Viewpoint: The end of the beginning of the drive to an HIV-preventative vaccine: A view from over 20 years." *The Lancet*, 366 (2005):1894–1898.

Garnett, G.P. and Baggaley, R.F. "Treating our way out of the HIV pandemic: Could we, would we, should we?" *The Lancet*, 373(9657) (3 January 2009).

Garrett, L. "Council on Foreign Relations Global Health Update." 10 January 2011.

Gedye, L. "Health sector 'terribly sick'." *The Mail and Guardian*, 13 August 2007.

Geffen, N. "What do South Africa's AIDS statistics mean?" A TAC briefing paper, 7 August 2006. Available at www.tac.org.za.

General Assembly fifty-ninth session agenda item 55, "Follow-up to the outcome of the Millennium Summit." 2 December 2004.

Genschel, P. and Zang, B. "Die Zerfaserung von Staatlichkeit und die Zentralität des Staates." *Aus Politk und Zeitgeschichte* (26 November 2007): 20–21.

Gentleman, A. "Indian Law on Generic Drugs is Upheld." *The International Herald Tribune*, 6 August 2007.

Gerson, M. "The AIDS Relief Miracle." *The Washington Post*, 12 March 2008.

Gevisser, M. *Thabo Mbeki: The Dream Deferred.* Jeppestown: Jonathan Ball Publishers (Pty) Ltd., 2007.

Gill, E. "Semen makes HIV more deadly." *The Mail and Guardian*, 28 January 2008.

Govender, P. "AIDS Wipes out SA's Teachers." *Sunday Times*, 4 November 2001.

Grill, B. and Hippler, S. *Gott, AIDS, Afrika: Das tödliche Schweigen der katholischen Kirche.* Bastei Lübbe, 2009.

Grimm, M. "AIDS-Epidemie in Entwicklungsländern." *Aus Politik und Zeitgeschichte*, 48 (26 November 2007).

Guha-Sapir, Debarati. "The Gates Foundation: Looking at the Bigger Picture." *The Lancet*, 374(9685) (18 July 2009): 201–202.

Gumede, W. "South Africa: Tread Carefully." In *The Africa Report: An Insight into Africa, An Outlook on the World.* Paris: Group Jeune Afrique, October–December 2007.

Gumede, W. "Thabo Mbeki, The most powerful man in Africa." *Time 100*, 2005.

Gumede, W. *Thabo Mbeki and the Battle for the Soul of the ANC.* Cape Town: Zebra Publishers, 2005: 91.

Haacker, M. "The Impact of HIV/AIDS on Government Finance and Public Services." In *The Macroeconomics of HIV/AIDS* (ed.) Haacker, M. Washington, DC: International Monetary Fund, 2004.

Haffajee, F., Tabane, R. and Forrest, D. "'Do I look like I've got horns?' Interview with Thabo Mbeki." *The Mail and Guardian*, 13 December 2007.

Hamilton, L. and Viegi, N. "The Nation's Debt and the Birth of the New South Africa." Work in progress (September 2007), *Cambridge Journal of Economics* (February 2009 revised submission).

Hansor, S. "South Africa's Worldview." *The Council on Foreign Relations* (15 November 2007). Available at www.cfr.org.

Harle, J. "Review: The Political Management of HIV and AIDS in South Africa." *Justice Africa* (29 November 2006). Available at www.justiceafrica.org.

Harrison, V. "Abbot to Lower Price of HIV Drug." *Pharmaceutical Business Review Online*, 11 April 2007.

Harsch, E. "Aid to Africa in jeopardy?" *The Mail and Guardian*, 20 January 2009.

Health for All: Justice for All: A Global Campaign for a Framework Convention on Global Health. Joint Action Learning Initiative on National and Global Responsibilities for Health.

Hein, W. "Global Governance und die Schaffung nachhaltiger Entwicklungsstrukuren." In Senghaas, D. and Roth, M. (eds) *Global Governance für Entwicklung und Frieden: Perspektiven nach einem Jahrzehnt.* Bonn: Stiftung Entwicklung und Frieden, 2006: 219–239.

Hein, W. and Wogart, J.P. "Global Health Governance and the Poverty-Oriented Fight of Diseases: Conclusion." In *Global Health Governance: Institutional Change and the Interfaces between Global and Local Politics in the Poverty-Oriented Fight of Diseases* (Research Report) (ed.) Hein, W., Bartsch, S., Calcagnotto, G., et al. Hamburg: GIGA, 2006: 513–523.

Hein, W., Bartsch, S. and Kohlmorgen, L. "Introduction: Globalization, HIV/AIDS and the Rise of Global Health Governance." In *Globalization, HIV/AIDS and the Rise of Global Health Governance.* London: Palgrave Macmillan, 2007.

Heise, A. "How to create a growth-oriented market constellation for South Africa." Working Papers on Economic Governance, Department of Economics and Political Science at Hamburg University (March 2007).

Herbst, J. *States and Power in Africa*. Princeton, New Jersey: Princeton University Press, 2000.

Hermann, R.M. "Novartis Before India's Supreme Court: What's Really At Stake?" *Intellectual Property Watch*, 2 March 2012. Available at: http://www.ip-watch.org/2012/03/02/novartis-before-india%E2%80%99s-supreme-court-what%E2%80%99s-really-at-stake/.

Horton, R. "The global financial crisis: An acute threat to health." *The Lancet*, 373, 31 January 2009: 355–356.

Horton, R. and Das, P. "Comment: Putting prevention at the forefront of HIV/AIDS." *The Lancet*, 372 (2008): 421–422.

Hösle, V. *Morals and Politics*. Notre Dame: University of Notre Dame Press, 2004.

Iliffe, J. *A History: The African AIDS Epidemic*. Athens, Ohio: Ohio University Press, 2006.

International Commission on Intervention and State Sovereignty (ICISS), "The Responsibility to Protect." Ottawa: International Development Research Centre, 2001.

Izugbara, C.O. Book Review of "The Politics of AIDS in Africa" by Patterson, A.S. African Studies Association, April 2007, available through ProQuest Information and Learning Company.

Jackson, R. *Quasi-States: Sovereignty, International Relations and the Third World*. Cambridge, 1990.

Jackson, R. *Sovereignty*. Cambridge: Polity Press, 2007.

Jacobson, C. "SA Energy Crisis Sends Rand Tumbling." *The Mail and Guardian*, 20 February 2008.

Johansson, L.M. "Fiscal Implications of AIDS in South Africa." Department of Economics, Stockholm University (14 June 2006).

Kahn, M. "Some people may transmit weaker version of AIDS." *The Mail and Guardian*, 21 March 2008.

Kapp, C. "Barbara Hogan: South Africa's Minister of Health." *The Lancet*, 373(9660) (24 January 2009): 291.

Kapp, C. "Lingering Issues, South Africa Heads into Elections in a Sorry State of Health." *The Lancet*, 373(9660) (24 January 2009): 285–286.

Kapp, C. "New Hope for Health in South Africa." *The Lancet*, 372 (2008): 1207–1208.

Karim, Q.A. "Health and Human Rights: HIV treatment in South Africa: Overcoming impediments to get started." *The Lancet*, 363 (2004): 1394.

Keck, M.E. and Sikkink, K. "Transnational advocacy networks in international and regional politics." Blackwell Publishers, UNESCO, ISSJ (159/1999): 90–103.

Keck, M.E. and Sikkink, K. *Activists beyond Borders: Advocacy Networks in International Politics*. Ithaca and London: Cornell University Press, 1998.

Kenyon, G. "Hopes for African generics from Chinese credit." *The Lancet Infectious Diseases*, 10(5) (May 2010): 300.

Kerouedan, D. "Health and Development Financing in Africa." *The Lancet*, 374(9688) (8 August 2009): 435–437.

Kidder, T. "A Death in Burundi." *The New York Times*, 22 July 2009.

Kinetz, E. "Europe trade deal could hit Indian generic drugs." *The Associated Press*, 26 April 2010.

Knight, J.B. and Ganhi Kingdon, G. "Unemployment in South Africa, 1995–2003: Causes, Problems and Policies." *Journal of African Economics*, 16(5) (2007): 813–848.

Krasner, S. *Sovereignty: Organized Hypocrisy*. Princeton: Princeton University Press, 1999.

Kumarasamy, N. "Comment: Generic antiretroviral drugs—will they be the answer to HIV in the developing world?" *The Lancet*, 364 (2004): 3–4.

Lacey, M. "Vulnerable to H.I.V., Resistant to Labels." *The New York Times*, 7 August 2008.

LaFraniere, S. "New AIDS Cases in Africa Outpace Treatment Gains." *The New York Times*, 6 June 2007.

LaFraniere, S. "World Bank reports progress in sub-Saharan Africa." *The New York Times*, 15 November 2007.

Lagakos, S.W. and Gable, A.R. "Challenges to HIV Prevention—Seeking Effective Measures in the Absence of a Vaccine." *New England Journal of Medicine*, 358(15) (10 April 2008): 1543–1545.

Lambach, D. "Der Staat zwischen Repression und Versagen: Minderheitspolitik, Staatszerfall und Nation-Building." In Senghaas, D. and Roth, M. (eds) *Global Governance für Entwicklung und Frieden: Perspektiven nach einem Jahrzehnt*. Bonn: Stiftung Entwicklung und Frieden, 2006: 195–218.

Laubscher, J. "Polokwane, ANC and the Budget" *Fin24*, 12 February 2008. Available at www.fin24.co.za.

Leach-Lemens, C. "HIV fall in Zimbabwe due to deaths and behaviour change, not migration." *Aidsmap*, 4 June 2010.

Leclerc-Madlala, S. "We will eat when I get the grant: Negotiating AIDS, poverty and antiretroviral treatment in South Africa." *African Journal of AIDS Research*, 5(3) (2006): 14–20.

Lisk, F. *Global Institutions and the HIV/AIDS Epidemic*. New York: Routledge Global Institutions, 2009.

Maj-Lis Follér and Håkan Thörn (ed.) *The Politics of AIDS: Globalization, The State and Civil Society*. New York: Palgrave Macmillan, 2008.

Mamdani, M. "Beyond Settler and Native as Political Identities: Overcoming the Political Legacy of Colonialism." *Comparative Studies in Society and History*, 43(4) (October 2001): 651–664.

Manuel, T. "Polokwane Briefing: Not in My Father's House." *The Mail and Guardian*, 13 December 2007.

Mathews, J.T. "Power Shift." *Foreign Affairs*, January/February 1997.

Mbeki, T. "Address at the University of the State of Bahia, Brazil." 14 December 2000. Available at http://www.anc.org.za/ancdocs/history/mbeki/ [accessed 20 July 2009].

Mbeki, T. "Address by Deputy President Thabo Mbeki: Declaration of Partnership against AIDS." 9 October 1998. Available at http://www.anc.org.za/ancdocs/history/mbeki/ [accessed 20 July 2009].

Mbeki, T. "Address of President Thabo Mbeki at the 59th Session of the United Nations General Assembly." New York, 22 September 2004.

Mbeki, T. "Address on World AIDS Day." 1 December, 1999. Available at http://www.anc.org.za/ancdocs/history/mbeki/ [accessed 20 July 2009].

Mbeki, T. "Remarks at the first meeting of the Presidential Advisory Panel on AIDS." 6 May 2000. Available at http://www.anc.org.za/ancdocs/history/mbeki/ [accessed 20 July 2009].

Mbeki, T. "State of the Nation Address of the President of South Africa." Speech to Joint Sitting of Parliament, 8 February 2008.

Mbeki, T. "We will resist the upside-downing of Africa." Available at www.anc.co.za.

Mbeki, T. Letter from the President, *ANC* Today, 5(40): 7–13 October 2005.

Mbeki, T. Speech at Davos, 2001, point 5. Available at http://www.anc.org.za/ancdocs/history/mbeki/ [accessed 20 July 2009].

McCoy, D., Kembhavi, G., Patel, J. and Luintel, A. "The Bill & Melinda Gates Foundation's grant-making programme for global health." *The Lancet*, 373(9675) (9 May 2009): 1645–1653.

McGreal, C. "Mbeki admits he is still AIDS dissident six years on." *The Guardian Unlimited*, 6 November 2007.

Mcinnes, C. "Security and Conflict" *International Affairs HIV/AIDS Special Issue*, 82(2) (2006): 315–326.

McNeil, D.G. Jr., "A Time to Rethink AIDS's Grip." *The World*, 25 November 2007.

McNeil, D.G. Jr., "After Departure, No Leader for U.S. AIDS Program." *The New York Times*, 31 January 2009.

McNeil, D.G. Jr., "Rare Treatment is Reported to Cure AIDS Patient." *The New York Times*, 14 November 2008.

McNeil, D.G. Jr., "UN cuts estimate of AIDS cases by 16%." *The International Herald Tribune*, 20 November 2007.

McNeil, D.G. Jr., "WHO official criticizes Gates Foundation 'cartel' on malaria research." *The New York Times*, 18 February 2008.

Messner, D. and Nuscheler, F. "Das Konzept Global Governance—Stand und Perspektiven." In Senghaas, D. and Roth, M. (eds) *Global Governance für Entwicklung und Frieden: Perspektiven nach einem Jahrzehnt*. Bonn: Stiftung Entwicklung und Frieden, 2006: 18–81.

Millennium Development Goals, Goal 6, "Combat HIV/AIDS, Malaria and other Diseases." United Nations, 2000. Available at http://www.un.org/millenniumgoals/aids.shtml.

Molt, P. "Zur Afrikastrategie der Europäischen Union." *Aus Politik und Zeitgeschichte*, 48 (26 November 2007).

Momberg, E. "Development Bank releases shocking statistics on AIDS in SA." *Sunday Independent*, 4 May 2008.

Montaner, J.S.G., Hogg, R., Wood, E., et al. "Viewpoint: The case for expanding access to highly active antiretroviral therapy to curb the growth of the HIV epidemic." *The Lancet*, 368 (2006): 531–536.

Morris, K. "Loss of Patients from HIV Programmes a Global Issue." *The Lancet Infectious Diseases*, 8(12) (December 2008): 742–743.

Motasim B., Maartens, G., Mandalia, S., et al. "Cost-Effectiveness of Highly Active Antiretroviral Therapy in South Africa." *The Lancet*, 359: 2059–2064.

Müller, R. "Wo Souveränität endet." FAZ, 16 May 2008.

Mundell, J. "HIV Prevention in Africa: A Complex Interplay between Religion, Culture, Tradition and Science." *Consultancy Africa Intelligence* (May 2009). Available at www.consultancyafricaintelligence [accessed: May 2009].

Mutume, G. "Health and 'intellectual property': Poor nations and drug firms tussle over WTO patent provisions." *Africa Recovery*, 15(1–2) (June 2001): 14.

Nath, K. and Mandelson, P. "Doha round: It's not only what we trade, but how." *The International Herald Tribune*, 5 July 2006.

Nattrass, N. "Now in fiction: the president on AIDS." *The Mail and Guardian*, 23 July 2007.

Nattrass, N. "South Africa's 'Roll-Out' of Highly Active Anti-Retroviral Therapy: A Critical Assessment." *JAIDS Journal of Acquired Immune Deficiency Syndromes*, 43(5) (2006): 618–623.

Nattrass, N. "Trading off Income and Health: AIDS and the Disability Grant in South Africa." *Journal of Social Policy*, 35(1) (2005): 3–19.

Nattrass, N. *Mortal Combat: AIDS Denialism and the Struggle for Antiretrovirals in South Africa.* Scottsville: University of KwaZulu-Natal Press, 2007.

Nattrass, N. *The Moral Economy of HIV/AIDS.* Cambridge: Cambridge University Press, 2004.

Navario, P. "PEPFAR's biggest success is also its largest liability." *The Lancet*, 374(9685) (18 July 2009): 184–185.

Navario, P. "Zimbabwe's Second Wave?" *Huffington Post*, 19 May 2010.

Ndou, C. "Doc who supported Nozizwe suspended." *The Mail and Guardian*, 24 August 2007.

Nef, J. *Human Security and Mutual Vulnerability: The Global Political Economy of Development and Underdevelopment.* Second Edition. Ottawa, Canada: International Development Research Centre, 1999.

Nishtar, S. and Pablos-Mendez, A. "The global financial downturn—imperatives for the health sector." *The Lancet*, 373(9658) (10 January 2009): 124.

Nyamnjoh, F.B. "Globalizations, Boundaries, and Livelihoods: Perspectives on Africa." *Philosophia Africana*, 6(2) (2002): 6.

Ooman, N., Berstin, M. and Rosenzweig, S. "The Numbers Behind the Stories—PEPFAR Funding for Fiscal Years 2004 to 2006." HIV/AIDS Monitor: Center for Global Development, 2008.

Oster, E. "Routes of Infection: Exports and HIV Incidence in Sub-Saharan Africa." Preliminary and Incomplete, University of Chicago and NBER, 4 April 2007.

Patterson, A. Draft of unpublished manuscript on "Christianity in Africa," obtained via personal correspondence August 2010.

PEPFAR [President's Emergency Plan for HIV/AIDS Relief]. Available at www.pepfar.gov [accessed 12 May 2012].

Perry, M. "Medical 'brain drain' hindering AIDS battle." *The Mail and Guardian*, 23 July 2007.

Peter, T., Blair, D., Reid, M. and Justman, J. "DART and laboratory monitoring of HIV treatment." *The Lancet*, 375(9719) (20 March 2010): 979.

Pharaoh, R. and Schoenteich, M. "AIDS, Security and Governance in South Africa. Exploring the Impact." Occasional Paper No. 65. Johannesburg: Institute for Security Studies, 2003.

Pieterse, J. "The foreskin strikes back (uncut): Male circumcision as a viable HIV 'prevention technology'?" Unpublished, 2006.

Piller, C. and Smith, D. "Gateses' charitable gifts have unintended consequences." *Tribune Newspapers: Los Angeles Times*, 16 December 2007.

Pisani, E. "AIDS Treatment in Brazil: Success beyond Measure?" *The Lancet*, 374(9685) (18 July 2009): 191–192.

Poku, N. and Whiteside, A. (eds) *The Political Economy of HIV and AIDS*. Aldershot: Ashgate, 2004.

Poku, N. and Whiteside, A. "25 years: Challenges and prospects." In *International Affairs HIV/AIDS Special Issue*, 82(2) (Oxford: Chatam House, March 2006).

Poku, N.K. "AIDS in Africa: An Overview." *International Relations*, 15(6) (2001): 5–14.

Poku, N.K. "Financing: Improving aid." *International Affairs HIV/AIDS Special Issue*, 83(2) (2006): 346.

Poku, N.K. "Report from Africa: Population, Health, Environment, and Conflict." ECSP Report Issue 12 (2007).

Pope Benedict XVI's Address to the UN General Assembly. *The New York Times*, 18 April 2008.

Posel, D. "Sex, Death and the Fate of the Nation: Reflections on the Politicization of Sexuality in Post-Apartheid South Africa." *Africa*, 75 (2005): 125–153.

Potter, D. "State Responsibility, Sovereignty, and Failed States." Refereed paper presented to the Australasian Political Studies Association Conference, University of Adelaide (Australia), 29 September–1 October 2004.

Powers, K.A., Poole, C., Pettifor, A.E. and Cohen, M.S. "Rethinking the heterosexual infectivity of HIV-1: A systematic review and meta-analysis." *The Lancet Infectious Diseases*, 8 (2008): 553–563.

Prins, G. "The Political Economy of HIV/AIDS in South Africa." Talk delivered at University of Pretoria and personal correspondence with author, 2004.

Quinn, A. "SA launches revamped Aids plan." *The Mail and Guardian*, 14 March 2007.

Rau, B. "The politics of civil society." *International Affairs HIV/AIDS Special Issue*, 82(2) (March 2006).

Revanga, A., Over, M., Masaki, E., et al. "The Economics of Effective AIDS Treatment: Evaluating Policy Options for Thailand." The World Bank, *Health, Nutrition, and Population Series 37449*, 2006.

Risse, T. "Paradoxien der Souveränität. Die konstituive Norm, auf der die heutige Staatenwelt gründet—dass nämlich Staaten souverän sind—gilt uneingeschränkt nicht mehr. Was heisst das?" *Internationale Politik* July/August (2007): 40–47.

Risse, T. "Regieren in Räumen begrenzter Staatlichkeit." (Berlin: SFB-Governance Working Paper Series No. 5, 2007).

Risse, T. and Lehmkuhl, U. "Governance in Räumen begrenzter Staatlichkeit." *Aus Politk und Zeitgeschichte*, 48 (26 November 2007).

Risse, T., Ropp, S.C., Sikkink, K. (eds) *The Power of Human Rights: International Norms and Domestic Change*. Cambridge: Cambridge University Press, 1999.

Risse-Kappen, T. *The Power of Principles: International Human Rights Norms and Domestic Change* Cambridge: Cambridge. University Press, 1995.

Rosen, S., Feeley, F., Connelly, P. and Simon, J. "The Private Sector and HIV/AIDS in Africa: Taking Stock of Six Years of Applied Research." Powerpoint presentation by Center for International Health and Development, Boston University, at International AIDS Economics Network Symposium International AIDS Conference Toronto, Canada (August 2006).

Rosen, S., Sanne, I., Collier, A. and Simon, J.L. "Rationing antiretroviral therapy for HIV/AIDS in Africa: Choices and consequences." *PLoS Med*, 2(11) (2005): e303.

Rosenau, J. and Czempiel, E.-O. (eds) *Governance without Government: Order and Change in World Politics*. Cambridge: Cambridge University Press, 1992.

Rosenau, J.N. "Governance, order, and change in world politics." In *Governance without Government: Order and Change in World Politics* (ed.) Rosenau, J. and Czempiel, E.-O. Cambridge: Cambridge University Press, 1992.

Rosenthal, E. "Recall of HIV/AIDS drug has many in poor nations in distress." *The International Herald Tribune*, 22 July 2007.

Rotberg, R.I. "Failed States, Collapsed States, Weak States: Causes and Indicators." In *State Failure and State Weakness in a Time of Terror* (ed.) Rotberg, R.I. Washington, DC: Brookings Institution, 2003.

Russell, A. "Five-year plan to halve Aids in S Africa." *The Financial Times*, 13 March 2007.

Russell, A. *Bring Me My Machine Gun: The Battle for the Soul of South Africa, from Mandela to Zuma*. Hutchinson, forthcoming 2009.

Samodien, L. "AIDS Sees Plunge in Growth Rate of SA's Population." *Cape Argus*, 4 July 2007.

Saxer, M. "The Politics of Responsibility to Protect." FES Briefing Paper 2, in Dialogue on Globalization, April 2008.

Schmitt, C. *Political Theology: Four Chapters on the Concept of Sovereignty*, trans. Schwab, G. Chicago: University of Chicago Press, 1985.

Schmitt, C. *The Concept of the Political*, Trans. Schwab, G. Chicago: University of Chicago Press, 1996: 48–49.

Schulz-Herzenberg, C. *A Lethal Cocktail: Exploring the Impact of Corruption on HIV/AIDS Prevention and Treatment Efforts in South Africa.* Institute for Security Studies and Transparency International Zimbabwe (2007).

Seekings, D. "Is there a Responsibility to protect? An Ethical Evaluation of the Responsibility to Protect." The Normal Patterson School of International Affairs, Carleton University. Available at http://www.carleton.ca/e-merge/docs_vol5/articles/article_Seekings.pdf [accessed 22 September 2010].

Seepe, S. "Unpacking Mbeki: Villain and victim." *The Mail and Guardian*, 30 September 2008.

Seers, D. *Dependency Theory: A Critical Reassessment.* London: Frances Pinter (Publishers) Ltd, 1981.

Šehović, A.B. "Development Dependence: Assuming Responsibility." Consultancy Africa Intelligence, 15 February 2010. Available at www.consultancyafrica.com.

Sen, A. "Why and how is health a human right?" *The Lancet*, 372(9655) (13 December 2008): 2010.

Shanker, T. "Command for Africa is Established by Pentagon." *The New York Times*, 5 October 2008.

Shrire, R. "Thabo's Republic: Robert Shrire's 1998 article on Mbeki." *Leadership Magazine* November 2008, reprinted and available at www.politicsweb.co.za.

Singh, J.A. "Comment: Why AIDS in South Africa threatens stability and economic growth in other parts of Africa." *The Lancet*, 364(2004): 1919–1920.

South African Business Coalition against HIV/AIDS (SABCOHA), "The Impact of HIV/AIDS on Selected Business Sectors in South Africa, 2005." A Survey Conducted by the Bureau for Economic Research (BER) (2005).

South African Constitutional Assembly, "Constitution of the Republic of South Africa." Act 108 of 1996 (8 May 1996). Available at http://www.info.gov.za/documents/constitution/1996/a108-96.pdf [accessed 22 September 2010].

South African Department of Health, "South African National HIV Prevalence, HIV incidence, Behaviour and Communication Survey 2005."

Sparks, A. *Beyond the Miracle: The Story of the Rise and Fall of Apartheid.* Jeppestown, South Africa: Jonathan Ball Publishers, 2003.

Sparks, A. *The Mind of South Africa* (New York: Alfred A. Knopf, 1990).

Sparks, A. *Tomorrow is Another Country: The Inside Story of South Africa's Negotiated Settlement.* Jeppestown, South Africa: Jonathan Ball Publishers, 2003.

Spät, K. "Inside Global Governance: New Borders of a Concept." *Critical Perspectives on Global Governance* (CPGG). Available at http://www.cpogg. org/paper%20amerang/Konrad%20Spaeth.pdf [accessed 28 July 2009].

Stablum, A. "HIV time bomb under the mining industry." *The Mail and Guardian*, 11 July 2007.

Steinberg, J. *Sizwe's Test: A Young Man's Journey Through Africa's AIDS Epidemic.* New York: Simon & Schuster, 2008.

Stiglitz, J. "Schaedliche Pharma-Patente." *Financial Times Deutschland*, 16 March 2007.

Stiglitz, J. "Trade agreements and health in developing countries." *The Lancet*, 373 (31 January 2009): 363–365.

Stiglitz, J. *Making Globalization Work*. New York: W.W. Norton & Company, 2006.

Stillwaggon, E. "What's Cooking." Centre for the Study of AIDS at the University of Pretoria in South Africa annual review (2006).

Stokes, B. "South Africa Striving." *The National Journal*, 3 February 2007.

Stolberg, S.G. "Obama Seeks a Global Health Plan Broader Than Bush's AIDS Effort." *The New York Times*, 6 May 2009.

Stolberg, S.G. and Nizza, M. "G-8 AIDS proposal is criticized, but Putin breaks ice." *The New York Times*, 8 June 2007.

Susser, I. *AIDS, Sex, and Culture: Global Politics and Survival in Southern Africa.* West Sussex, UK: Wiley-Blackwell, 2009.

Sutcliffe, C.G., von Dijk, J.H., Bolton, C., et al. "Review: Effectiveness of antiretroviral therapy among HIV-infected children in sub-Saharan Africa." *The Lancet Infectious Diseases*, 8 (2008): 477–489.

Swidler, A. "Local management of global demands." *International Affairs HIV/ AIDS Special Issue*, 82(2) (March 2006).

Tabane, R. "Shaken but not stirred." *The Mail and Guardian*, 10 October 2008.

Takemi, K., Jimba, M., Ishii, S., et al. Task Force on "Challenges in Global Health and Japan's Contribution." Trilateral Commission Plenary Meeting, 25–28 April, 2008, Washington, DC.

Taljaard, R. "If Those in Power Do Not Listen Nor Care, They Are Failing the Constitution." *Cape Argus*, 2 August 2007.

Taljaard, R. "Think Again: South Africa." *The Mail and Guardian*, April 2009.

Taylor, A.L. and Gostin, L.O. "International Recruitment of Health Personnel." *The Lancet*, 375(9727) (15 May 2010): 1673–1675.

Terreblanche, S. *A History of Inequality in South Africa 1652–2002.* Pietermaritzburg: University of Natal Press, 2002.

Tetzlaff, R. "Global Governance: die lautlose Steuerung internationaler Interdependenz." In Senghaas, D. and Roth, M. (eds) *Global Governance für Entwicklung und Frieden: Perspektiven nach einem Jahrzehnt.* Bonn: Stiftung Entwicklung und Frieden, 2006: 82–103.

Timberg, C. "In South Africa, a Dramatic Shift on AIDS Treatment, Prevention Get New Emphasis as Deputy President Takes Key Role." *The Washington Post Foreign Service*, 27 October 2006.

Timberg, C. "Rethinking AIDS Strategy after a String of Failures. In Wake of Cancelled Vaccine Study, Some Experts are Reemphasizing Proven, Low-Tech Prevention Methods." *Washington Post Foreign Service*, 1 November 2007.

Timberg, C. "Speeding HIV's Deadly Spread: Multiple, Concurrent Partners Drive Disease in Southern Africa." *The Washington Post Foreign Service*, 2 March 2007.

Trewhela, P., "A Note on the ANC." *Everfaster News*, 17 February 2008.

Trewhela, P., Sampson, A. and Gordimer, N. "Looking Back Six Years—to Mbeki." *New York Review of Books*, 10 August 2006.

Tutu, D. "Taking the responsibility to protect." *The International Herald Tribune*, 19 February 2008.

Ulbert, C. "The Effectiveness of Global Health Partnerships: What Determines their Success or Failure?" Paper presented at the 49th Annual ISA Convention. San Francisco, CA: Institute for Development and Pease (INEF), University of Duisburg-Essen, 26—29 March 2008.

UNAIDS, "2008 Report on the Global AIDS Epidemic." August 2008.

UNAIDS, "AIDS Epidemic Update 2006."

UNAIDS/WHO, "AIDS Epidemic Update: December 2005." Available at http://www.unaids.org/epi/2005/doc/report_pdf.asp.

United Nations General Assembly resolution 60/262, "Political Declaration on HIV/AIDS." 15 June 2006.

United Nations General Assembly resolution S-26/2, "Declaration of Commitment on HIV/AIDS." 27 June 2001.

Van Vurren, H. "Motlanthe and the challenge of democratic governance." *The Mail and Guardian*, 1 October 2008.

Von Schoen-Angerer, T. and Limpananont, J. "Correspondence: US pressure on less developed countries." *The Lancet*, 358 (2001): 245.

Wagner, W. "Global Governance: Überlegungen zum Konzept und Anrregungen für die Forschung." In Senghaas, D. and Roth, M. (eds) *Global Governance für Entwicklung und Frieden: Perspektiven nach einem Jahrzehnt*. Bonn: Stiftung Entwicklung und Frieden, 2006: 131–153.

Wawer, M.J., et al. "Circumcision in HIV-infected men and its effect on HIV transmission to female partners in Rakai, Uganda: A randomised controlled trial." *The Lancet*, 374(9685) (18 July 2009): 229–237.

Weisman, S.R. "World Bank Calls on Sovereign Funds to Invest in Africa." *The New York Times*, 3 April 2008.

Wellings, K., Collumbien, M., Slaymaker, E., et al. "Series, Sexual and Reproductive Health. Sexual behavior in context: a global perspective." *The Lancet*, 369 (2006): 1706–1728.

Whiteside, A. "Development: failures of vision." *International Affairs HIV/AID Special Issue*, 82(2) (Oxford: Chatam House, March 2006).

Whiteside, A., de Waal, A. and Gebre-Tensae, T. "AIDS, Security and the Military in Africa: A Sober Appraisal." *African Affairs*, 105/419 (Advanced access published: 18 January 2006): 201–218. Available at http://www.

justiceafrica.org/wp-content/uploads/2006/06/Whiteside_etal_AIDSmilit06.
pdf [accessed 22 September 2010].

Willan, S. "HIV/AIDS, Democracy and Governance in South Africa." GAIN Issue
Brief No. 1, 2004. Available at www.justiceafrica.org.

Wines, M. "AIDS activist Nozizwe Madlala-Routledge keeps her convictions but
loses her job." *The New York Times*, 7 September 2007.

Wines, M. "Influx from Zimbabwe to South Africa Tests Both." *The New York
Times*, 23 June 2007.

Wines, M. "South Africa Strike Foreshadows Political Contest." *The New York
Times*, 13 June 2007.

Wissink, H. "History and Development of Policy Studies and Policy Analysis."
In *Improving Public Policy* (ed.) Cloete, F. and Wissink, H. Pretoria: Van
Schaik, 2000.

Wogart, J.P., Calcagnotto, G., Hein, W. and von Soest, C. "AIDS, Access to
Medicines, and the Different Roles of the Brazilian and South African
Governments in Global Health Governance." *GIGA* (2008).

Wood, E., Braitstein, P., SG Montaner, J., et al. "Extent to which low-level use of
antiretroviral treatment could curb the AIDS epidemic in sub-Saharan Africa."
The Lancet, 355 (2000): 2095–2100.

Wroughton, L. "World Bank launches new AIDS strategy for Africa." *The Mail
and Guardian*, 29 November 2007.

Young, O.R. "The Effectiveness of International Institutions: Hard cases and
Critical Variables." In *Governance without Government: Order and Change in
World Politics* (ed.) Rosenau, J. and Czempiel, E.-O. Cambridge: Cambridge
University Press, 1992: 160–194.

Zacher, M.W. "The decaying pillars of the Westphalian temple: Implications for
international order and governance." In *Governance without Government:
Order and Change in World Politics* (ed.) Rosenau, J. and Czempiel,
E.-O. Cambridge: Cambridge University Press, 1992: 58–101.

Zuger, A. "Book Review: AIDS in Africa: Rising Above the Partisan Babble." *The
New York Times*, 3 July 2007.

Zürcher, C. "Gewollte Schwäche. Vom schwierigen analytischen Umgang mit
prekärer Staatlichkeit." In *International Politik* (September 2005): 13–22.

Zvomuya, P. "Rating the Impact of AIDS." *The Mail and Guardian*, 2
November 2007.

Interviews and Personal Correspondences

African Institute of Corporate Citizenship, Johannesburg, South Africa, 2005–2006.

Ambassador Richard Barkley, deputy chief of mission, Pretoria, South
Africa 1985–1988, 11, 13 and 15 February 2008.

Ambassador Thomas Wheeler, resident South African diplomat (ret.), researcher, South African Institute of International Affairs (SAIIA), Johannesburg, 18, 21 and 22 January 2008.

American Chamber of Commerce in Johannesburg's HIV and AIDS Committee 2003–2006.

Dr Lynne Webber, virologist, Lancet Laboratories, Johannesburg, 2005.

Dr Viviane Brunne, Population Unit of the UN Economic Commission for Europe (UNECE), January 2009.

Fanyana Shirburi, former reporter for the *Sowetan,* former director of policy and government relations, DaimlerChrysler 2006**,** 7 September, 19 October, and 5 December 2007.

Gene Cunningham, US military, 1 February 2008.

Johan Calitz, senior demographer at DIB/DBSA, Cape Town, 27 May 2008.

Kalafong Hospital, north of Pretoria, November 2004.

Lee Hamilton, former US Congressman and ICISS expert panelist, 4 September, 2008.

Lt. Col. Richard Skow, US Army Attaché, US Embassy Pretoria, 2005.

Mariette van Beek**,** former World Bank specialist, Africa, 24 January 2008.

Okey Nwanyanwu, US Centers for Disease Control, Pretoria, South Africa, 2005.

Professor Franklyn Lisk, University of Warwick, UK, May/June 2009.

Professor Larry Gostin, O'Neill Institute for National and Global Health Law, Georgetown University, 2011–2012.

Professor Patrick Bond, University of KwaZulu-Natal, 22 January 2008.

Professor Ruben Sher, virologist, Johannesburg, 8 March 2005, and Professor Sher's private notes.

Professor Solomon Benetar, University of Cape Town (ret.), 2007 and 2008.

Professor Vittorio Hösle, University of Notre Dame, 22 January 2008.

Steven Smith, PEPFAR representative, US Embassy, Pretoria, South Africa at American Chamber of Commerce 2005, Johannesburg, South Africa.

Index